EUROPEAN HEALTH CARE REFORM

ANALYSIS OF CURRENT STRATEGIES

WHO Library Cataloguing in Publication Data

European health care reform : analysis of current strategies / edited and written by
 Richard B. Saltman and Josep Figueras

 (WHO regional publications. European series ; No. 72)

 1.Health care reform 2.Delivery of health care - trends 3. Financing, health
 4.Health services accessibility 5.Europe I.Saltman, Richard B. II.Figueras, Josep
 III.Series

 ISBN 92 890 1336 2 (NLM Classification: WA 541)
 ISSN 0378-2255

WHO Regional Publications, European Series, No. 72

EUROPEAN HEALTH CARE REFORM

ANALYSIS OF CURRENT STRATEGIES

Edited and written by
Richard B. Saltman & Josep Figueras

World Health Organization
Regional Office for Europe
Copenhagen 1997

ISBN 92 890 1336 2
ISSN 0378-2255

PRINTED IN SPAIN

Contents

Figures and tables

Foreword

Many governments in the WHO European Region are reviewing their health care systems and the suitability of their existing approaches to financing, organizing and delivering health care services. Yet health care reform is inherently a normative as well as an economic and organizational activity. Pressures to achieve better expenditure control and/or greater productivity and efficiency need to be balanced against deeply rooted moral imperatives to maintain universal access to necessary care, and to improve the equity with which services are distributed across social classes. Reform measures will be judged not only by short-term savings to public budgets but also by their ability to promote health and to generate health gain for the entire population in line with WHO's health for all strategy. These normative dimensions are equally as important in the restructured health systems of central and eastern Europe and the Commonwealth of Independent States as in the widening health reform activities in western Europe.

Since the early 1990s, the WHO Regional Office for Europe has conducted an extensive programme of activities in support of reform development and implementation, including the establishment of a knowledge base and information system on reform, the development of networks to exchange experiences and support decision-makers, and the provision of direct advisory support on policy and competence building in individual countries.

The Regional Office commissioned a study on recent experience in health care reform in the European Region. The study was structured as an analysis of critical challenges that confront national health policy decision-makers in the second half of the 1990s. It was conceptual as well as empirical in approach, combining epidemiological, economic, organizational and managerial perspectives on the current status of health systems in both the eastern and western parts of the Region. The

This book draws heavily on commissioned papers written by a team of academic and policy experts. The work was conducted under the direction of Constantino Sakellarides, Director of the Department of Health Policy and Services at the WHO Regional Office for Europe.

The contributors are (in alphabetical order): Olusoji Adeyi, Jørgen Steen Andersen, Anders Anell, Drazen Babic, David Banta, Howard Barnum, Adèle Beerling, José Luis Bobadilla, Ferenc Bojan, Jacques Bury, Michael Calnan, Sally Campbell, Gnanaraj Chellaraj, David Chinitz, André-Pierre Contandriopoulos, Nick Doyle, Nigel Edwards, Ainna Fawcett-Henesy, Hernán Fuenzalida-Puelma, Milagros García-Barbero, Juan Gervas, Ellen Goldstein, Claire Gudex, Lázló Gulásci, Bernhard Güntert, Janoz Halik, Chris Ham, Petr Háva, Martin Hensher, Frank Honigsbaum, David Hunter, Dominique Jolly, Panos Kanavos, Gyula Kincses, Simo Kokko, Joseph Kutzin, Marju Lauristan, Ellen Leibovich, Kimmo Leppo, Jane Lethbridge, Alistair Lipp, Christopher Lovelace, Hans Maarse, Michael Marek, Martin McKee, Elias Mossialos, Vicente Ortún, Anastas Philalithis, Alexander Preker, Thomas Rathwell, Lise Rochaix, Francis Roger France, Jolanta Sabbat, Serdar Savas, Joan Sedgwick, Igor Sheiman, Jan Sørensen, Kirsten Stæhr Johansen, Frans Stobbelaar, Ellie Tragakes, Agis Tsouros, Koos Van der Velden, Mikko Vienonen, Gill Walt, Morton Warner, Jürgen Wasem, Ursula Werneke, Miriam Wiley and Cezary Wlodarczyk. The full list of authors and paper titles is given in the Annex.

study's findings are based on over 30 background papers written by an extensive team of scholars and practitioners from all parts of Europe, as well as from Canada, the World Bank and WHO.

This volume presents the major findings of the study. The full set of background papers written by the project team will become available in a further publication in 1997.

The aim of this book is to provide a broad overview of the health and health sector challenges faced by policy-makers in the European Region, and to review the available evidence on the impact of key reform strategies. The book's approach is to present a concise yet substantive perspective on those selected areas. Readers can thus benefit from the extensive research that has been conducted on each topic of discussion. It should be noted that this volume is not intended to provide policy-makers with a set of specific recommendations. Rather, it is designed to synthesize the background evidence, which can help provide a foundation for further national health policy development.

A draft of this book, and a separate summary of its conclusions, laid the foundations for detailed discussions and recommendations at the WHO Conference on European Health Care Reforms, held in Ljubljana, Slovenia, in June 1996. The Conference adopted the Ljubljana Charter on Reforming Health Care, which is available separately. The main conclusions of the Conference are also available in the official report.

The Ljubljana Conference has set the stage for an intensified initiative by the Regional Office in the area of health care reform that could be of major importance for health providers, citizens, patients and scholars alike. It is hoped that this new initiative will assist policy-makers in surmounting the challenges they face as European health care systems prepare themselves for the next generation of service to their citizens.

J.E. Asvall
WHO Regional Director
for Europe

Valuable contributions and advice on several sections of the book were provided by Martin McKee. Many inside and outside WHO provided helpful comments, including: Iain Chalmers, Antonio Duran, Cees Goos, Alex Gromyko, Deborah Hennessy, Rüdiger Krech, Suszy Lessof, Serguei Litvinov, Christopher Lovelace, Tom Marshall, Casten von Otter, Anna Ritsatakis, Mikko Vienonen, Jan de Vries, Bart Wijnberg, Erio Ziglio and Herbert Zöllner.

The text was edited by Annabelle May, Frank Theakston and Mary Stewart Burgher. Zvonko Hocevar was responsible for data management. He and Phyllis Dahl jointly headed the production team, which comprised Kathryn Winther, Doris Holst, Gill Paludan-Müller, Rafael Paz-Fernandez, Charlotte Brandigi and Sheila Duke. The text was typeset by Wendy Enersen, and Sven Lund undertook the cover design and page layout.

Preparation of the chapter on implementation of reforms was aided by contributions from participants in a workshop on management of change. These included, in addition to staff from the Health Policy and Services Department, Gunnar Griesewell, Bradford Herbert, Ieva Marga, Alex Preker, Tom Rathwell, Francisco Sevilla Perez, Igor Sheiman, Per Axel Svalander, Ondrej Typolt, Gill Walt and Bart Wijnberg. Special thanks go to the Organisation for Economic Co-operation and Development (OECD) for the data on health services in western European countries, to the World Bank for the data on health care expenditure, and to the Epidemiology, Statistics and Health Information unit at the Regional Office for providing a special update of the health for all database.

Introduction

Over the last two decades, health policy in Europe has become increasingly concerned with the growing costs of care. The aging of the population, higher levels of chronic disease and disability, the increased availability of new treatments and technologies, and rising public expectations have all exerted upward pressure on overall health-related expenditure.

Most European countries have responded with a series of measures to control these cost pressures. Organizational arrangements originally conceived to improve equity, access and health status have increasingly been constrained by the concern for effective cost-containment. In western Europe, successful expenditure controls at the macro (system) level in the early 1980s have given way in the 1990s to additional efforts to restrain spending growth at the micro (institutional) level. In central and eastern Europe (CEE) and the Commonwealth of Independent States (CIS),[1] the Soviet system of cost-constraint based on macro-level health budgeting on a "residual basis" has been replaced by efforts to increase funding in a time of economic transition, and parallel concerns have emerged about the efficient use of scarce resources.

This clash between, on the one hand, the moral imperative of maintaining solidarity and the social good character of health care and, on the other, the fiscal imperative of cost control has been the driving force behind much of the health policy debate across Europe in the 1990s. Several countries have expressed concern about the impact of specific cost-containment measures on equity and health status. Indeed, a substantial part of the present health reform discussion revolves around the links between social solidarity and cost-containment. Must cost-containment inherently and necessarily damage solidarity, defined in terms of health status and equity of access, as some public health professionals believe? Alternatively, are increased efficiency and effectiveness in the use of scarce health sector resources essential to preserving solidarity, as some economists believe?

The impact of this reform debate on health policy can now be seen across Europe. Many western European countries are reviewing their health care systems in search of alternative strategies for financing and delivering services more efficiently and equitably. Some, such as Germany and the United Kingdom, have formally adopted comprehensive reform programmes. Elsewhere, limited reform strategies have been introduced to deal with specific problems. In the eastern part of the Region, the reform phenomenon has been triggered by the political changes that followed the fall of the Soviet system in the late 1980s. Some reform models and ideas have been transferred across national boundaries. For instance, the reform of the National Health Service (NHS) in the United Kingdom, based on a notion of competitive contracting imported from the United States, has in turn influenced the content of health

---

[1] Throughout most of this book, data on the CEE countries include those on Estonia, Latvia and Lithuania, the remainder of the eastern part of the Region comprising the CIS countries. The exception is the overview of health trends in Europe on pages 15–24 of Chapter 1, in which data on the Baltic states are combined with those on the CIS countries to give a single figure for the newly independent states (NIS) of the former USSR.

care reforms in several countries in both the western and eastern parts of Europe. To date, there is little empirical evidence concerning the effectiveness of many reform policies, not just in those countries on the receiving end, but also in countries championing such strategies. In certain instances, the debate has been driven more by ideology and rhetoric than by evidence of benefits. Although many of these limitations are likely to persist, current trends can be expected to continue in the second half of the 1990s, as more western European countries introduce reform programmes and the eastern part of the Region continues the recently initiated reform process.

Defining reform

The term "reform" has become increasingly popular during the last few years. In spite of the wide use of this concept, there is no consistent and universally accepted definition of what constitutes health sector reform. Different policy-makers and analysts attribute different meanings and connotations to this concept. In some cases, national policy-makers and politicians have sought to magnify small changes in health system organization by labelling them "reforms".

It is useful to distinguish structural reforms from incremental changes. Cassels *(1)* defines health sector reform as activities concerned with changing health policies and the institutions through which these are implemented. Redefining policy objectives alone is not enough. To deal with health sector constraints, there is a need for institutional reform with changes to existing institutions, organizational structures and management systems. Thus, health care reform is concerned with "defining priorities, refining policies and reforming the institutions through which those policies are implemented" *(1)*.

Health care systems, however, typically experience a continuous process of day-to-day operational change. Normal evolutionary and incremental system changes should be differentiated from fundamental structural reforms. Following this approach, a recent report by the Organisation for Economic Co-operation and Development (OECD) distinguishes countries according to whether they are undergoing evolutionary reforms or radical structural reforms. The report points out, however, that the distinction between evolutionary and structural change is somewhat arbitrary and subjective *(2)*. While reform is often understood as a political concept that involves a top-down process of structured change, important structural and organizational shifts often take place without any deliberate intervention by governments, being influenced by other factors such as the introduction of new technology or economic scarcity.

Looking at the process dimension, Berman *(3)* argues that, for reform to occur, changes must aim to achieve a series of policy objectives. Yet there is evidence that some reform programmes have been set in motion without a clear set of objectives. In terms of the duration of the process, Berman contends that reform should consist of sustained long-term change rather than a "one-off" event.

Given that both the approaches to reform and the number and diversity of measures included in "reform" packages vary substantially between countries, analysts seeking to evaluate them should specify the definition adopted and distinguish between its distinct components. Reforms are typically not debated and decided on as a single homogeneous entity but as a package of different measures, each of which needs to be evaluated separately. The relative importance of issues varies between different countries, and therefore the design and objectives of each reform programme will vary similarly.

Box 1 summarizes the key elements of a definitional framework that can be used to characterize specific health sector reforms. Reform is defined as a process that involves sustained and profound institutional and structural change, led by government and seeking to attain a series of explicit policy objectives.

Box 1. Key elements of health care reform

Process
- Structural rather than incremental or evolutionary change
- Change in policy objectives followed by institutional change, rather than redefinition of objectives alone
- Purposive rather than haphazard change
- Sustained and long-term rather than one-off change
- Political top-down process led by national, regional or local governments

Content
- Diversity in the measures adopted
- Determination by country-specific characteristics of health systems

---

These elements suggest a variety of questions. What types of connection exist between change and reform? Can a series of changes aggregate into reform? Can certain strategic changes trigger a period of more major structural reform? Alternatively, can certain strategic changes act as obstacles to more thorough reforms? Can reforms be led by local initiatives without a purposive, political, top-down process? The answers to these questions are unclear; the evidence presented in this volume may help to suggest solutions.

The organization of the book

This volume offers an overview of the complex issues currently confronting health policy-makers in Europe. In pursuit of this objective, it incorporates a variety of different analytical perspectives. It is both conceptual and empirical, and addresses relevant policy issues in both the western and eastern sections of the WHO European Region. It seeks relevant evidence from a number of different academic disciplines:

epidemiology, public health, economics, political science, organizational behaviour and management theory.

The book is organized under four broad headings. The first, represented by Chapter 1, focuses on the *pressures for reform*, and reviews the central factors that define the context in which health care reform is being pursued. The most influential of these include a society's cultural values and the macroeconomic requirements of an increasingly global economy, demographic changes and the role of medical technology, as well as specific health sector concerns in terms of health status and health gain and in terms of the structure and organization of the sector itself.

The next section focuses on current reform strategies. Chapter 2 deals with four *integrating themes* that cut across the reform landscape. These themes are: the changing roles of state and market; decentralization to lower levels of the public sector or to the private sector; patient empowerment, rights and choice; and the evolving role of public health.

Chapters 3–6 assess a number of *key policy strategies* that countries have adopted or proposed, or are considering. Reform strategies can be categorized according to a variety of analytical perspectives, including objectives (e.g. whether they are aimed at achieving equity, effectiveness or efficiency), health system components (e.g. whether they affect the funding, allocation or delivery of services) and health sector actors (e.g. whether they focus on the patient, the third-party insurer, the third-party purchaser or the service provider). Strategies can also be categorized according to traditional economic factors, such as their effect on supply and demand. The approach adopted here classifies the evidence on the impact of different policy interventions into four categories, drawing on a mix of these perspectives. The first group consists of strategies that address resource scarcity, mainly by containing aggregate spending (Chapter 3). The second group brings together strategies that affect health care funding, seeking to maintain universal access and financial sustainability by acting on third-party insurers (Chapter 4). The third group includes strategies for achieving a more effective reallocation of financial resources from third-party purchasers to service providers, in accordance with health service objectives and priorities (Chapter 5). The final group includes strategies that act directly on service providers to achieve more cost-effective and higher quality care (Chapter 6).

Following this review of strategies, the book turns to the *process of implementation*. Chapter 7 utilizes analytical tools drawn from political science to examine why some reforms are introduced successfully while others, however well designed, never materialize. The analysis identifies a series of key factors that national policymakers may wish to consider when they design implementation schedules for future reforms. Finally, in Chapter 8, these somewhat disparate perspectives are drawn together in a number of conclusions, encapsulated in the phrase *the way forward*.

1 The Pressures for Reform

The widespread nature of health care reforms suggests that they are generated by broad secular trends that cross national boundaries. Two broad types of factor have played an important role. First, various pressures from outside the health sector affect the basic framework within which health-related policies are formulated. In many cases, health care reforms are not isolated phenomena, but instead form part of wider structural efforts to reform various state-supported welfare programmes and other social sectors. The reform process is influenced by political, ideological, social, historical, cultural and economic factors, all of which need to be taken into consideration in understanding the context of pressures for reform.

A second set of pressures relates to existing health and health sector problems. These include specific challenges to the health of the population of Europe, along with implications for the models of health services required, as well as increasing pressures on health spending and a number of organizational and structural challenges.

The context for health reform

A health system's present structure and capacity for future change reflect a wide variety of contextual factors. Societal norms and values influence the central principles of the system, as well as the desire for reform. A nation's level of economic development influences the level of disposable resources available for health services (4). Intersectoral factors such as housing stock, social insurance, nutrition and environmental pollution also have important effects. The role of education, particularly the number of individuals with sophisticated management training, and the penetration and quality of information technology systems will also influence a health system's capacity for serious and sustained reform (5).These contextual factors are reviewed here under three headings: the defining role of values, the reality of macroeconomics, and demographic and social pressures.

THE DEFINING ROLE OF VALUES

Across Europe, the technical resources that comprise a health system are configured in a variety of different ways. Some of these differences are historical; others reflect more recent political or financial decisions. All these arrangements are strongly influenced by the underlying norms and values of the wider society. Health care services, like other human service systems, mirror the deeply rooted social and cultural expectations of society as a whole.

Core norms

One key indicator of a society's normative values involves the very nature of health care itself. Some societies view it as a predominantly social or collective good, whereby all citizens benefit when an individual receives needed curative as well as preventive service. Social solidarity is a related value, whereby the costs of care are intentionally cross-subsidized from young to old, from rich to poor and from the healthy to the sick, to ensure that all members of society receive the care that they need. Other societies, influenced by the radical market-oriented thinking of the 1980s, increasingly perceive health care as a commodity that can be bought and sold on the open market. This position emphasizes the technical and dynamic efficiency that market incentives can instil into health services provision, and the contributions that these incentives are believed to make towards restraining future spending growth. While the concept of health services as a market commodity has been discussed in some policy-making circles, however, it has not been adopted as the basis for policy formulation in any European country (6).

A second set of deeply rooted norms concerns the role of the state in the health sector, and with it the roles of voluntary, self-regulating organizations and the public. In some European countries, the state has traditionally played a major part in developing the health sector, typically in both the financing and delivery of services. In other European contexts, the state has taken a lower profile, with health systems that are predominantly run by self-regulating associations of insurers and providers. Where this strong state role has existed in western Europe, it has been legitimized by free democratic elections, and it directly reflects the popular will. In the CEE and CIS countries, however, a strong state role is associated with the former regimes, and national policy-makers are now engaged in a concerted effort to create more balanced government and nongovernmental arrangements. Policy-makers in these countries also hope these new arrangements will encourage citizens to cast off the personal passivity learned in the past and play a more active role in issues concerning their own health and health care.

A third societal norm is accountability. A health care system is responsible to a number of different political, social and economic constituencies. As a consequence, one can speak of five different types of health system accountability: ethical, professional, legal, political and financial. While every system has elements of all five, typically one or two will predominate – reflecting the values that are central to a particular national health system (7). Here, too, as with the fundamental nature of health care and the role of the state, expectations about accountability define the parameters of feasible and sustainable health sector reform.

Constructing health sector values

Looking beyond these specific core values, one finds that health systems are part of a broader process by which societies decide on which values to prioritize and institutionalize. From this process-oriented perspective, the difficulties faced by democratic societies in reforming their health care systems are tied to the complex relations that exist between society's values, the norms adopted in order to put those values into operation, and the existence of individuals who are autonomous yet dependent on those values. In this context, the reform of health care systems cannot be reduced to a mechanical exercise that consists of implementing a rational plan to improve the effective use of resources. More fundamental issues are at stake than simply financial retrenchment. It is a question of maintaining a health care system perceived by the public as a central element of society's core values, while simultaneously introducing necessary changes so as not to mortgage society's survival. This requires a difficult process of negotiation between the key actors defined by each society's history, traditions and culture.

The stability of large social systems such as health care is a result of the coherence that exists between society's values (known as the dominant belief system) and the social and physical structure of health care institutions. This structure is composed of the processes, laws and regulations that define how resources and authority are distributed in the health sector (8), as well as the volume and type of resources available. These resources and the manner in which they are organized are a direct reflection of society's values.

The dominant belief system

The concept of the dominant belief system does not signify that there exists a unique system of beliefs and values shared by all. Rather, the concept implies that the continuing daily tension between differing values and beliefs in a society possesses a certain stability. This tension between divergent values can best be understood by separating them into four groups: values, understanding phenomena, allocation of resources and methods of regulation. The relationships between these factors constitute the symbolic structure that allows actors to interpret the world and to give it meaning (9).

VALUES

In most democratic societies, three major values are in tension with each other: equity, individual autonomy and efficiency.

Equity refers to a collective concern for individual justice. Equity can be defined, in very general terms, as an appreciation of what (collectively) people believe is just to distribute equally between individuals or groups (10).

Individual autonomy is one of the central values of the health care system, and of the social sphere in general. It is currently taken as a synonym for independence and freedom, in contrast to the collectivist view of society defined by the concept of equity. The notion of autonomy has a variety of meanings, however, including self-determination, individual freedom, independence, self-rule, acting according to one's own principles, or following one's own plan of life (11). It includes two basic concepts: autonomy of action (the possibility of acting in a voluntary and intentional manner) and the capacity to act independently (relying on one's own judgement and with the necessary resources to achieve a desired result).

Efficiency is the desire to maximize a social entity (health or access to care) in the most economical way possible. Every definition of efficiency corresponds to a particular sub-principle for resource allocation. It is useful to distinguish three levels of efficiency: technical, allocative and social. Efficiency, however, is not in itself a sufficient definition of an allocation mechanism. In keeping with the above definition of equity, examining the nature of efficiency can lead one to define several different allocation principles.

UNDERSTANDING PHENOMENA

An understanding of phenomena such as life, health, sickness, death, pain and their determinants is a way of interpreting the objectives of the health care system. This perspective evolves over time *(12–14)* and is not uniform. The concept of health incorporates realities that are very different and cannot be superimposed.

Thus, if one chooses to describe a population's health by indicators constructed around the concept of mortality (life expectancy or standardized mortality rates) one cannot see health as it is perceived by individuals who are in pain or worried about being sick. If the latter perspective is chosen, however, one ignores biological functions (on the level of organs, tissues, cells or molecules) that modern diagnostic methods can identify and that biological technology makes it possible to treat.

ALLOCATION OF RESOURCES

This factor concerns the perception of the role and functions of different individuals working in the health care sector, and of the allocation of resources between sectors. On the one hand, this reflects the opinions prevailing in society about the responsibilities and positions that professionals must hold, the resources they must acquire and the education they must attain. On the other hand, it reflects the optimal allocation of public resources between health and health care and, within health care, between prevention and cure, between hospital and ambulatory care, and between the public and private sectors of the health care system.

METHODS OF REGULATION

The interaction between actors in health care delivery is defined by one of four basic regulatory models found in most parts of society. These are the technocratic model, the professional self-regulating model, the market-based model and the democratic model. Each model emphasizes a different set of values. The dominant model selected for use with a given health care system reflects the priorities chosen by society as a whole.

In the technocratic model, trained "experts" guide the system, relying on their specialized knowledge and their dominant position in political and economic institutions *(15)*. This regulatory approach, also called the "command-and-control planning model" *(16)*, is based on normative analysis produced by experts responsible for structuring, monitoring and assessing the activities of the health care system. This model implies direct state intervention in operating the health care system, in order to achieve rationalization and to limit shifts in policy goals caused by actors' irrational behaviour *(15)*.

In the professional self-regulatory model, physicians[2] are at the centre of the health care system and the utilization of health resources depends on their decisions. Acting as patients' agents, they have access to all information concerning their needs and are expected to provide care on this basis. This model assumes that control over the health care system must be delegated to the medical profession. Given the

---

[2] The term "physician" is used here generically to denote all medical practitioners irrespective of specialization. The term "doctor" is used as appropriate to connote a specific relationship to patient care.

imbalance of information and knowledge in their favour, the central role of physicians in determining resource use and the absence of any real legal framework to control medical practice, limits to abuse can only be set by the medical profession itself. This control is exerted through education and training that ensures standardized skill acquisition. It is also exerted through a strong professional code of ethics that emphasizes medical practice based on the patient's needs, avoiding both over-utilization and underutilization of services. Control of medical practice is further influenced by professional socialization to certain ethical norms.

In the market-based model, regulations are established in competing markets in accordance with supply and demand, and on condition that certain constraints are accepted. This type of regulation leads to what may be considered a Pareto-optimal allocation of resources,[3] in the sense that it is impossible to change it without penalizing at least one economic agent. Mainly because of its normative and ideological aspects, this is a powerful model. The approach is based on a doctrine that affirms the autonomy of the market and therefore considers that government intervention in economic affairs must be minimal.

In the democratic model, each citizen possesses the right and has the responsibility to influence sociopolitical decisions and actions in society. This democratic right can be exercised directly or indirectly. Usually it is exercised indirectly, through either elected or appointed representatives. The democratic model links the population into the process of formulating needs, problems, priorities and solutions to the management and administration of the health care system.

Institutionalizing health sector values

The above review implies that there is rarely, if ever, one model to which everyone can subscribe. In reality, there are interlinked belief systems connected by discussions that, at a particular moment in time, crystallize into a discrete, concrete set of organizational forms. These organizational forms become the legal, administrative and physical structure of the dominant value system, defining how material resources are allocated and how authority and power (what Bourdieu *(17)* calls symbolic capital) are distributed *(8)*.

These organizational structures produce a vast array of incentives, constraints, obligations and norms that, at any given moment, reinforce a specific set of values, perceptions and beliefs. The social and material structure produces a "field of incentives" similar to a magnetic force field, in which actors struggle to transform the existing order to serve their own interests *(17)*.

If one can imagine that the organizational structure is a reflection, at a given moment, of both the equilibrium and the tension that exist between the beliefs and perceptions of the various actors in the system, it is also plausible that the organization and symbolic structures have different evolutionary rhythms. As time passes, one can imagine a disjunction between the two. The greater the break, the more the previous organizational forms are perceived as inadequate, and the system enters a

---

[3] Pareto improvement means improvement in the welfare of one individual without adversely affecting the welfare of others (Alfredo Pareto, Professor of Economics at Lausanne University, d. 1923).

crisis situation. This can be resolved by transforming a particular organizational form without disturbing the equilibrium of forces in tension that characterizes the system as a whole. It is also possible, however, that this crisis is more profound if it affects one or more of the four factors that structure these symbolic representations. In this situation, marginal changes to organizational structures are not enough to resolve the crisis; deeper transformations are needed. This may well be the situation that prevails in a number of developed countries today *(18)*.

THE REALITY OF MACROECONOMICS

The structure and status of the overall national economy are a similarly important factor for the character of health reform. National, regional and municipal governments in many countries are under severe financial pressure. In western Europe, the member states of the European Union (EU) are cutting back public spending in order to reduce their budget deficits to the target set by the Maastricht Treaty for joining the proposed European Monetary Union. Growing unemployment and social welfare costs have strained local government budgets. More generally, economists have argued that, for western European countries to remain competitive in a globalizing world economy, their public sector spending levels must be reduced in order to free capital for private investment *(19)*. These macroeconomic pressures suggest that publicly financed and/or operated health systems may well face retrenchment, regardless of how efficiently or effectively they perform.

In the CEE countries, although several years of negative economic growth have now been replaced by improvements in overall gross domestic product (GDP), current levels of production have only returned to their 1989 levels in Poland (Table 1). In the CIS countries, 1996 economic productivity is estimated to be barely more than half of that in 1989. These reduced levels of GDP reflect the painful economic restructuring that is under way, and help to explain the sharp fall in state revenue available to the health sector.

DEMOGRAPHIC AND SOCIAL PRESSURES
An aging population

One important development throughout the Region appears to be the further aging of the population. The percentage of people over 65 years of age, especially the very old, will continue to rise. Although the use of health services by the elderly varies by country and cohort, governments are concerned that higher numbers of elderly citizens will need a greater volume of health care services, and that overall spending rates will increase. This is further explored below, in the section on implications for health services (pages 24–28).

Technological developments

The development of both invasive and noninvasive clinical innovations has increased over the past decade. For reasons of safety, efficiency, quality of care and prestige, as well as of patient satisfaction, health care providers find themselves under pressure to adopt the latest available medical techniques. Even when new

Table 1. Economic growth in the CEE and CIS countries, 1990–1996[a]

Country	Annual percentage change in real GDP (1989 = 100)						Real GDP (1989 = 100)	
	1990	1991	1992	1993	1994	1995 (estimate)	1996 (projection)	1995 (estimate)	1996 (projection)
Albania	−10	−28	−10	11	9	9	5	77	81
Armenia	−7	−11	−52	−15	5	7	7	38	40
Azerbaijan	−12	−1	−23	−23	−21	−8	−4	38	36
Belarus	−3	−1	−10	−11	−12	−10	−5	61	58
Bulgaria	−9	−12	−7	−2	2	3	−4	76	73
Croatia	−9	−20	−10	−4	1	2	5	65	68
Czech Republic	−0	−14	−6	−1	3	5	5	85	90
Estonia	−8	−11	−14	−9	−3	3	3	64	66
Georgia	−12	−14	−40	−39	−35	2	8	18	20
Hungary	−4	−12	−3	−1	3	2	2	86	87
Kazakstan	−0	−13	−13	−12	−25	−9	1	45	46
Kyrgyzstan	3	−5	−19	−16	−27	1	2	50	51
Latvia	3	−8	−35	−16	1	−2	1	51	52
Lithuania	−5	−13	−38	−24	1	3	2	40	41
Poland	−12	−7	3	4	5	7	5	99	103
Republic of Moldova	−2	−18	−29	−1	−31	−3	4	38	39
Romania	−6	−13	−9	1	4	7	5	84	88
Russian Federation	−4	−13	−15	−9	−13	−4	3	55	53
Slovakia	−3	−15	−7	−4	5	7	6	84	89

Table 1. (contd)

Country	Annual percentage change in real GDP (1989 = 100)							Real GDP (1989 = 100)	
	1990	1991	1992	1993	1994	1995 (estimate)	1996 (projection)	1995 (estimate)	1996 (projection)
Slovenia	-5	-8	-5	1	5	4	3	91	94
Tajikistan	-2	-7	-29	-11	-22	-13	-7	40	37
The Former Yugoslav Republic of Macedonia	-10	-12	-21	-8	-4	-2	3	54	56
Turkmenistan	2	-5	-5	-10	-20	-10	0	60	60
Ukraine	-3	-9	-10	-14	-23	-12	-7	46	43
Uzbekistan	2	-1	-11	-2	-4	-1	-1	83	82
CEE and CIS average	-5	-12	-10	-5	-6	0	1	68	68
CEE average[b]	-7	-11	-4	1	4	5	4	87	90
CIS average[c]	-4	-12	-14	-9	-14	-5	-3	54	52

[a] Data for 1989–1995 represent the most recent official estimates of out-turns as reflected in publications from the national authorities, the International Monetary Fund, the World Bank, OECD, PlanEcon and the Institute of International Finance. Data for 1995 are preliminary actuals, mostly official government estimates. Data for 1996 represent projections of the European Bank for Reconstruction and Development (EBRD).

[b] Estimates for real GDP represent weighted averages for Albania, Bulgaria, Croatia, the Czech Republic, Estonia, Hungary, Latvia, Lithuania, Poland, Romania, Slovakia, Slovenia and The Former Yugoslav Republic of Macedonia. The weights used were EBRD estimates of nominal US $ GDP for 1995.

[c] Here taken to include all countries of the former USSR except Estonia, Latvia and Lithuania. Estimates for real GDP represent weighted averages. The weights used were EBRD estimates of nominal US $ GDP for 1995.

Source: European Bank for Reconstruction and Development (20).

procedures are less expensive (such as laparoscopic surgery or cardiac imaging), they typically entail substantial capital costs for new equipment and renovated facilities, and sometimes involve higher operating costs for additional personnel. Advances in information technology also demand investment in hardware and training, particularly if market-oriented competitive incentives push purchasers and providers to set prices for services.

Expectations of citizens and patients

Citizens in all parts of Europe are demanding a more patient-oriented approach to the delivery of health care services. In western Europe, patients' rights movements are growing, and governments in countries with tax-funded systems are under popular pressure to reduce waiting times and remove other scheduling obstacles. Providers are also expected to offer high-quality services, in line with international standards. In the CEE and CIS countries, patients have strong views on the need for choice and quality in health services, often backing up these demands with out-of-pocket payments to providers.

Political requirements

Politicians often look for quick or short-term solutions to policy problems, to coincide with electoral cycles. They also try to identify reforms that fit with broader ideological themes suitable for election campaigning. In both eastern and western Europe, past policy decisions have frequently been tailored to these requirements.

Corporate management strategies

Starting in the 1980s, reform decisions in the health sector began to take into account the latest thinking about management in private corporations. Strategies such as decentralizing to entrepreneurial subunits, outsourcing and re-engineering – all approaches that flatten traditional hierarchies and create team-based management – have influenced the design of health sector reforms in the 1990s.

The reform predicament: health and health sector challenges

While the specific contextual factors that trigger health care reforms have varied from country to country, the underlying problems in the health systems themselves tend to be quite similar. This is true despite strikingly dissimilar conditions in eastern and western Europe. Incorporating the broad contextual pressures noted above, a set of dilemmas specific to health and the health sector have led national policy-makers to opt for major structural reforms.

HEALTH CHALLENGES

The changing pattern of disease in Europe is one factor driving change in the configuration of health services at both the micro and macro levels. The expansion of services for sexually transmitted diseases in the wake of the rise in HIV infection and AIDS is an example of the former *(21)*. The latter is typified by concerns about the long-term financing of health services in the light of aging populations and the rising level of chronic disease. This section provides an overview of some of the major trends in health in Europe; first, however, it is necessary to consider the ways in which patterns of disease can be described.

Measuring health and disease

Two issues must be considered. The first is how the relative contribution made by various conditions to the overall burden of disease can be measured. The second is how these data can be used to describe trends over time, and hence to forecast how they might change further in the future.

There are various approaches to this. The simplest is a measure of mortality, such as crude or age-standardized death rates. This will show, for example, what the leading causes of death are. The number of years of life lost due to premature death is a further variation on this theme *(22)*. It can take several forms, such as the recalculation of life expectancy in the absence of deaths from a particular cause, or the potential years of life lost; the latter typically involves adding the differences between the age of death from each disease and a figure chosen to represent the normal life span, usually 65 or 75 years. This can be further refined by techniques such as differential weighting to allow for variations in the social value of life at different ages *(23)*.

These measures have been used to show how, for example, when measured in terms of years of life lost, the major threats to health in the CIS differ between the European republics (where they are largely noncommunicable diseases such as ischaemic heart disease, lung cancer and chronic obstructive pulmonary disease) and the central Asian republics (where these causes are supplemented by communicable diseases and reproductive disorders) *(24)*.

A complementary approach involves measuring the burden of disease that does not result in death. This has traditionally been done with readily available measures such as days lost from work, but it is increasingly recognized that the numerous variables involved limit the value of such measures. Other approaches include surveys of the number of people with long-standing illness; these can be refined by including a wide range of health status measures *(25)*. Health care reformers may also wish to ensure that the priorities implied in reform measures maximize the benefits that can be achieved for a given input of resources. To do so, they must place a value on different health states. The different measures used are based on the idea that a year of life in less than perfect health should be valued as less than one year of quality- or disability-adjusted life by applying a weighting factor derived from surveys. Perhaps the best known examples are the quality-adjusted life-year (QALY) *(26)* or disability-adjusted life-year (DALY) *(27)*. The former uses weightings allocated to health states, normally in a two-dimensional matrix encompassing distress and disability, while the latter allocates weights to six different levels of disability.

The second issue is how to forecast future trends in levels of disease. As with all forecasting, this involves making certain assumptions that existing trends will be projected into the future. The standard technique for forecasting disease patterns is age period cohort analysis, in which trends in each age group are examined separately. The results can then be linked with information on projected population numbers to gain some idea of how diseases might behave in the future. This approach, although producing valuable insights, is tenable only in the short term. It can, however, be supplemented by techniques such as Delphi methods, which allow expert opinion to be synthesized to identify possible changes that might be expected based on analogy rather than on pre-existing trends) and scenario analysis, in which different assumptions about the future can be tested.

This information can be combined with evidence of the likelihood of various strategies achieving particular results, as well as the costs of doing so. A good example is contained in the 1993 *World development report* of the World Bank *(28)*, where the cost per DALY of a range of health strategies was estimated. There is a variety of tools available to support this type of analysis, the most widely used of which is the Dutch PREVENT model *(29)*.

Health trends in Europe

For the purposes of the overview presented in this section, the WHO European Region is considered in terms of three major blocs: the EU countries, the CEE countries and the newly independent states (NIS) of the former USSR.[4] It is important, however, to recognize that, while there are general trends in the patterns of disease in different parts of the Region, the use of aggregate data inevitably obscures what is a highly complex picture, both between and within countries *(30)*.

Starting with overall trends in mortality, the most striking finding is the divergence in life expectancy between these three parts of the Region (Fig. 1 and 2).

Between 1980 and 1994, male life expectancy at birth in the EU increased by 3.1 years from 70.7 to 73.8; for females, it increased by 3.2 years from 77.4 to 80.6. By contrast, in CEE countries, the figure for males increased by only 0.6 of a year, from an already low value of 66.7 to 67.3 years; the increase for females was 1.8 years, from 73.5 to 75.3 years. The situation in the NIS is the most disturbing, with life expectancy at birth actually falling: for men by 1.6 years from 62.2 to 60.6 years, and for women by 0.6 of a year from 72.5 to 71.9 years.

As noted above, these aggregate figures conceal considerable national diversity. For example, life expectancy is generally greater in countries in the south of each of the regions. Furthermore, even within western Europe, some countries – such as Denmark – experienced very little increase in life expectancy over the period *(31)* while the previously rapid improvement in Spain slowed down after 1981. In the CEE countries, the Czech Republic and Poland have experienced recent reversals of long-term downward trends in life expectancy, while Hungary has not. In the NIS,

---

[4] The data given in this section are taken from the Regional Office's health for all database, in which statistics on the CIS countries and the Baltic states are combined to give a single NIS figure (see footnote 1, page 1). More detailed information from the database is readily available from the Epidemiology, Statistics and Health Information unit, WHO Regional Office for Europe, Scherfigsvej 8, DK-2100 Copenhagen Ø, Denmark. The database may also be consulted on or downloaded from the World Wide Web at http://www.who.dk/country/country.htm.

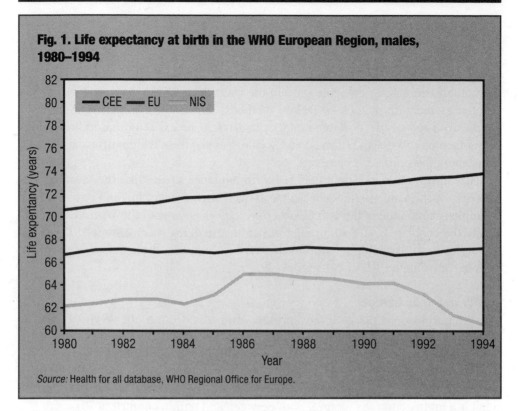

Fig. 1. Life expectancy at birth in the WHO European Region, males, 1980–1994

Source: Health for all database, WHO Regional Office for Europe.

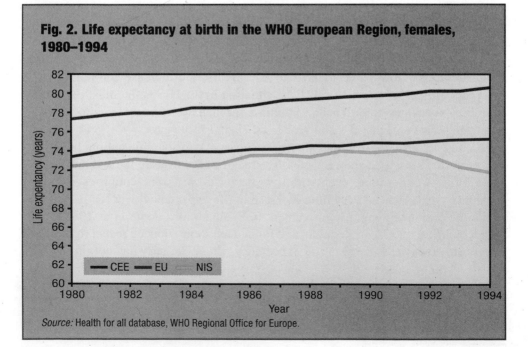

Fig. 2. Life expectancy at birth in the WHO European Region, females, 1980–1994

Source: Health for all database, WHO Regional Office for Europe.

the Russian Federation has experienced a particularly serious deterioration in male life expectancy at birth, losing 7 years between 1986 and 1994. As shown in Fig. 1 and 2, there have also been differences in trends over time, with a dramatic improvement in life expectancy in the NIS after 1985 (widely attributed to the campaign against alcohol at that time) that has subsequently been reversed (Fig. 3).

In any ranking of leading challenges to health in Europe, cardiovascular diseases feature strongly. They cause half of all deaths and a third of all permanent disability in the Region, and are therefore responsible for a substantial proportion of total health care costs. Death rates vary widely within the Region and, as with life expectancy, the trends are diverging (Fig. 4 and 5). There are also large differences between the rates in males and females; this is partly explained by the protective effect of female hormones, which delay the onset of disease until after the menopause, but also by the lower level of tobacco consumption by women in many countries.

In the EU countries between 1981 and 1993, the age-standardized death rate from ischaemic heart disease among men aged 0–64 years decreased from 77.2 to 52.0 per 100 000 population. In females, there was also a decrease from 16.8 to 12.2. In the CEE countries, however, the figure for males increased from 86.2 in 1981 to 106.9 in 1993, with a smaller increase for women from 22.2 to 27.8 per 100 000. As with life expectancy, the situation in the NIS is significantly worse, with an increase among men from 153.9 per 100 000 in 1981 to 215.2 in 1993; the corresponding figures for

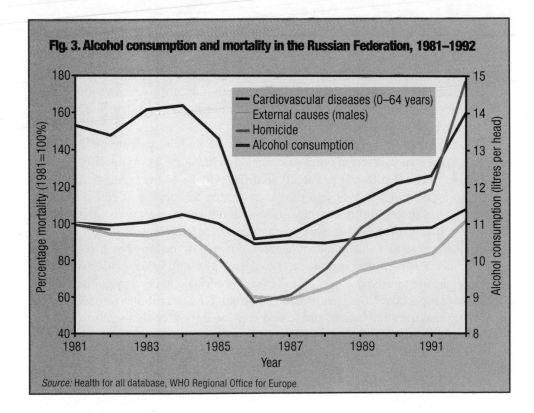

Fig. 3. Alcohol consumption and mortality in the Russian Federation, 1981–1992

Legend:
— Cardiovascular diseases (0–64 years)
— External causes (males)
— Homicide
— Alcohol consumption

Y-axis (left): Percentage mortality (1981=100%)
Y-axis (right): Alcohol consumption (litres per head)
X-axis: Year

Source: Health for all database, WHO Regional Office for Europe.

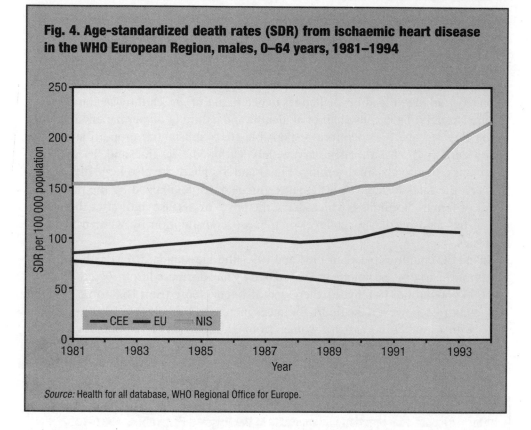

Fig. 4. Age-standardized death rates (SDR) from ischaemic heart disease in the WHO European Region, males, 0–64 years, 1981–1994

Source: Health for all database, WHO Regional Office for Europe.

women are 47.1 and 62.6. Thus, in this age group, the death rates from ischaemic heart disease among NIS citizens are now between four and five times those in the EU. Cardiovascular diseases account for approximately half of the difference in life expectancy between eastern and western Europe.

Cancer is the second greatest cause of death in the Region, accounting for 20% of all deaths. The many different types of cancer, and the corresponding differences in risk factors, mean that trends in each type differ widely. Many types of cancer are related to aspects of lifestyle and thus preventable to varying degrees, although certain genetic susceptibilities render some individuals at greater risk than others. The role of lifestyle is most clearly demonstrated by tobacco consumption, which is an important cause of a wide range of cancers, not only of the lung but also of several other organs. Furthermore, it may act synergistically with other causes of cancer, such as exposure to asbestos and, in the case of cervical cancer, human papillomavirus. Other aspects of lifestyle are also important. Diet contributes to cancer of the gastrointestinal tract and breast, and sexual activity, through viral infection, contributes to cancer of the cervix.

Nevertheless the leading avoidable cause of cancer in Europe is tobacco smoking (Fig. 6). Lung cancer rates offer a marker for the consequences of juvenile smoking, and in the CEE countries and the NIS the aggressive marketing by tobacco companies will

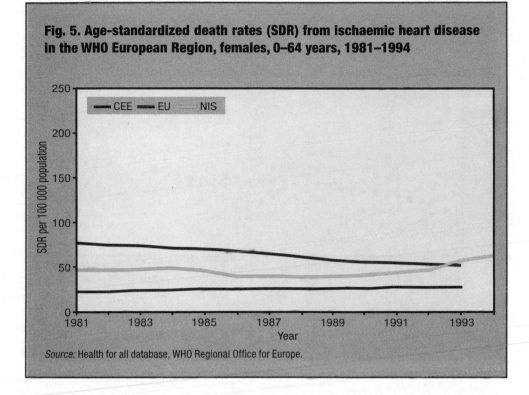

Fig. 5. Age-standardized death rates (SDR) from ischaemic heart disease in the WHO European Region, females, 0–64 years, 1981–1994

Source: Health for all database, WHO Regional Office for Europe.

have major health consequences in the future. As with heart disease, there are large differences both between different parts of the Region and between men and women. In each part of the Region, death rates are much lower in women than in men, reflecting their somewhat later adoption of smoking on a large scale. There are inevitably large national variations, partly reflecting cultural differences, and the gap between the sexes is rapidly closing in some countries, such as Denmark.

Overall, there was a small decrease in the death rates from lung cancer in males aged 0–64 years in the EU between 1981 and 1993, from 34.1 to 32.2 per 100 000 population. In contrast, death rates increased slightly among women: from 5.7 to 6.7 per 100 000. There were far greater increases in the CEE countries: from 41.3 to 53.4 per 100 000 in men, and from 5.5 to 8.2 per 100 000 in women. A similar pattern is seen for men in the NIS, with an increase from 46.2 to 50.0 per 100 000, although there was a slight decrease among women, from 5.1 to 4.8 per 100 000.

External causes of death, such as accidents, homicide and suicide, are the third greatest cause of death in the Region, and they are the second largest contributor to the gap in life expectancy at birth between eastern and western Europe. They particularly affect adults in their thirties and forties, and thus have a disproportionate impact on families and on industrial productivity. They have risen dramatically in the NIS, partly due to the increasing violence, the relaxation of previous occupational safety measures, and the growing psychological stress, which, in turn, contributes to increasing levels of alcohol consumption. The age-standardized death

Fig. 6. Estimates of smoking prevalence in the WHO European Region, early 1990s

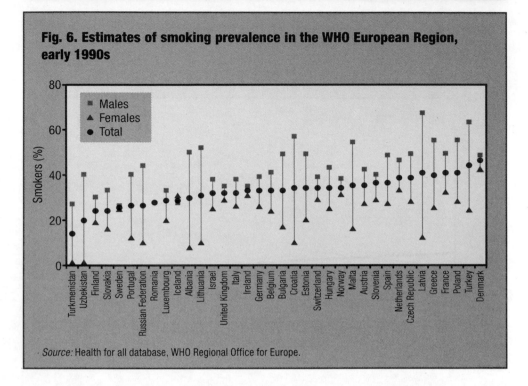

Source: Health for all database, WHO Regional Office for Europe.

rate for this category, encompassing all ages, fell in the EU from 56.9 per 100 000 in 1981 to 46.6 in 1993. It rose only slightly in the CEE countries, although from an already higher level, i.e. from 76.4 to 80.2 per 100 000. There was a greater rise in the NIS, again from a high level, from 131.7 to 164 per 100 000 over the same period (Fig. 7).

As the above statistics indicate, there has been a dramatic deterioration in health in many of the CEE countries and the NIS. Although some underlying factors, such as those related to lifestyle, are the same as in the west, they are of quite a different order of magnitude. Changes of this size inevitably have major consequences for the need for health care, and for patterns of disease.

There is still much debate about the reasons for the failure of the CEE countries and the NIS to match the increases in life expectancy seen in western Europe *(32)*. Certain issues, however, emerge as important. Overall, the high levels of cardiovascular diseases in the CEE countries and the NIS make the largest contribution to east–west differences in life expectancy at birth, followed by external causes of death and respiratory diseases (Table 2). As noted earlier, however, there are important differences between countries. Accidents and violence, as well as liver cirrhosis – all strongly related to alcohol consumption – play an important role in the European republics of the NIS and in Hungary but somewhat less so in, for example, Poland, where a campaign against alcohol consumption in the early 1980s halted a previously increasing trend in alcohol-related diseases.

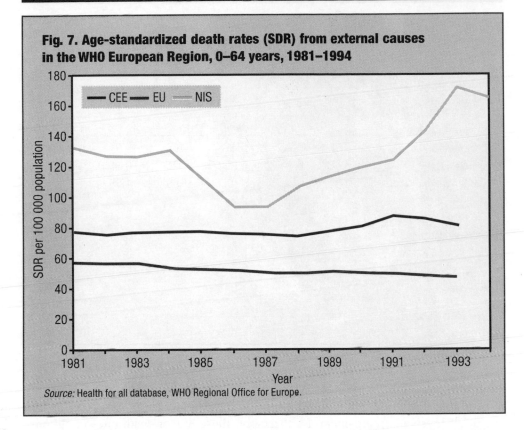

Fig. 7. Age-standardized death rates (SDR) from external causes in the WHO European Region, 0–64 years, 1981–1994

Source: Health for all database, WHO Regional Office for Europe.

Tobacco consumption presents a further major challenge, with death rates from lung cancer in men already well in excess of those seen in most western European countries. As there is an interval of many years between starting smoking and developing lung cancer, the very high rates of smoking currently seen in these regions suggest that the health services of the twenty-first century will face an enormous burden from this disease.

Diet is also likely to be an extremely important factor, with generally low levels of nutrition in the CEE countries and the NIS *(33)*. Again, there is recent evidence of national diversity: the decreasing consumption of animal fats and increasing consumption of fruit and vegetables in, for instance, Poland are not seen to the same extent in Hungary. Detailed examination of the trends in patterns of diseases identifies other problems that are not yet a major concern, but where there are steady long-term upward trends – various forms of cancer, for example.

Concentrating on specific diseases entails the risk, however, that important underlying factors will be ignored. Western Europe has been engaged in a long-running debate about whether increased levels of ill health among the poor can be entirely explained by their exposure to higher levels of risk factors, or whether social position and socioeconomic status contribute. There is now convincing evidence that social factors are important, most notably from the British Whitehall study in which

Table 2. Factors contributing to the gap in life expectancy between the CEE countries and NIS and western European countries

Cause of death	Additional life expectancy in western Europe by age group				
	< 1 year	1–34 years	35–64 years	≥ 65 years	All ages
Infectious and parasitic diseases	0.3	0.1	0.08	−0.01	0.47
Cancer	0	0.05	0.25	−0.35	−0.05
Cardiovascular diseases	0	0.07	1.36	1.85	3.28
Respiratory diseases	0.68	0.2	0.15	−0.5	0.97
Digestive diseases	0.02	0.03	0.08	−0.04	0.09
External causes	0.04	0.64	0.71	0.03	1.41
Undefined conditions	−0.1	0.01	0.04	0.18	0.12
Other diseases	0	0	−0.02	−0.2	−0.22
All causes	0.93	1.09	2.63	1.4	6.06

Source: Health for all database, WHO Regional Office for Europe.

the health status of civil servants was followed for long periods (34). This study showed that death rates were higher among officials in lower grades, and this was true at all levels of employment. Furthermore, these higher death rates could only partly be explained by known risk factors, such as diet and tobacco consumption (35). Similarly, there is a growing body of evidence that inequalities in wealth are important determinants of differences in mortality between (36) and within countries (37,38). Finally, the fear of unemployment and the insecurity that accompanies it are also important predictors of ill health. Although research on this issue in the CEE countries and the NIS is still relatively sparse, there is evidence that those at the margins of society and in relative poverty in the CEE countries – divorced men, for example – have been most adversely affected (39) and that stress is playing a significant part in the high levels of mortality (40).

The emergence of new infectious diseases and the resurgence of old ones also have substantial implications for health services in Europe. Probably the best known example of a new disease is HIV infection and AIDS. The incidence of AIDS varies widely within Europe, reflecting the numerous factors, including cultural differences, that influence exposure to risk factors. The highest incidence is currently in France, Italy and Spain. In some countries, the rate of increase is beginning to slow down, largely as a consequence of health promotion policies, but in others it is continuing to accelerate. Furthermore, the pattern of underlying risk factors is also changing (Fig. 8).

AIDS is only one example of the increasing threat from infectious diseases. The breakdown of previous control measures in the NIS has contributed to the reappearance of diseases such as diphtheria and cholera, while the incidence of tuberculosis is increasing throughout the Region.

The present pattern of disease in Europe has several implications for health sector reform. The first is the need to recognize that health services *per se* can have only a relatively limited impact on the major causes of ill health in the European Region. Health status is largely determined by the interaction of four linked factors: genetic susceptibility, behaviour and lifestyle, socioeconomic status and environmental conditions *(42)*.

The second implication is that reformed health systems must incorporate mechanisms for tackling the major threats to health. In particular, there is a need for strong public health services with the ability to monitor trends in diseases and to support the development of integrated programmes to deal with them. How this can be achieved

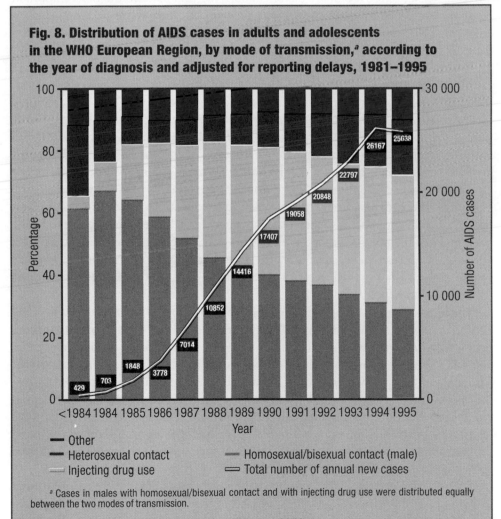

Fig. 8. Distribution of AIDS cases in adults and adolescents in the WHO European Region, by mode of transmission,[a] according to the year of diagnosis and adjusted for reporting delays, 1981–1995

— Other
— Heterosexual contact
— Injecting drug use
— Homosexual/bisexual contact (male)
— Total number of annual new cases

[a] Cases in males with homosexual/bisexual contact and with injecting drug use were distributed equally between the two modes of transmission.

Source: European Centre for the Epidemiological Monitoring of AIDS *(41)*.

is discussed in detail in the section on reforming public health services in Chapter 2 (see pages 69–78).

The third implication is that, as patterns of disease change over time, health services will need to respond to these changes and not remain trapped in structures designed for a time when disease patterns were quite different.

CHANGING PATTERNS OF HEALTH: IMPLICATIONS FOR HEALTH SERVICES

Patterns of disease have continually changed. Ten thousand years ago, the occupants of the first cities in Sumeria and the Indus Valley faced newly emerging infections arising from their increased contact with domesticated animals *(43)*. As human activity has evolved, old diseases have disappeared and new ones have emerged. As mentioned earlier, the populations of Europe currently face a rather particular pattern of disease. There are many factors underlying this pattern, the most important being the challenge of aging populations, changes in diet and lifestyle, new and re-emerging infectious diseases, and – especially in the CEE countries and the NIS – the effects of economic decline and widening differentials in income.

Health services have regularly responded to new challenges. In the nineteenth century the new diseases of urbanization, such as cholera, typhoid and tuberculosis, led to the development of public health services and sanatoria. More recently, the spread of HIV infection and AIDS has stimulated the development of health promotion activities and services directed at sexually transmitted diseases. While the record of responses to abrupt changes in patterns of disease has often been good, however, results have been less satisfactory in the face of longer-term trends.

The changing demography of the European population is producing a substantial challenge to health services (Fig. 9). When individuals reach retirement age, their need for health care begins to increase, and it accelerates once they are over 75. The percentage of the population in these age groups is increasing in all parts of Europe, although increases will be especially great in southern and western Europe. This has implications both for total need for health care and for the pattern of diseases contributing to it.

The increased need for health care has important resource consequences. In many countries, this is compounded by falling birth rates, so that the number of working people able to contribute to health care funds will decrease just as need is increasing, and when other demands for social welfare, such as pensions, are also increasing. The scale of this problem will vary. Some countries, such as the United Kingdom, will be affected relatively mildly, but others, like Germany, will face substantial challenges. While the long-term trends are still difficult to predict, the dramatic decline in birth rates in many CEE countries and NIS is also likely to prove a problem, since a smaller economically active population will be available to support growing numbers of elderly people.

Patterns of disease will also continue to change. In particular, there will be further growth in the number of people suffering from heart disease, cerebrovascular disease, cancer, dementia and, especially among women, fractures. It will no longer be sufficient for health services to respond reactively to these conditions. As research

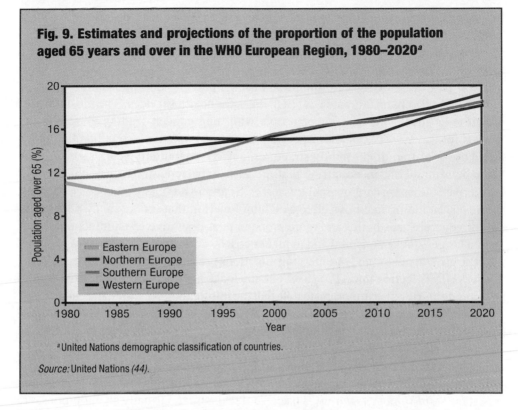

Fig. 9. Estimates and projections of the proportion of the population aged 65 years and over in the WHO European Region, 1980–2020[a]

Legend:
- Eastern Europe
- Northern Europe
- Southern Europe
- Western Europe

[a] United Nations demographic classification of countries.

Source: United Nations *(44)*.

develops on the effectiveness of specialized programmes to tackle the major causes of disease, health services will have to reconfigure themselves accordingly with, for example, regionalized cancer services, dedicated multidisciplinary stroke units *(45)* and integrated packages of care that involve orthopaedic surgery, geriatric medicine and rehabilitation for patients with fractured hips. A further consequence of aging is that an increasing number of people will suffer from multiple disorders, thus receiving a wide range of treatments with potential for interaction. This presents health services with new challenges, and emphasizes the need to move away from a model of care that is based on individual physicians to one involving multidisciplinary teams.

Changes in diet and lifestyle also present serious challenges to health services. For many years, longevity has been greater in the countries of southern Europe than in other parts of the Region, even within groups of countries that are otherwise broadly similar. For example, life expectancy at birth in Greece and Spain has exceeded the average for the EU, that in Albania has exceeded the average for the CEE countries, and that in the Caucasian republics has exceeded the average for the NIS. This is largely believed to be due to differences in diet *(46)*. Although the exact mechanisms remain a matter of debate, the greater life expectancy appears to be directly related to high levels of consumption of fresh fruit and vegetables *(47)*. Unfortunately, the situation is changing in those countries that have historically enjoyed this advantage. The spread of northern European diets to countries such as Spain and especially the growing consumption of "fast foods" containing high levels of animal fat are likely to lead to increasing levels of heart disease and to other diet-related diseases such as breast cancer. It may become necessary, for example, to reassess the need for screening programmes in southern European countries with previously low levels of breast cancer.

The growth in tobacco consumption in some parts of Europe is another way in which lifestyle changes create new challenges for health services. The most obvious result is an increasing number of people with lung cancer, leading to greater demands for cancer services and, where the increase is taking place in parallel with a breakdown of traditional family structures, a need for palliative care services. The growth of smoking in countries that are also experiencing dietary change will exacerbate the rise in cardiovascular diseases. Smoking has many other consequences, however, including insidious effects on lung function that render many people less fit for general anaesthetics and more prone to post-operative chest infections, leading to longer stays in hospital and to higher costs.

The growth of new and re-emerging infections presents a further challenge. Some, such as HIV infection and AIDS, have already led to a reorientation of health services in some countries. It is important to note that the implications of the emergence of HIV have not been confined to services for sexually transmitted diseases, but have affected nearly all aspects of health care, including approaches to hospital infection control and the screening of blood products. Others are less well known. The growth of multiresistant bacteria in hospitals is likely to have major consequences for the way in which hospital services are provided. Already, some patients infected with methicillinresistant *Staphylococcus aureus,* a bacterium resistant to virtually all antibiotics, are seen in some countries as too dangerous to admit to hospital and are being treated at considerable expense in their own homes. In some countries, the lack of appropriate, enforced antibiotic policies is causing large increases in the rates of hospital-acquired infections and consequently adding to both length of stay and costs. The risks from certain hospital-acquired infections are already forcing some countries to reassess the ways in which they provide health care, leading in particular to the transfer of some interventions to settings other than hospitals. This trend is also being reinforced by efforts at cost-containment, as well as by a growing volume of research suggesting that many interventions are as effective in non-hospital settings.

The growth of infectious diseases, however, is not confined to patients already in hospital. As noted above, the breakdown of public health measures in the NIS has contributed to the re-emergence of poliomyelitis, diphtheria, cholera and malaria, with important implications for public health and primary health care (PHC) services (Fig. 10 and 11). All of Europe is facing an increasing incidence of tuberculosis, a disease many thought had almost disappeared. The emergence of a variant resistant to most common drugs is especially worrying, necessitating new approaches such as the supervised administration of medication and the prescription of expensive second-line drugs.

The preceding paragraphs give some examples of the changes in disease patterns that European health systems are confronting. These changes will affect countries' ability to sustain existing levels of provision, as well as the way in which services are

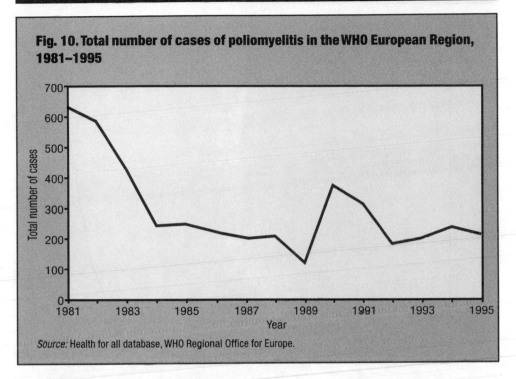

Fig. 10. Total number of cases of poliomyelitis in the WHO European Region, 1981–1995

Source: Health for all database, WHO Regional Office for Europe.

provided. Various factors often come together to exacerbate particular challenges. The likelihood of a growing need for stroke services is one example, owing partly to an aging population but also, in some countries, to changes in diet, particularly the reduced consumption of fresh fruit and vegetables that are recognized to have an important protective effect. The need will be further accentuated, especially in southern Europe, by the consequences of the breakdown of the extended family structure.

This changing environment carries considerable implications for health care reform. In many countries, the existing structures and incentives are based on a historical pattern of disease that is no longer dominant. This is intrinsically bound up with the evolving body of research on the effectiveness of treatment for specific diseases. Both of these factors mean that traditional hospital care, with treatment regimes based on a narrow medical model and with a wide range of diseases treated in general wards, is no longer appropriate. New structures and packages of incentives should reflect the demands currently facing providers, and not reinforce obsolete models of care. This, in turn, makes it essential that those involved in health sector reform should incorporate into their debates evidence about trends in disease patterns and their implications for health services, using the approaches described above in the section on health challenges (pages 13–24).

Finally, incorporating the changing patterns of disease into debate has a further set of implications for those involved in health care reform. It is clear that many of the diseases that will contribute most to the burden of ill health in the coming decades are caused by factors outside the formal health sector. If they are to be most effective,

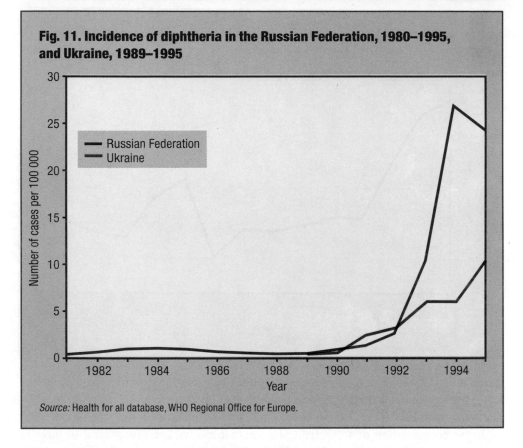

Fig. 11. Incidence of diphtheria in the Russian Federation, 1980–1995, and Ukraine, 1989–1995

Source: Health for all database, WHO Regional Office for Europe.

cost-containment strategies should address demand in terms of both the numbers of people seeking care and of the health system's ability to return them rapidly to the community.

To do so, they must ensure that reformed health systems have a strong public health component that can analyse trends in disease, identify explanations, and propose and monitor effective responses. These responses are likely to require coordinated activities, including the development of healthy public policies, prevention, the strengthening of PHC and the reorientation of hospital services. This will require effective support and trained individuals with an understanding of epidemiology, of health care evaluation and of approaches to changing professional behaviour. Without intersectoral action that can address the major underlying causes of ill health, the growing burden of disease will compromise efforts to achieve other government objectives, such as economic growth.

PRESSURES ON HEALTH EXPENDITURE

Existing statistical series suggest a set of general trends in health spending in both the western and eastern parts of the Region. Each part needs to be discussed separately, in order to reflect the substantial historical and economic differences between the two.

The size, scope and underlying meaning of current levels of health care expenditure in Europe can be controversial. Different groups of national policy-maker – in particular those in health and finance ministries – tend to interpret the same figures differently. These different interpretations typically reflect the national policy objectives that the two ministries believe should be given priority. Furthermore, a variety of different statistical series can be cited, not all of which point in precisely the same direction. In terms of the percentage of GDP spent on health, the shrinkage of overall GDP during the 1990–1993 recession in western Europe can create the illusion of increased health sector expenditure. In the CEE and CIS countries, expenditure statistics do not include informal and/or unreported payments to health care providers or for pharmaceuticals. Moreover, current trends do not reflect the possible future impact of an aging population, with higher levels of demand for services as well as for new technology. Ultimately, therefore, available statistics on aggregate health spending can serve as only one contribution to the more fundamental discussion in each country about the values and functions that its national health care system should pursue.

The methodological approach employed to calculate levels of health care expenditure differs between countries. These differences often lead to disparate results and constitute a major obstacle when seeking to compare levels of health care expenditure. Whenever possible, sources have been used that apply the same methodology across countries. In Fig. 12, for western European countries and for most CEE countries, the data came from the OECD and the World Bank, respectively. Health expenditure is less comparable for CIS countries and for three CEE countries, for which health expenditure was obtained from different sources.

Health spending in western Europe

In 1994, in terms of US dollar purchasing power parities (US $PPP) per head of population, the highest-spending country in western Europe was Switzerland (US $2294), with an expenditure nearly four times that of Greece (US $598) and ten times that of Turkey (US $223). Austria, France and Germany spent between US $1800 and US $2000 per head, which is roughly one third above the western European average of US $1419 (Fig. 13).

When spending is expressed as a percentage of GDP, similarly large disparities are revealed. In 1994, Austria and France had the highest levels of expenditure with 9.7% of GDP devoted to health care, followed by Switzerland, Germany, the Netherlands, Italy, Finland, Israel, Belgium, Iceland and Ireland, all of which had percentages above the western European average of 7.7%. At the other end of the spectrum, Turkey and Greece spent 4.2% and 5.2% of GDP, respectively, on health care. Differences in the level of expenditure are partially explained by levels of national income, but relatively wealthy countries such as Denmark, Luxembourg and the United Kingdom spend less on health care as a proportion of GDP than poorer countries such as Portugal (see Fig. 12).

In western Europe, the broad trends in aggregate health care expenditure can be divided into three distinct periods. The first was the 1960s and 1970s, when health

Fig. 12. Total expenditure on health as a percentage of GDP in the WHO European Region, 1994

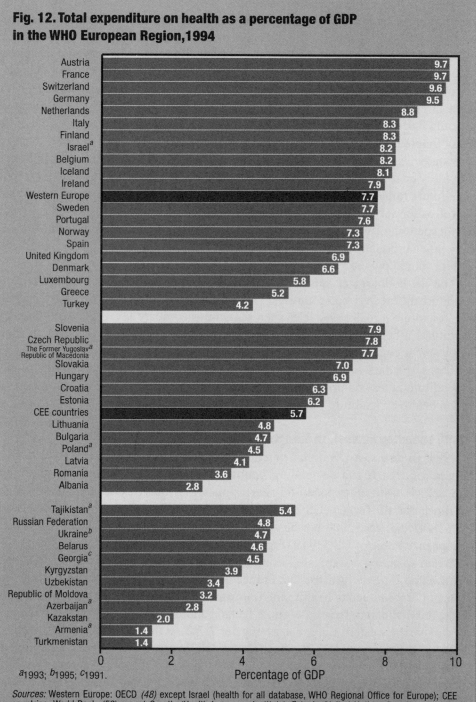

Austria 9.7
France 9.7
Switzerland 9.6
Germany 9.5
Netherlands 8.8
Italy 8.3
Finland 8.3
Israel[a] 8.2
Belgium 8.2
Iceland 8.1
Ireland 7.9
Western Europe 7.7
Sweden 7.7
Portugal 7.6
Norway 7.3
Spain 7.3
United Kingdom 6.9
Denmark 6.6
Luxembourg 5.8
Greece 5.2
Turkey 4.2

Slovenia 7.9
Czech Republic 7.8
The Former Yugoslav[a] Republic of Macedonia 7.7
Slovakia 7.0
Hungary 6.9
Croatia 6.3
Estonia 6.2
CEE countries 5.7
Lithuania 4.8
Bulgaria 4.7
Poland[a] 4.5
Latvia 4.1
Romania 3.6
Albania 2.8

Tajikistan[a] 5.4
Russian Federation 4.8
Ukraine[b] 4.7
Belarus 4.6
Georgia[c] 4.5
Kyrgyzstan 3.9
Uzbekistan 3.4
Republic of Moldova 3.2
Azerbaijan[a] 2.8
Kazakstan 2.0
Armenia[a] 1.4
Turkmenistan 1.4

0   2   4   6   8   10
Percentage of GDP

[a]1993; [b]1995; [c]1991.

Sources: Western Europe: OECD *(48)* except Israel (health for all database, WHO Regional Office for Europe); CEE countries: World Bank *(52)* except Croatia (Health Insurance Institute), Estonia (United Nations Development Programme *(53)*) and Latvia (Ministry of Health); CIS: ministries of health except Armenia and Belarus (United Nations Development Programme *(53)*), Georgia (health for all database, WHO Regional Office for Europe), Kyrgyzstan (Ministry of Finance), Tajikistan (State Committee for Statistics and Economic Situation) and the Russian Federation (MedSocEconInform Institute).

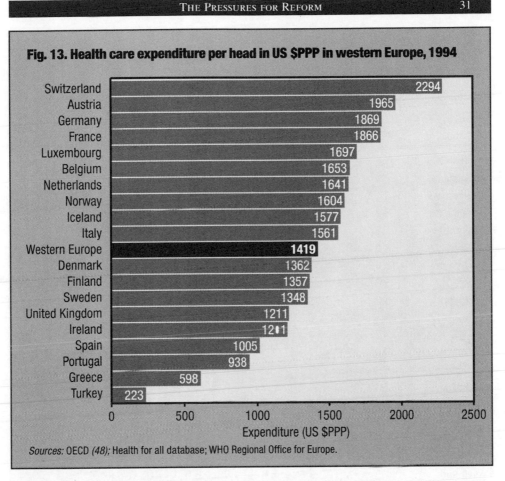

Fig. 13. Health care expenditure per head in US $PPP in western Europe, 1994

Country	Expenditure (US $PPP)
Switzerland	2294
Austria	1965
Germany	1869
France	1866
Luxembourg	1697
Belgium	1653
Netherlands	1641
Norway	1604
Iceland	1577
Italy	1561
Western Europe	1419
Denmark	1362
Finland	1357
Sweden	1348
United Kingdom	1211
Ireland	1201
Spain	1005
Portugal	938
Greece	598
Turkey	223

Sources: OECD *(48);* Health for all database; WHO Regional Office for Europe.

spending rose at a relatively rapid pace both in absolute terms and compared to percentage growth of GDP generally *(49)*. The second period was in the 1980s, in which health care spending in most countries was broadly stable *(50,51)*. This stability reflected governments' adoption of macro-level expenditure controls in response to the economic consequences of the oil crises of 1973 and 1978, and the consequent "stagflation" of the early 1980s. In most countries, this overall macroeconomic stability lasted until the early 1990s (see Table 3).

The third period began in 1991 with a severe recession across Europe and a small but significant upturn in aggregate expenditures. The cost of pharmaceuticals was one factor contributing to this increase, and this has in turn become the subject of considerable cost-containment initiatives of late.

In some countries, the overall percentage increase was as much statistical as real, partly reflecting a fall in overall GDP and thus in the denominator of the ratio that expresses the percentage of GDP given over to health. Finland provides an extreme example of this pattern: aggregate health spending grew from 7.4% in 1989 to 9.3% in 1992, largely as a result of a 16% reduction in total GDP over those three years. The data also reflect anomalous events in Germany (with the accession of the German Democratic Republic and its substantially less expensive health care system to

Table 3. Total expenditure on health as a percentage of GDP in western European countries, 1970–1995

Country	Year									
	1970	1975	1980	1985	1990	1991	1992	1993	1994	1995
Austria	5.4	7.3	7.9	8.1	8.4	8.5	8.9	9.4	9.7	9.6
Belgium	4.1	5.9	6.6	7.4	7.6	8.0	8.1	8.3	8.2	8.0
Denmark	6.1	6.5	6.8	6.3	6.5	6.6	6.7	6.8	6.6	6.5
Finland	5.7	6.4	6.5	7.3	8.0	9.1	9.3	8.8	8.3	8.2
France	5.8	7.0	7.6	8.5	8.9	9.1	9.4	9.8	9.7	9.9
Germany	5.9	8.1	8.4	8.7	8.3	9.0	9.3	9.3	9.5	9.5
Greece	3.4	3.4	3.6	4.1	4.3	4.3	4.5	4.6	5.2	–[a]
Iceland	5.0	5.8	6.2	7.3	7.9	8.1	8.2	8.3	8.1	8.1
Ireland	5.3	7.6	8.7	7.8	6.7	7.0	7.3	7.4	7.9	–
Italy	5.1	6.2	6.9	7.0	8.1	8.4	8.5	8.6	8.3	7.7
Luxembourg	3.7	5.1	6.2	6.1	6.2	6.2	6.3	6.2	5.8	–
Netherlands	5.9	7.5	7.9	7.9	8.4	8.6	8.8	9.0	8.8	8.8
Norway	4.6	6.1	6.1	5.9	6.9	7.2	7.4	7.3	7.3	–
Portugal	2.8	5.6	5.8	6.3	6.6	7.1	7.2	7.4	7.6	–
Spain	3.7	4.9	5.7	5.7	6.9	7.1	7.2	7.3	7.3	7.6
Sweden	7.1	7.9	9.4	8.9	8.6	8.4	7.6	7.6	7.7	7.7
Switzerland	5.2	7.0	7.3	8.1	8.4	9.0	9.4	9.5	9.6	–
Turkey	2.4	2.7	3.3	2.2	2.9	3.4	2.9	2.6	4.2	–
United Kingdom	4.5	5.5	5.6	5.9	6.0	6.5	7.0	6.9	6.9	6.9

[a] Not available.

Source: OECD (48).

the Federal Republic of Germany) and in the United Kingdom (the 1991 reforms, which were accompanied by a substantial increase in spending) (54), as well as efforts by the socialist government in Spain to widen access to health care.

It should also be noted that in certain countries health spending fell substantially in both real and percentage terms in the first half of the 1990s. In Sweden, a combination of tight public budgets, the introduction of competition between public providers, and the shift in 1992 of responsibility for elderly residential care out of the health sector, produced a drop of 1.2% of GDP in total health expenditure – from 8.6% in 1990 to 7.7% in 1995 (Berleen, G., personal communication, 1996). A similar fall is under way outside the European Region in another high-cost country (Canada) where, after peaking at 10.3% of GDP in 1993, health spending dropped to 9.7% in 1994 and to below 9.5% in 1995 (Fedyk, F., personal communication, 1996).

Public expenditure is still the dominant source of health financing in most western European countries. In 1993, public expenditure accounted on average for three quarters of total health expenditure. The proportion is higher in Norway (93.3%), followed by Luxembourg, Belgium, Iceland, the United Kingdom, Sweden and Denmark, where more than 80% of total health expenditure is derived from public sources. Portugal had the lowest share of public expenditure with 55.5%.

Countries differ markedly in their allocation of expenditure between inpatient care, outpatient care and pharmaceuticals. Some of these differences can be explained by organizational and financial arrangements. In 1993, for the countries where data are available, outpatient care consumed almost half of aggregate health expenditure in Luxembourg and over 30% in Belgium, Denmark, Switzerland and Finland, while in Spain it was less than 15%. The share increased significantly in Denmark during the 1980s.

Remuneration of health employees in the period 1987–1994 accounted for between 40% and 57% of total health spending in Denmark, Finland, Greece, the Netherlands, Spain, Sweden and the United Kingdom. The method of remunerating physicians is important in determining whether additional pressure is exerted on health budgets (for example, fee-for-service as opposed to capitation payment), but the numbers of physicians that enter the market are more important. Physicians' salaries and total employment in the health sector are rising, but the share of salaries as a percentage of total health spending remained the same or decreased over the period 1987–1994, while other components (particularly pharmaceuticals and technology) increased their share.

Spending on pharmaceuticals is the most dynamic component of health expenditure, with growth rates higher than those of both GDP and total health expenditure in most countries. In Europe, France and Germany spend the most on pharmaceuticals; in Germany they account for 17% of total health spending. Governments have attempted to control pharmaceutical expenditure through a variety of mechanisms: price controls, reference price systems, positive and negative lists, patient co-payments, generic prescribing, the "de-listing" of products, and the control of pharmaceutical companies' profits. These strategies are explored in more depth in Chapter 5.

Trends in expenditure in CEE countries

In 1994, the percentage of GDP spent on health in the CEE countries ranged from 2.8% in Albania to 7.9% in Slovenia (Fig. 12). Although these levels are lower on average than in western European countries, CEE countries spend a greater share of national income on health care than might be predicted, given their income level. This proportion has increased during the transition to open economies. Despite the severe contraction (or moderate expansion in the best of cases) in real growth in GDP over the period 1987–1994, real health expenditures either grew faster or contracted more slowly than GDP.

There are two groups among the CEE countries, as classified by expenditure trends. Countries spending the highest proportion of GDP on health (6–8%) are those that have historically relied on, or recently adopted, a national health insurance system financed by payroll taxation. This includes Croatia, Slovenia and The Former Yugoslav Republic of Macedonia as well as the Czech Republic, Hungary and Slovakia. In these countries, the shift towards national health insurance has led to a marked and sustained increase (2.0–2.5%) in the share of GDP devoted to health and, in most of them, an increase in real public spending on health. A second group of CEE countries includes those still predominantly relying on general revenue to finance health care, such as Albania, Bulgaria, Latvia, Lithuania, Poland and Romania, which are spending between 3% and 5% of GDP on health. In some cases the share crept upwards in the period 1989–1994, but there was not the marked increase that followed the introduction of insurance in neighbouring countries. Of course, these statistics do not include informal payments to hospitals and physicians, or cash transactions for pharmaceuticals.

Contrary to expectations, the switch to national health insurance has not resulted in a shrinking revenue base for health. Insurance contributions have not been substituted for general revenues; instead, they have supplemented those revenues, thus increasing total public resources for health. Some of this increase may reflect the transformation of previously informal payments into official ones, however. Given existing contribution rates, the extent of formal employment in the sector and the mandate for universal coverage and broad benefit packages, the insurance funds in many countries now have structural deficits. Thus, general budgetary subsidies have been necessary to sustain desired levels of health spending.

This real increase in health spending was partially by design. For instance, policy-makers chose to augment physicians' incomes, as part of a larger trend towards increasing returns to those with higher levels of education. This was the case in Hungary, where capitation payments for PHC providers were introduced on top of existing salaries. The swift rise in the share of GDP for health also reflects the inadequate attention paid to the structure of financial incentives for health care providers and patients. This became apparent in the fiscal crises that followed dramatic increases in health insurance costs in the Czech Republic, Hungary and Slovakia. In the rush to introduce "western-style" health insurance, insufficient thought was given to setting limits on basic insurance coverage, to defining actuarially appropriate premiums, or to establishing payment mechanisms with incentives for efficiency and cost containment.

The CEE countries that experienced severe economic contraction saw roughly proportional reductions in real public spending on health. Once economic growth resumed, however, public spending on health tended to bounce back to pre-transition levels, even before full economic recovery. Referred to as the "Rule of Eighty", this applied to Bulgaria, Romania and Slovakia. All three countries had proportional reductions in real spending on health in the period 1990–1993. In 1994, GDP recovered to around 80% of its 1990 level, while public spending on health fully recovered its previous level. This indicates that governments face political pressures to restore real spending on health once the economy recovers. These pressures reflect popular expectations of maintaining universal access to care and comprehensive coverage, as well as the desire to catch up with western European standards.

Expenditure on health personnel has not been shielded from overall spending cuts. Real spending on personnel has followed the general trend for public spending on health. Countries that maintained or increased overall health spending also maintained or increased spending on personnel. In Hungary, for instance, real public spending on health sector personnel rose by nearly 20% after the introduction of health insurance, suggesting that one explicit goal of insurance – to increase physicians' incomes – was achieved. In countries where real public spending on health fell, however, expenditure on health personnel fell by as much or more. For instance, in Albania, Croatia and Lithuania, public spending on the health workforce fell by 60–70% in real terms between 1990 and 1994. In some countries, groups such as pharmacists and dentists have moved to the private sector, thus accounting for some of the spending reductions, but in most countries the bulk of the health personnel have remained in the public sector. This suggests that, as for other types of state-owned enterprise, adjustment in the health sector has occurred through the erosion of real wages rather than mass reductions in personnel. As in other types of enterprise, retaining workers at low wages without sufficient working capital – in this case for drugs, medical supplies, utilities and so on – results in low productivity and low morale, and leads in turn to inefficiencies and low-quality services. In many countries, public sector physicians supplement their salaries through informal payments, but hard data on the extent of this activity are scarce or nonexistent; estimates in some countries start at 30% of official salaries.

Spending on pharmaceuticals as a share of recurrent public expenditure on health varies from less than 10% in The Former Yugoslav Republic of Macedonia to more than 40% in the Czech Republic and Romania. Change in the relative share during the transition has also varied from country to country, declining in Poland and in The Former Yugoslav Republic of Macedonia, rising in Albania and Croatia, and remaining stable in Bulgaria, Hungary and Romania. Using GDP deflators, public spending on drugs in the period 1990–1994 declined in most countries whose economies were contracting, with the notable exception of Croatia. Drug spending held relatively steady in Hungary and Romania, while increasing dramatically in Bulgaria and Croatia. This variation can be explained by a mix of factors that apply to these countries in different degrees: changes in the relative prices of drugs associated with varying degrees of economic liberalization and reliance on imports, recourse to foreign assistance for vaccines and drugs, and planned and unplanned shifting of costs to the private sector. These issues are explored in Chapter 5.

All CEE countries have dramatically reduced capital spending during the transition. In the late 1980s, capital investment as a share of total public expenditure on health ranged from 4% to 15% in the countries studied. In several countries, including Albania and Poland, capital spending declined in real terms throughout the 1980s and early 1990s. Not surprisingly, real expenditure for public investment fell the least in countries with the mildest economic problems, such as the Czech Republic and Hungary, and most in the countries of the former Yugoslavia, owing to the regional conflict. This uniform decline in real capital investment was a response to fiscal crises that undermined operational expenditure on basic health services. In a few countries, it appears that investment spending on health began to recover in 1994. In the medium term, however, these countries will need massive investment to replace and upgrade equipment and facilities, which are often outmoded or near the end of their useful lives.

CEE countries have opted to retain predominantly publicly funded health systems; no movement towards large-scale private funding has taken place. Rather, these countries are following the pattern of western Europe where, as noted above, public or statutory funding accounts on average for three quarters of total expenditure. Data on private health expenditure in the CEE countries are sparse, but extrapolation from recent household surveys in several countries suggests that out-of-pocket spending ranges from 2% to 30% of the total, mainly for purchasing drugs in the private pharmaceutical market. A growing number of countries have introduced cost-sharing arrangements, or intend to do so in the near future, but revenues from this source usually account for less than 5% of the health total.

Trends in expenditure in CIS countries
Levels of expenditure in CIS countries from different years are shown in Fig. 12. There are very few comparative data on the components of health expenditure and trends during the economic transition. There appears to have been a sharp decline in publicly financed health spending, however, both in real terms and as a share of GDP, corresponding to the overall collapse of the state apparatus.

HEALTH SECTOR CHALLENGES
Beyond challenges to health and the health sector and pressures on health expenditure, there are also a substantial number of structural and organizational challenges in how countries in the Region finance and deliver health services.

Limitations to health gain
As the above discussion of health status suggests, the existing financing and delivery systems do not maximize health gain. Many policy-makers believe that it is necessary to shift the allocation of funds from curative to preventive care, and from secondary and tertiary to primary care, but may have been thwarted by existing configurations of power and resources. Cooperation between the health sector and the housing, agriculture, nutrition, job training and other key sectors with an influence on health remains insufficient in many countries. In western Europe, continuity of care between the hospital and PHC sectors, as well as between health and social care providers, remains inadequate. In the CEE and CIS countries, overexpanded hospital systems consume too high a proportion of the available finances, while a low level of competence and excessive personnel hinder the preventive efforts of the sanitary–epidemiology services.

Rising inequities in health care
Concern about existing inequities in health services – in terms of access to necessary, good-quality care – has been replaced by cost-containment as the top

health-related priority in many countries. Data cited above suggest that inequities are growing even in countries where, formally, health system structures provide universal access to services. Commentators attribute at least part of such increases to the consequences of market-oriented competitive reforms (55–57). Alternatively, a newly published study draws on international data to suggest that inequality of income distribution, the structure of organizational workplace hierarchies and the degree of work autonomy may be key explanatory factors in the distribution of health inequities across populations (34).

In the CEE and CIS countries, the rapid fall in real value of public sector health budgets, the high cost of private insurance for the elderly and the poor, and the emergence of overt fee-for-service care in hospitals and health centres have pushed millions of citizens out of the health care system. Many countries that have developed social insurance arrangements have not been successful in retaining access for their less well-off citizens. In the extreme case of Georgia, only 10–15% of all medically necessary care is being financed through the national health insurance mechanism, while payment for most other services is left to individuals, if they have sufficient personal funds.

Inadequate cost–effectiveness (allocative efficiency)

A growing body of research has raised questions about the appropriateness and/or cost–effectiveness of various clinical procedures. Although clinicians have long speculated that 20–30% of all delivered clinical services are medically ineffective, advances in the fields of technology assessment and economic evaluation have made it possible to begin to determine exactly which services should be restricted.

Beyond the clinical effectiveness of care, questions can be raised about the overall usefulness of increasing health spending in western European societies that already spend 7–10% of their GDP on health. These opportunity cost or social utility issues are further complicated by changing aggregate parameters defined by increased numbers of elderly people and by changes in the wider economy. Several northern European governments have commissioned reports on the dilemmas presented by the issues of rationing and possible explicit priority setting in clinical and/ or preventive services (58).

Inefficient health system performance (technical efficiency)

Health policy decision-makers in both western and eastern Europe have come to believe, for different reasons, that their health systems are not performing efficiently at the micro level. In western Europe, expenditure constraints were previously focused on the aggregate system level, with insufficient emphasis laid on micro-level behaviour. There was evidence of poor coordination between providers and across subsectors, a lack of adequate information about the costs and quality of services, inadequate management of capital resources, and insufficient and/or inappropriate micro-level management of operational budgets. Analysts believe that all these factors have produced more expensive delivery systems that are less capable of producing care of an appropriate quality. In the CEE and CIS countries, in addition to similar efficiency-related concerns at institutional level, substantial "under-the-counter" payments to providers have created distortions in the patterns of service delivery. Among other dilemmas, providers' official salaries were too low to stimulate efficient work; disposable supplies, pharmaceuticals and capital equipment were woefully inadequate; and maintenance of existing buildings and equipment was minimal *(28)*.

Service quality

One important result of the focus on micro-level activities has been an increasing concern with quality. Researchers have found wide variations in the utilization of particular procedures, and in the outcomes achieved. In the United States, small-area variation studies have demonstrated that the decisions of clinicians in different areas regarding patients presenting with identical complaints could vary by as much as 40% *(59)*. Quality has assumed increasing importance, both as a measure of value for money – for example, reducing readmission and infection rates – and as a strategic instrument in a period of increased competition among hospitals. Quality is also emerging as an important issue in patient satisfaction surveys. The CEE and CIS countries are facing particularly acute challenges, owing to the poor state of their medical equipment and facilities.

Choice and accountability

Patients in both eastern and western Europe have become increasingly restive. They are no longer willing to be passive objects of the service delivery system. Rather, they are increasingly insistent that they – not health personnel, health planners or politicians – should be perceived as the subject of the health system.

Patient empowerment has several dimensions. One concern is patients' rights with regard to health care services. Patient choice is a second dimension. In some countries, this has meant choice of physician and treatment facility for PHC or hospital care *(6)*. In a few western European countries and an increasing number of CEE and CIS countries, choice has been extended to the selection of a private insurance carrier. A third pressure on health systems involves patients' participation in clinical decision-making. A fourth source of pressure on national decision-makers has been the increasing use of private sector providers. In the CEE and CIS countries, patient empowerment issues have created strong pressures on government policy-makers.

2 Integrating Reform Themes

In response to contextual changes and health and health sector challenges, countries have developed a wide variety of strategies for policy intervention at different levels of the health system. Underlying these different strategies and mechanisms, it is possible to identify a number of broad themes that affect all levels of the health system. For analytical purposes, these policy responses can be summarized in terms of four integrating themes that can be observed across Europe as national policy-makers have sought to achieve their objectives. The four are: the changing roles of the state and the market in health care; decentralization to lower levels of the public sector, or to the private sector; greater choice for and empowerment of patients; and the evolving role of public health.

The changing roles of state and market in health care

In the late 1980s, many European governments began to re-examine the structure of governance in their health systems. In countries where the state has traditionally been the central actor in the health sector, the presumption of public primacy, along with a strong state role in nearly every dimension of health sector activity, is being reassessed. National policy-makers in countries of northern Europe, the Mediterranean region and central and eastern Europe have felt compelled by a combination of economic, social, demographic, managerial, technological and ideological forces to review existing authority relationships and structures. In countries where the state has played a less central role in the health sector, mainly acting to set out ground rules and to referee between quasi-public, statutory and/or private insurers and providers, a similar process of reassessment is under way, although from a different starting point.

While the pressure for change has been felt unevenly across the different parts of Europe, there appears to be a set of parallel trends regarding governance. Some state functions have been decentralized within the public sector to regional and/or municipal authorities. Other functions have been given over to private management and, particularly in CEE and CIS countries, to private ownership. Conversely, some countries where the state plays a less central role have seen an increase in regulatory intervention in various subsectors of their systems.

The responsibility for planning and allocating resources has been one of the most important issues raised. Western European countries have developed diverse organizational patterns in the structures of their health-related services, facilities, institutions and workforces. The mix of public, quasi-public, statutorily regulated private, private non-profit and private profit-making bodies in each national health system reflects a country's particular history, customs and culture, as well as the existing balance of political and economic power. In the CEE and CIS countries, planning was wholly the responsibility of state agencies. The present decade has brought change to these organizational patterns. Based on new expectations, as well as new possibilities, existing arrangements are coming under scrutiny and alternative arrangements are being debated, proposed and adopted.

The greatest pressure for change has been in the relative role of the private sector in operating and, in some countries, financing health care services. While the popular media and some political figures have simplified this issue into "state versus market", in practice the issues are substantially more complicated (60). There is no single, simple concept of market that can be adopted for use in a health system. Rather, market-style mechanisms include a number of different specific instruments such as consumer sovereignty (patient choice), negotiated contracts and open bidding. They can be adopted in markets organized on different principles: on price, on quality or on market share. Markets can, in turn, be introduced into different sectors of the health system: in health care funding, in one or more subsets of the production of health services (among and/or between hospitals, nursing homes, physicians and social services personnel) and/or in the allocation instruments that distribute funds to service providers (61). Competitive incentives can be brought to bear on the behaviour of physicians, nurses, support personnel or home care personnel. In practice, then, there is not one decision but a series of decisions to make. Rather than a monolithic commitment to one of two abstractions – state or market – both western and eastern European health systems confront a range of smaller decisions.The decision-making process needs to be not only strategic but also practical in nature, and as a result it typically involves a multitude of approximations, if not compromises.

In some instances, the decision taken has been to combine elements of both models – to mix an increased use of market-style incentives with continued ownership and operation of facilities by the public sector. This hybrid approach has been given a number of different names: internal market (62), public competition (63), provider market and quasi-market (64). The design and implementation of this type of publicly designed and administered market has played an important role in health reform in Finland, Italy, Spain, Sweden and the United Kingdom, as well as in various CEE and CIS countries.

The application of market-style mechanisms to the health sector is fraught with both conceptual and practical dilemmas. Conceptually, health care is considered by many academics (except neoclassical economists) to be a social good, in which the provision of services to each individual is also valuable to the community as a whole. This view has, in turn, formed part of the traditional consensus in most European societies about the importance of solidarity and universal coverage in the design of health care financing systems. Market-style incentives, however, are by their nature based on the assumption that every service is a commodity, suitable for sale in the open market. Further, the classical concept of a market requires a clear distinction between the demand side (the buyer) and the supply side (the seller). Yet modern health care comprises a four-part relationship involving patient, physician, hospital and payer (65). Thus, the application of market incentives to health care will by necessity focus on one or another submarkets rather than being comprehensive in character.

Two additional dilemmas should be mentioned concerning the application of market theory to health care. First, physicians are simultaneously suppliers of services (to patients) and demanders of services (from hospital staff), which adds another layer of complexity to simple market-oriented assumptions. Second, neoclassical economic theory assumes that cross-subsidies between different categories of payer and client are inefficient and unfair, yet the social function of a responsible health care system involves substantial cross-subsidies: from young to old, from rich to poor and from the healthy to the sick.

The mythical capabilities sometimes attributed to market strategies are more subtle, but potentially more misleading. Policy-makers sometimes seem seduced by powerful imagery from the United States, in which the supposed supremacy of the lone rational individual appears to be real rather than a socially devastating illusion. The notion that market mechanisms always have superior decision-making outcomes than public planning may seem equally enticing the farther one sits from the societal consequences. Resisting the siren call of the "myth of the individual" and the "myth of the market", however, requires credible alternative models of reform.

The practical dilemmas involved in introducing competitive mechanisms into health care provision are equally daunting. Market relations, by their very nature, require real prices. Yet the development of real (i.e. litigable) prices in health care is extremely expensive.

The role that market-style mechanisms can or should play in a socially responsible health system remains controversial. Fifteen years of intense debate have followed the publication of the first major academic study on this issue (66). Opponents of reliance on market-style incentives have raised strong arguments against their introduction. In the opinion of several well respected analysts, market mechanisms necessarily create conditions in which vulnerable populations – particularly the less well-off – will not receive equal access to quality services (55,57). Concerns have been voiced about the likelihood that market-oriented individualism will erode the collective responsibility that underpins the legitimacy of the European welfare state (56). The introduction of market mechanisms in the funding of health systems, replacing single-source or collectively associated payers with multiple competing private insurers, has been criticized as economically, clinically and socially counterproductive (61,67). Using market mechanisms to replace district-level management has also been questioned as a strategy for a socially accountable delivery system (68–70).

The two western European countries whose market-oriented reforms have received the most international attention – Sweden and the United Kingdom – have pulled back in the last year from reliance on competitive incentives as the driving force for health sector reform. In Sweden, the defining word at both national and county levels has become "cooperation", and there has been a resurgence of interest in county-based planning as well as in national regulation (particularly concerning pharmaceutical expenditures). In the United Kingdom, the current Secretary of State for Health has taken pains to emphasize the traditional responsibilities of health authorities, and attention is turning towards the logic of long-term contracts based on a high level of trust (71–73).

The ability of competitive mechanisms to increase efficiency and reduce costs, not just in the health sector but in total public spending, is an important issue for national policy-makers. In the health sector, there is substantial concern that the transaction costs of contract-based relationships (the cost of pricing services, negotiating contracts and litigation) can, if not constrained, outweigh real improvements in operating efficiency. Serious questions also have been raised about the duplication of capital equipment and expensive installations that market competition can generate. A further issue concerns the extent to which overall budget savings from contracting, particularly when previously publicly operated services are let to private providers, come predominantly from reduced wages and benefits (especially pension payments) paid to health sector support workers, thus reducing wages and benefits to an already low-paid sector of the workforce *(60)*.

As part of the broad changes currently under way at the level of system governance, ministries are also confronted with redefining their own tasks and responsibilities. Health ministries have responded to these pressures for change in a variety of ways.

The most basic question – primarily raised in the CEE and CIS countries but also in Greece, Israel and Spain – has concerned the appropriateness of ministries retaining the day-to-day responsibilities for operating provider institutions. This is a sensitive question, in that change often affects the status and job security of the medical staff who work in these institutions. Such changes are essential, however, to free officials to focus on broader issues of national strategy and health system development.

State regulation is a related issue. It has expanded beyond traditional command-and-control measures to incorporate new market-derived arrangements based on incentive. Here, it is important to note that the contribution of both regulatory and competitive measures depends on how they are configured and introduced. Regulatory measures have demonstrated their effectiveness in a number of areas, most recently in the control of pharmaceutical expenditure. Regulation, however, is only a valuable idea when, first, it can reasonably be expected to achieve its intended objective and, second, when it can do so without creating major economic and financial distortions in the structure and quality of the services delivered. To achieve these goals regulation needs to be flexible, and it should accommodate the multiple differences – technical, geographical and demographic – that can exist across a democratic society within the limitations imposed by national law. Most importantly, effective regulation should be concerned with monitoring and evaluating outcomes, not with stipulating inputs.

Similarly, competitive measures should be carefully designed to achieve their intended objective. As most economists recognize, there is no room for unrestrained market activity in the provision of a social good such as health care. Hence the use that policy-makers have made of market mechanisms has been successful where it has incorporated tight monitoring and evaluation, as well as clear standards for market participants. Indeed, the decision to adopt a more incentive-oriented framework in one or other subsector of a health system does not require less government activity, but different activity. Some researchers have concluded that governments have to be more competent to supervise contracting and other market-style arrangements than to run services directly *(74)*.

Reorganizing the system: decentralization, recentralization and privatization

Decentralization is a central tenet of health sector reform in many European countries. It is seen as an effective means to stimulate improvements in service delivery, to secure better allocation of resources according to needs, to involve the community in decisions about priorities, and to facilitate the reduction of inequities in health. Rapid advances in information systems have helped to increase the technical feasibility of decentralization.

Decentralization is attractive because it is difficult for the central administration to be close enough to the users of services to make appropriate and sensitive responses to expressed preferences. There is widespread disillusion with large, centralized and bureaucratic institutions. In almost every country, the same drawbacks of centralized systems have been identified: poor efficiency, slow pace of change and innovation, and a lack of responsiveness to changes in the environment that affect health and health care. The susceptibility of centralized systems to political manipulation is also seen as a cause for concern (although decentralization is not automatically a solution to this problem).

Various objectives have been cited as a rationale for decentralization. It has been seen as an important political ideal, providing the means for community participation and local self-reliance, and improving the accountability of government officials. For instance, increased local control can result in more responsiveness to local needs, improved management of logistics and greater motivation for local officials, thus facilitating the implementation of reforms. It also has been seen as a way of transferring responsibility for development from the centre to the periphery, and consequently as a way of spreading the blame for any failure to meet local needs. Decentralization can offer physicians opportunities to increase their income through dealings with more amenable local or private sector decision-makers.

Historically, many western European countries have had strong systems of local government. In some cases, central government powers developed somewhat later than those of local government. A number of countries have inherited structures that provide a wide range of services that are financed by local funds. Central governments, however, have increasingly tended to place restrictions on local government. Achieving equality of public services throughout the country has been common objective in expanding central government powers. Central government policies, regulations, and specific and general grants have been used to reallocate resources geographically. In the first half of the 1990s, faced with economic recession and the need to restrain overall public spending, some central governments have sought to limit local discretion further.

CONCEPTS OF DECENTRALIZATION

Decentralization can be defined as the transfer of authority, or dispersal of power, in public planning, management and decision-making from the national level to subnational levels or, more generally, from higher to lower levels of government (75).

Decentralization places responsibility for making decisions at the lowest possible level of the organization. At one extreme, in completely decentralized institutions, all decisions would be made at the lowest operational level: where possible, at the point of application. At the other extreme, in wholly centralized institutions, all decisions would be made at the highest level of management. In the real world, organizations do not exist in pure form at either end of that continuum, but operate at various points between the two extremes.

Similarly, most health care systems are not consistently organized according to one particular model. Certain elements or subsectors may be more or less decentralized or centralized. Until recently, for example, Sweden's health care system was centrally administered (though only from the regional level downwards) yet most dental care is provided privately. In Germany, curative health services are formally decentralized, yet the monitoring and regulation of hundreds of health insurance funds through a small number of agencies at *Land* level has certain characteristics that resemble those of a centralized system.

Furthermore, the precise balance between centralization and decentralization can shift over time. In Kazakstan, measures taken directly after national sovereignty was declared in 1991 to decentralize control over financing of the health system to the regions (*oblasts*), soon resulted in widening disparities between the wealthy and poor parts of the country. Consequently, in 1995, it was proposed to recentralize authority over health financing within the government in a new agency called the National Health Insurance Fund *(76)*.

TYPES OF DECENTRALIZATION

Various types of decentralization can be identified *(77,78)*. Four main ones – deconcentration, devolution, delegation and privatization – are briefly described here. The distinction between these is essentially their legal status. Other factors (such as financial authority, means of representing the local community and geographical conditions) also are important in classifying types of decentralization.

Studies of decentralization frequently include privatization. This, however, has been questioned on the grounds that transferring authority to the private sector constitutes the adoption of quite a different system of organizing and managing activities, rather than a shift between various forms of organization and distribution of responsibilities in a single system *(79)*. Decentralization and privatization are conceptually two different processes that may or may not be interrelated. It is probably more accurate to regard the transfer of authority and functions from the public to the private sector as a process of privatization. Nevertheless, privatization is included here as a form of decentralization, although it is substantially different from the others. The issue becomes further complicated where there is a public–private mix, and public bodies become purchasers of care that may or may not be provided privately (through either profit-making or non-profit organizations).

A summary of the different types of decentralization is given in Table 4.

Deconcentration (administrative decentralization) refers to the redistribution of administrative responsibilities within the existing structure of central government:

Table 4. Types of decentralization

Type of decentralization	Definition
Deconcentration (administrative decentralization)	Decision-making is transferred to a lower administrative (civil servant) level
Devolution (political decentralization)	Decision-making is transferred to a lower political level
Delegation	Tasks are allocated to actors at a lower organizational level
Privatization	Tasks are transferred from public to private ownership

Source: Borgenhammer *(80).*

only administrative, not political, authority is transferred to one or more lower levels. This has been termed the "ministerial" model, whereby administrative responsibilities are handed over to local offices of central government ministries *(81).* Since deconcentration involves the transfer of administrative rather than political authority, it is seen as the least extensive form of decentralization. Possibly owing to its less radical nature, deconcentration has been the most frequently used form of decentralization.

Local administration set up under deconcentration can be one of two different types. In the vertical pattern of local administration, local staff are responsible to their own ministry. The second type of local administration may be referred to as the integrated or prefectoral form. In its most extreme form, a local representative of central government responsible to one ministry (e.g. the ministry of the interior or of local government) is responsible for the performance of all government functions in that area. The sectoral government ministries exercise only technical supervision over their staff. An example of deconcentration is given in Box 2.

Box 2. An example of deconcentration: Poland

In Poland, a major reform of public administration was carried out in 1990 as one step in the process of political transformation away from the centralized model. The provincial (*voivodship*) authorities acquired substantial power. At this level, they engaged in planning, made decisions about the structure of health institutions, and allocated funds within centrally agreed budgets. A provincial health officer was selected and employed by authorities operating at this level. In practice, the Ministry of Health lost its capacity to influence the health service.

Source: Golinowska & Tymowska *(82).*

In implementing devolution (political decentralization), central governments relinquish certain functions to different or new organizations outside their direct control. Devolution means strengthening or creating subnational levels of government that are substantially independent of the national level with respect to a defined set of functions. These are typically regional or local governments.

Devolution thus implies a more radical restructuring of health service organization than deconcentration. Two major issues arise. First, health makes heavy demands on recurrent spending, yet local governments have restricted opportunities for raising revenue. One trend, therefore, has been to keep health service financing out of local government control, as health services have become too expensive for them to maintain. On the other hand, if costs are covered by central government grants to local agencies, then this implies dependence and a reduction in local autonomy. This situation, particularly in budgets covering actual expenses, gives health services an incentive to overspend and become inefficient. Second, devolution may complicate efforts to integrate primary, secondary and tertiary services and to set up regional structures. Examples of devolution are given in Box 3.

In delegation, the emphasis is on transferring to an authority the ability to plan and implement decisions without direct supervision by a higher authority. This form

---

Box 3. Devolution

Example: Sweden

Sweden (population about 9 million) provides an example of a tax-based health care system in which the responsibility for financing and organizing services is devolved to the regional administrative level in the form of 26 democratically elected county councils. These councils receive some of their income through government grants and a national social insurance system but, more importantly, they have the right to levy a proportional income tax directly on the population. Furthermore, the county councils are authorized to structure most aspects of health service delivery in their respective geographical regions. Most health care facilities, and almost all hospitals, are owned and operated by the county councils. In short, three key words can be used to describe the overall structure of health services in Sweden. First, decision-making is *decentralized* to local public authorities, i.e. the county councils. Second, each county council has a *monopoly* when it comes to the delivery of health services in its own region. Third, the county councils own and operate their own facilities, and have thus *integrated* the responsibility for financing and providing care.

Source: Anell *(83)*.

Example: Spain

In Spain, 1986 legislation created the national health system and laid down the principles and framework for the future. In 1981, the first devolution of the social security health care network (INSALUD) services to Catalonia took place, followed by Andalusia (1984), the Basque Country and Valencia (1988) and Navarra and Galicia (1991). With this process, a highly centralized model of health care administration at national level came to an end. The governments of the autonomous communities are responsible for the management of the health services to their regional parliaments, which pass and control the regional health care budgets. The main source of financing is a block grant transferred by the national government according to agreed objective criteria. Devolution was administratively and politically very important. Although it has reformed many aspects of the health services, however, its impact on the organization and managerial modernization of the system is far from evident some ten years later, especially when compared with original expectations.

Source: Freire *(84).*

Cautious devolution: Poland

In 1993, the Polish government embarked on the next step of the reform of public administration initiated three years earlier. Its chief objective was substantially to strengthen authorities at local level, whose influence on health matters was very limited. These authorities were appointed autonomously by local councils, whose members were chosen in open elections. In the framework of the pilot project, which started in 1994, 43 large cities were invited to take the responsibility for running health care establishments. This resulted in the transfer of decision-making power from provincial to local authorities in 28 cities, inhabited by more than 20% of the country's population. The experiment is continuing, so it is too early to evaluate the results.

Source: Hunter et al. *(85).*

Extreme example: Finland

Finland has a health care system financed mainly by taxation, with most health services provided by public service providers. Administratively, it is a fairly complex multi-level system, in which it is the responsibility of 460 local authorities (municipalities) to organize the delivery of services. The government has a role in planning, supervising and financing (about 50%) services. The self-government of the municipalities, with democratically elected representation and the right to levy local taxes, has existed for more than 100 years, and the overall political tendency has been to delegate more power to them. The large-scale administrative reforms introduced throughout the Finnish public sector in the late 1980s and early 1990s aimed to give the municipalities even more freedom and responsibility to organize their services, with a minimum of directives from the centre. At the macro level, this reform aspired to push back the frontiers of public regulation and control spending, and at the micro level to expose public agencies to more competition, cost-containment and innovation in organizing their activities. By replacing the cost-based state grant system in 1993 with block grants based on objective criteria of demographic and financial information, municipalities now have an opportunity to reallocate the state subsidies in response to local needs and political will.

Source: Martikainen & Uusikylä *(86).*

of decentralization relates only to defined tasks, not to all activities. The attraction of delegation is that it allows government regulations to be bypassed and management to be more flexible. If the management of an entire nationalized health service were delegated to a parastatal organization, the health ministry's role would be confined to strategic and policy issues. Examples of delegation are given in Box 4.

Privatization involves the transfer of government functions to a nongovernmental organization, which may be a private profit-making company or a non-profit voluntary

---

Box 4. Delegation

Example: Hungary

As the health insurance system (established in 1991) was developed in Hungary, aspects of both decentralization and centralization were present. The establishment of an independent health insurance fund and the transfer of the state's financing role to a self-regulating system of health insurers were major achievements in the decentralization process. On the other hand, as the whole health care system is now financed by a single agency, one might perceive it as centralization. Decentralization and regionalization were both strongly emphasized by the government's 1994 programme, but implementation was never begun. For instance, it was stated that a significant aspect of continuing health care reform was regular coordination between the various actors in the health services, and therefore that a National Health Council and regional health councils should be established. These councils would be special institutions to mediate between social interests. These bodies were never set up, however, and the Ministry of Welfare's approach to the reorganizing of the hospital structure favoured overcentralization.

Source: Orosz *(87)*.

Example: Italy

Italian public health care was traditionally organized under a system of compulsory social insurance. The reform of 1978 drastically changed the situation, transforming service provision from a worker's entitlement to a citizen's right. It suppressed the plethora of separate funds and established a new, uniform structure based on the regions and local health units. In the 1980s, this new institutional framework began to reveal two serious shortcomings: overpoliticization and a lack of rational financial incentives.

Another reform was carried out in 1992. The first major change was a thorough transformation of the administrative structure of local health units. These were made into "public enterprises" and given organizational autonomy and responsibility. They are no longer run by political committees but by a general manager, who is appointed by the regions on the basis of professional qualifications and whose contract is renewable every five years. Larger hospitals can now establish themselves as independent "public hospital agencies" with autonomous organization and administration. They operate with balanced budgets, and surpluses can be used for investment and staff incentives. Unjustified deficits can result in the loss of their autonomous status.

Source: Ferrera, M., unpublished data, 1994.

Deconcentration combined with delegation: the United Kingdom
The National Health Service reforms in the United Kingdom were introduced in 1991. Decentralization was a key theme from the outset: a hybrid of deconcentration and delegation. Devolution was ruled out at an early stage, with the retention of subnational authorities appointed by the Secretary of State for Health. Elected health authorities, or the integration of health services with local government, were not considered serious options. The reforms sought decentralization by introducing an internal market in which purchasers and providers were separated, with providers encouraged to take up trust status. This allowed hospitals and community services greater freedom than if they had remained as directly managed units under the control of the health authorities. Trust boards are accountable to the Secretary of State for Health, so the link to the centre remains. The "wild card" – or "winning hand" – of the reforms has been general practitioner fundholding, whereby certain practices over a particular size have volunteered to hold budgets for purchasing some health care services. The government is actively promoting this model, because it considers fundholding to be a particularly successful feature of the reforms.

Source: Hunter *(88).*

agency. It may refer to the provision or the financing of services, or to both *(89)*. In practice, there are many different combinations of these two elements. It should also be noted that privatizing previously public services does not necessarily involve changes in the actual provision of health care. Privatization is often adopted only for support functions such as maintenance, cleaning, transport and catering.

Privatization is the ultimate form of decentralization, in that it is intended to replace direct public authority over decision-making with privately capitalized firms. The central benefits of privatization are seen to flow from introducing market incentives for greater efficiency and higher quality into the management of health care institutions *(90)*. In addition, fiscally pressed governments see privatization as a way of enticing private capital into the health sector, and thus reducing demands on scarce public investment funds. An example of privatization in the Czech Republic is given in Box 5.

The disadvantages of privatization are, however, considerable. Private management and invested capital require financial returns that are consistent with those obtainable in other private markets. The pressures involved in achieving these returns can result in abandoning the social good character of health services and intentionally discriminating against sick and vulnerable groups who require care *(63)*. Recent experiences with private competitive insurance in the Czech Republic, Israel *(92)*, the Russian Federation, and, to a lesser degree, the Netherlands *(67)* have confirmed observations from the United States that private insurers have powerful financial incentives to engage in adverse risk selection *(93)*. On the production side, in a worst-case example from Sweden, a commercial laboratory was found to be intentionally sending fabricated blood test results to physicians as a way of maintaining a high turnover *(94)*. Privatization can often lead to recentralization as privately managed companies consolidate to gain economies of scale. An example of privatization difficulties in Hungary is given in Box 6.

Box 5. An example of privatization: the Czech Republic

The Czech Republic embarked on rapid privatization of pharmacies. Anybody was allowed to start and own a pharmacy, and licences were available – at a high price – from the "Pharmacists' Chamber". The aim was to improve the availability of drugs, and to allow market forces and competition to influence prices. The mandatory health insurance scheme was intended to cover the expenses of prescription drugs, but there was a policy for individual out-of-pocket responsibility for each prescription and a reference price beyond which a subsidy was no longer paid. As a result, the number of pharmacies has grown considerably, especially in bigger cities, and all drugs are now available. There is a tendency, however, to stock only the more expensive drugs. If a GP prescribes a cheaper drug, the pharmacies have a habit of changing this for a more expensive brand, and patients have to pay the difference.

Prior to 1990, some 110–180 pharmaceuticals were registered annually. Following the deregulation of drug imports in 1990, the number of registrations has increased drastically. In 1991, 1992 and 1993 there were 827, 1344 and 1356, respectively. Now there are more than 10 000 brand names on the drug market. Total spending on drugs approximately doubled between 1991 and 1993.

Sources: Rubaš *(91)*; Marx, D., unpublished data, 1993.

Box 6. An example of privatization difficulties: Hungary

After the political changes in Hungary in 1990, the government perceived no significant difference between the world of business and health care services. One of the main slogans of the reforms was that "the privatization of business corporations shall be carried out simultaneously with the privatization of health care services". Reality, however, has proved much more complex than theory. The relationship between the health care business sector and the Hungarian Health Insurance Institute (established in 1991) is particularly delicate. The 1991 budget entitled the Institute to conclude contracts with private providers, but no details had been worked out as to which aspects should be considered when signing the contracts or how prices should be defined. Another complicating factor is that the premiums collected by the Health Insurance Institute do not cover the expenses of running the system. The government has agreed to cover the deficit through the state budget, but this is disputed and the deficit is now considerable (Ft 53 billion between 1992 and 1994).

Source: Orosz *(87)*.

If privatization is not to undermine wider health policies, national governments must accompany any decision to privatize with strengthened central regulatory controls. It is frequently noted that the country that allows the greatest private sector participation in health service delivery – the United States – has also built up the largest and most intrusive public regulatory apparatus. Physicians in the United States, for example, although private, must contend with concurrent and retrospective control – as well as possible judicial review – over each medical act they perform *(95)*. Conversely, recently independent CIS countries such as Kazakstan and Kyrgyzstan have found that privatization without regulation has left their health ministries with few levers to control the quality of care that patients receive. In short, while it may seem paradoxical, the more a health system relies on market mechanisms for financing and delivering care, the greater the regulatory control governments have found they must exercise *(61)*.

None of these four approaches to decentralization can be found in pure form. Countries employ different patterns simultaneously for different activities. In the United Kingdom, for instance, the organizational model is one of deconcentration, but the chain of command from centre to periphery is interrupted by appointed health authorities and by regional offices that are agents of the Secretary of State for Health. At the centre, the National Health Service (NHS) Executive functions as a form of delegated operational authority. The abolition of the intermediate level in 1996 (the 14 previous regional health authorities have been replaced by 8 regional offices, which have become arms of the NHS Executive) can be seen from two angles. Formally, the removal of an intermediate administrative tier decentralizes services. In practice, it could strengthen the power of central government, since local health authorities are too dependent on the government for their legitimacy to pose any real challenge. In reality, therefore, formal decentralization may be recentralization (see Box 7).

The outcome of devolution depends entirely on the strength of local government. Countries in which regional and/or local government management of health care is

---

Box 7. An example of recentralization: national health insurance in Kazakstan

The proposed new health insurance arrangements are de facto a declaration that financial decentralization to the *oblasts*, established by legislation in 1993, was a failure and should be reversed. For this reason, and because of the powerful position of the *oblasts* through the President under the new Constitution, implementation of the draft national insurance law is not a certainty.

Health insurance revenues will be collected by a newly established National Health Insurance Fund. This Fund will not be administered by the Ministry of Health, but by a separate state agency with responsibilities to three different ministries – finance, social affairs and health. The procedures through which the Fund will allocate its money are not entirely clear. The 1995 health insurance legislation provides for 10% of the Fund's revenues to be distributed by the Ministry of Health as an equalization fund, to provide additional resources to poorer *oblasts*. The most likely result is that only this 10% of health insurance revenues will flow into the Fund – indeed, wealthy *oblasts* are angry about losing control over even that amount. Under this arrangement, the remaining 90% of revenues would remain within the *oblast* in which it was raised, in a local *oblast* office of the Fund.

Source: Saltman & Akanov *(76)*.

successful have typically had this arrangement for a long time; local democracy cannot be put in place overnight. Transferring decision-making and executive power to weak administrative bodies could allow political factions to distort local democratic control for narrow political gain. These dilemmas are particularly acute in the CEE and CIS countries where, prior to the transition, local governments were understood to be only implementing bodies for national policies.

ADVANTAGES AND DISADVANTAGES OF DECENTRALIZATION

Decentralization is seen as a means of resolving the problems that have arisen in complex public bureaucracies. These organizations were criticized for being cumbersome, inefficient and insensitive to users' preferences.

Decentralized institutions have a number of advantages over centralized ones (96); they can:

- be more flexible, and can respond more rapidly to changing circumstances and needs;
- be more effective, as front-line workers are better able to identify problems and opportunities;
- be more innovative in the types of solution they adopt; and
- generate higher morale, more commitment and greater productivity in the workplace.

Some governments have sought to apply to public sector organizations management principles from the private sector. Known as the "new public management", this strategy emphasizes the centrality of competition and performance measurement. Table 5 summarizes the main expected results.

Table 5. Benefits of decentralization

Type of decentralization	Benefits
Deconcentration	Reduced need for central administrative bodies
	Local innovations implemented
Devolution	More local decision-making power and chance for more people to gain influence
	Less central power
Delegation	Faster implementation
Privatization	Independence of activities from politicians, who are thought to be incapable of making decisions and unclear about their role

Source: Borgenhammer (80).

Successful decentralization needs a specific social and cultural environment. Borgenhammer *(80)* has identified the following requirements: sufficient local administrative and managerial capacity; ideological certainty in implementation of tasks; and readiness to accept several interpretations of one problem. Institutions themselves also have to change: "Organizations that decentralize authority also find that they have to articulate their missions, create internal cultures around their core values, and measure results" *(96)*.

Decentralization can have negative effects, including fragmented services, weakening of central health departments, inequity, political manipulation in favour of particular interests or stakeholders, and a weakening of the status and position of the public sector.

The experience of many countries in recent years demonstrates that there are certain areas where decision-making power should not be decentralized. Four such areas can be identified:

- the basic framework for health policy
- strategic decisions on the development of health resources
- regulations concerning public safety
- monitoring, assessment and analysis of the health of the population and health care provision.

The first of these four is a fundamental part of the state's activities; essential decisions should be restricted to the highest government level. Health policy invariably involves basic value choices that can affect many aspects of social life. These core strategic matters should therefore be governed by the same procedures as other public policy.

The second area is a key characteristic of the overall health system. Decisions about the resources to be devoted to health are strategic, in that they shape the future of the entire system. Such infrastructural concerns embrace personnel (training and accreditation, licensing), major capital development, expensive equipment, and research and development. These resource-related decisions require a broad overview to ensure an appropriate balance as well as the efficient use of scarce resources.

The third area concerns regulatory decisions that involve protecting the public interest. The regulation of new drugs and medical interventions, and the accreditation of providers, should be matters for central control. Experience in some CEE and CIS countries suggests that lower levels of authority may be more susceptible to corruption than higher levels.

The final area focuses on monitoring and evaluating the overall national health situation. Assessment of equity, health gain, efficiency, quality of care, consumer choice and patients' rights can be an efficient tool for influencing the behaviour of the decentralized units. Since, by definition, decentralization involves giving control over essential services to new decision-makers, it is essential to be able to monitor whether these new bodies are performing adequately. Publicizing the results of these evaluations can be a powerful disincentive to undesired behaviour.

The different forms of decentralization can each generate specific disadvantages. These are presented in Table 6.

Table 6. Risks of decentralization

Type of decentralization	Risks
Deconcentration	The "right hand" not always knowing what the "left hand" is doing Unacceptable variations in practice
Devolution	Lack of political control
Delegation	Less professionalism Difficulty in maintaining quality and efficiency if the decentralized units are too fragmented
Privatization	Emergence of private monopolies that may exploit their power (market failure)

Source: Borgenhammer *(80).*

Decentralization tends to incur costs in relation to the subsequent need for coordination. In decentralized institutions, it is typically more difficult to guarantee a sufficient level of uniformity of decision-making than in centralized ones. Economies of scale cannot be made, and sometimes both specialists and equipment are underutilized.

DECENTRALIZATION: KEY QUESTIONS
Any decision to decentralize raises three major issues:

- the level to which the decentralization should take place
- to whom authority should be decentralized
- the tasks that should be decentralized.

The choice of level of decentralization is important in terms of the centre–periphery relationship and, in particular, of the type of accountability adopted. The more local the level, the more concerns there are about scarcity of management skills, fragmented provision due to a large number of small operating units, and the difficulty of providing services efficiently for large populations. One solution is to establish a hierarchy with levels, such as regions and districts, between the centre and the periphery. Decentralization is in the eye of the beholder, however, and what may look like decentralization from a central perspective may appear quite different to a service user (see Box 8).

As to the question of to whom to decentralize, within a devolved system the local authority will be elected and accountable to its electorate (see Box 9). Where health policy and management remain the responsibility of central government, the deconcentrated organization may have some type of appointed board. Health boards can be seen as a way of making local health services more responsive to their local

> **Box 8. Decentralization/Centralization – to which level? Croatia**
>
> In the former Yugoslavia, where the health services were highly decentralized during the socialist regime but still suffered from inefficiency and poor organization, there were no illusions about what decentralization alone could achieve. Croatia, with 4.7 million inhabitants, decided to delegate financial responsibility from the local authorities to the National Health Insurance Fund, a single, highly centralized financial institution. This development was linked to careful and slow privatization, mainly of general practice but also creating competition among providers, introducing contracting and allowing patient choice. The main reason for the refusal to allow rapid privatization was that it would represent a high risk, because private physicians are less accessible to those on average or low incomes. The Croatian reforms are still too recent to allow any evaluation of their outcome, but it appears that the chaos and anarchy created by the former decentralization of health services have disappeared.
>
> *Source:* Oreskovic *(97)*.

communities, without actually devolving power to a local government structure or completely removing the line of accountability to the centre *(99)*. However, appointed boards have been criticized for having no democratic legitimacy, and for being administrative arms of the centre *(100)*. Even when responsibility is devolved to a local authority, central government typically retains, and exercises, considerable power through the appointments system and by other means. Accountability is firmly upwards, even if delegation is downwards. Decentralizing responsibilities while maintaining a degree of central influence appears to be the optimum form of decentralization for many countries. It is neatly summed up in the United Kingdom context in the title of a document published in late 1994, *Local freedoms, national responsibilities (101)*. Produced by the NHS Executive, it sought to establish the ground rules for the evolving internal market in health care services by striking an optimum balance of local freedoms compatible with a national approach that ensures equity and fair play.

Tasks to be decentralized include revenue raising, policy-making and planning, resource allocation, the funding of service provision, and interagency and intersectoral coordination. Revenue raising may be shared by the state with regional or local authorities, as in Finland and Spain, or may be entirely the responsibility of a regional authority as in Sweden, or of a quasi-public statutory body as in Germany and the Netherlands. Examples of task decentralization and its implications are given in Box 10.

Policy-making and planning are usually divided between the central and subnational levels, although the precise mix will vary between countries and over time. In general, local freedom in policy-making and planning is constrained by the need to operate in a centrally determined framework that seeks to establish priorities.

Decentralization is often favoured as a means of improving the coordination of services and activities at local level. It also reflects the recognition that health is more than health care, and that other agencies outside the health care system must be involved in reshaping the policy agenda.

Box 9. Decentralization – to whom? The Russian Federation

The objective of health care reform in the Russian Federation was to put more emphasis on PHC, and on improving the quality of medical services, decentralizing management, breaking the state monopoly on provision, and introducing some market elements through the adoption of patients' rights and choice and "a planned market". During the legislative process and debate in Parliament, however, these principles were reduced, amended, compromised and eventually unclearly formulated in legislation approved in June 1991. The legislation was amended in April 1993, but it nevertheless proved impossible to restore the original principles. An independent non-profit financial and credit institution – the Federal Fund of Mandatory Health Insurance – was established to ensure proper balance between different regions. The regional health insurance funds were established in order to collect the insurance premiums and to pay for the services provided to insured persons by medical facilities. Actual health insurance for individuals, however, is organized through private insurance companies. These sign contracts with employers and local authorities for the mandatory insurance of their workers, and purchase services from medical institutions and the private medical sector.

Experience during the first two years of implementing mandatory health insurance has shown that the insurance premium (3.6%) is too low; the actual expenses amount to 11.2%. The budget deficit is aggravated by the fact that, owing to their own budget deficits, local authorities cannot pay for the populations for whom they are legally responsible. Furthermore, the mandatory health insurance funds received certain reserves through the state budget but, instead of purchasing medical equipment or pharmaceuticals, they then turned themselves into commercial, profit-making businesses without consulting the health care institutions. As many institutions have not been able to sign contracts with the insurance companies, they still depend on the state budget for funding. Last, a considerable share of the collected funds has gone to setting up and running the insurance bureaucracy, and has never benefited patients.

The Russian Federation has embarked on a very complicated and bureaucratic health insurance system that provides an opportunity for private insurance companies to exploit the system for their own profit-making interests, without appropriate responsibility for the health care services they should be providing. Furthermore, difficulties in interpreting the legislation and its amendments have created a situation where there are different practices in different regions, thus creating inequity across the population.

Source: Tchernajvskii & Komarov *(98).*

EVALUATING DECENTRALIZATION

The outcome of decentralization has not often been evaluated in the light of health gain, equity, efficiency, quality of care and consumer choice. Decision-makers have typically taken it for granted that decentralization automatically brings about positive changes, and assumed that there is no need for evaluation. Furthermore, the

Box 10. Decentralization – which tasks?

Norway

The Norwegian block grant reform of 1980 replaced state reimbursements to hospitals by block grants allocated to counties according to objective criteria. The reform was accompanied by a general decentralization of budget authority to local level, and aimed to promote PHC, equalize the supply of health care across regions, and give counties the incentives to improve hospital efficiency. A decade later, the reform was reversed. The government imposed restrictions that reduced the budgetary discretion of the counties, and part of the block grant was made dependent on hospital performance. The government also issued a "waiting list guarantee", which stated that patients suffering from serious conditions were entitled to medical treatment within six months.

The block grant system did not fulfil the expectations of its architects, because it was based on the critical assumption (which turned out to be unrealistic) that governments would be willing to incur the political costs of enforcing financial constraints on counties. The new health policy gave priority to PHC. As county and hospital finances deteriorated and hospitals moved to the top of the political agenda owing to soaring waiting lists for elective surgery, however, the government repeatedly intervened to raise hospital performance and prevent ward closures, undermining the counties' incentive to do their job. The counties engaged in various forms of lobbying directed at the government, acting as advocates for their institutions rather than implementing agents for the state. For instance, in 1986, hospitals exceeded their budgets by 9% on average. Hence hospitals were still rewarded for rising costs, just as they were under the previous reimbursement system.

Hospitals and waiting lists are politically sensitive issues. Implementing an unpopular budget decision becomes much harder when it is widely recognized that the decision-maker is likely to receive additional grants that will make the decision unnecessary. Interventions by the government showed that the original block grant did not represent a fixed budget constraint for the counties. Unless county politicians exploited every opportunity to achieve higher grants, they would be held personally responsible for the consequences of tight budgets. The hospitals knew that budget decisions were part of the game between two tiers of government. Repeatedly, hospitals in financial trouble were rescued, either by the state or by the county. As the block grants evolved into a struggle between the two tiers, the government concluded that the financial system delegated too much authority to the counties. As a consequence, the government introduced new regulations that again strengthened the state's control over the counties.

Source: Carlsen *(102).*

Hungary

Political interference by the state can undermine the potential benefits of decentralization. In Hungary, the respective interests of the Health Insurance Institute and the Ministry of Welfare clashed at the end of 1993. Following the theory of self-government, the Health Insurance Institute should have been allowed to make decisions about concluding – or not concluding – contracts with health care service providers. The Minister of Welfare insisted,

Box 10 (contd)

however, that the Institute sign contracts with all the institutions it had previously financed. When the 1995 contracts came up, a small committee of four people, set up by the Ministry and the Health Insurance Institute, made suggestions about the content of the contracts. This behaviour contradicted the main objective of the reform, which was to remove the Ministry from the direct management of health care. It also contradicted a government decree in autumn 1994, which made proposals for structural changes towards decentralization through the regional councils.

Source: Orosz *(87).*

Sweden

Sweden's experience indicates that the delegation of responsibility always precedes the delegation of the corresponding authority. This was true for the first decentralization reform, from state to county level (1960s–1970s), as well as for the second (1980s) and third reforms (1990s), from higher to lower levels of county administration. In theory, the delegation of responsibilities and powers should go hand in hand; in reality, this is seldom the case. This pattern reflects politicians' need for caution: trying out the recipient of increased responsibilities first, before formal authority is delegated. From the agent's perspective, this strategy can be frustrating. The careful agent would rather receive power first, to make decisions without the corresponding responsibility to deal with any potential problems. These conflicts of interest partly explain the continuing tension between the centre and the periphery in any decentralization process. This tension should be recognized, and managed, in order to avoid unnecessary conflicts.

Source: Anell *(83).*

expected outcomes are often not well defined in advance. It would be a major step forward if policy-makers could define explicitly what kinds of improvement were expected from decentralization policies.

Whether the advantages of decentralization outweigh the possible disadvantages – notably fragmented and duplicated services as well as high transaction costs – is an issue that must be resolved by national policy-makers on a case-by-case basis. It is not uncommon to find that countries that have engaged in radical decentralization subsequently recentralize control over key elements of the system, typically health funding and professional standard setting. Privatization, however, has only rarely been viewed as a viable health policy strategy in western Europe, and it has been pursued in CEE and CIS countries unevenly and with considerable trepidation.

Empowerment, rights and choice

In addition to the objectives of equity, effectiveness and efficiency, European policy-makers are also grappling with the concept of patient empowerment. In the health sector context, this refers to a growing insistence that citizens be allowed a greater say in logistical matters (such as selecting their doctor and hospital) and in clinical matters (such as participating in elective medical decision-making). Increasingly, they are also asking to be allowed to participate in local policy-making when the state has made this possible through decentralization.

Ideas about citizen participation and patient choice in health care are in various ways linked with different philosophies about health care financing and organization. Some policy analysts have argued that taking citizens' collective views into account through increased participation in the decision-making process can democ-ratize health services, making the medical profession and the state more account-able *(61)*. This approach is typically associated with the view of health care as a "social good", as found in publicly operated health systems. In contrast, concern with individual choice is also associated with systems that emphasize market princi-ples such as competition. Patient choice in this instance is usually linked to the idea of consumer sovereignty, and the importance of systems being tailored to meet the "individual" demands of their users. These two different types of logic suggest that the notion of *participation* has been limited to patient *needs,* while the concept of *choice* of provider has traditionally been connected to patient *wants.*

This analysis is, however, incomplete. In some systems where market principles have been introduced, and "rationing" has become more explicit, the public and the community are also asked for their views about priorities. In this case, however, the emphasis is on the public being reactive rather than on proactive community partici-pation and representation in the policy-making process.

In a democratic–political approach, patient choice is construed as an exercise in democratic rather than commercial rights. Patient choice becomes a mechanism whereby individuals can exercise more influence over what happens to them inside a publicly operated system, typically through the choice of hospital and physician. Patient choice thus becomes a political characteristic in which patients, through their participation, help to legitimize the underlying authority of the service delivery system. From this perspective, patient choice is an important concept for examining users' approaches to health care systems, irrespective of whether they are privately or publicly funded.

One useful framework for examining approaches to participation *(103)* constructs a ladder of participation to describe the different degrees of power potentially avail-able to the consumer. These range from manipulation and therapy, through informa-tion, consultation and conciliation, to partnership and power, where decisions are made by citizens rather than by governments or service providers.

A similar system of classification differentiates the degrees of authority that can be considered to create "empowered patients" *(61)*. The continuum moves from the least to the most empowered position for the individual patient. It begins with moral persuasion (the ability only to ask to be heard), through formal political control, to the ability to control one's own organizational destiny. Requests from patients to have a physician's decision reviewed are at the least empowered end of the contin-uum. Moving along the scale are: legal remedies, the annual selection by patients of their insurance carriers, choice of physician and hospital without a direct link to the payment of providers, elected democratic control over finance and service provision, influence over type of treatment, and, finally, choice of physician and hospital but with links to the payment of providers. In this typology, the key to understanding empowerment is the degree of individual leverage over specific decisions on service delivery. To become empowered, therefore, patients have to wrest substantial control over budgetary authority and resource allocation away from managers and providers. The typology, therefore, focuses mainly on the individual and emphasizes the importance of patient choice and control over decisions.

There are, however, a number of unresolved issues associated with choice in health care. The first concerns whether choice is as important for users as some policy analysts believe. To what extent is choice important for all health care provision, or is it only important in certain areas such as maternity services? A related issue is whether, given the special characteristics of health care, users have access to enough information to make informed choices if they want to *(104)*. Finally, there is the question of inequality of access to choice: those with the most resources (finance, time and energy) are likely to have the greatest opportunity to make choices.

CITIZEN PARTICIPATION

Two key issues are, first, how the citizen's voice is heard in relation to the structure of health care in different countries and, second, how much authority and power citizens have in influencing decisions. Countries have taken various approaches at both collective and individual levels. In Finland, citizens have a formal influence through municipal health boards. The elected municipal council selects a health board consisting of the chief physician from the municipal health centre and a mix of local lay people representing citizens' views. The United Kingdom has adopted a different approach. While health authority members are not elected but nominated, and do not automatically include citizens' representatives, local community health councils have been in existence for 20 years. These are agencies set up specifically to represent citizens' interests in health care. Unlike in Finland, the members of these councils are not elected but appointed, and the councils tend to have an advisory and informative role. A more recent initiative put forward by the United Kingdom attempted to portray the new purchasing authorities and consortia as champions of the people. A number of mechanisms for consulting local communities were cited in *Local voices*, an advisory document produced by the NHS Executive *(105)*. Suggestions include the use of "focus groups" drawn from the local population, surveys and health forums. These suggestions were not incorporated into statutory mechanisms, and have only taken root sporadically.

The CEE countries have seen rapid development in the voluntary sector, including a variety of patient support groups. At the same time, the advent of independent media has given publicity to issues of patient participation and choice. In Poland, the important role played by the press has been reflected in the formation of a patients' rights movement.

One of the more successful reforms in Poland has been the establishment of local self-governing councils with health committees. Despite centralized financing and provision of health care, many local governments have taken over some health care responsibilities, typically with regard to PHC. In the majority of cases these responsibilities are delegated, together with the budget, and this limits empowerment. Local governments have to be consulted about the closure or establishment of health care facilities in their areas.

PATIENTS' RIGHTS AND QUALITY OF CARE

One common policy in a number of European countries has been the introduction of mechanisms for protecting patients' rights. While this does not necessarily involve public participation, it is an attempt to make health service provision more sensitive to aspects of patient demand. In Poland, for instance, an act passed in 1991 ensures that patients are entitled to: a level of care appropriate to current medical knowledge, information on their state of health, informed consent to or refusal of specific components of health care, privacy and dignity, and a peaceful and dignified death. In addition, when undergoing inpatient treatment, the patient has a right to personal telephone communication and correspondence with the outside world, to be nursed by family or friends, and to receive spiritual care. No provision was made for implementing these rights, however. A patients' rights charter is currently being developed, although as yet it has not become law.

In 1992, the United Kingdom introduced its Patient's Charter, setting out ten rights and introducing national and local standard setting as a device for improving the quality of care. The emphasis is on standards rather than legal rights, and thus the Charter's success will depend on the quality of the mechanisms and procedures developed to give substance to its principles, and the significance attached to these by those responsible for their implementation. Without effective mechanisms, the Charter can do little to empower citizens.

In contrast to the approach taken in Poland and the United Kingdom, Finland in 1993 defined patients' rights by law. This is a landmark in the development of legislation in Europe *(106)*. The law gives patients the right to good health and medical care and related treatment, access to care, information and self-determination. The status of minors, emergency treatment and the right to information and good clinical competence are also covered. Perhaps one of the more important aspects of the Finnish legislation is the role of the patients' ombudsman. Under the Finnish scheme, every health care institution must nominate an ombudsman who can be responsible for a number of local health care units. The ombudsman's role includes advising patients on all practical matters concerning the implementation of the law on patients' rights, and assisting patients in writing a complaint or application for compensation.

The Netherlands has taken the most comprehensive approach to patients' rights. Its legislation on medical contracts, which took effect in April 1995, spells out clearly the principal rights of patients *(107)*. The legislation treats the relationship between patient and physician as a "special contract" within civil contract law. This gives the individual patient a direct claim on the doctor, and the ability to enforce those rights through the courts, without relying on any further action by the government. The provisions of this legislation include informed consent, information, access to medical records and data, retention periods for medical data, confidentiality, the legal position of minors and of adults who are not capable of managing their own affairs, medical liability, the use of medical data and records, and the use of human tissue for research purposes *(107)*.

Italy has adopted a different approach, its Tribunal for Patients' Rights. The Tribunal is composed of ordinary citizens who voluntarily monitor the quality of health services, resolving patients' complaints and lobbying for more humane methods of administration. Representatives of the Tribunal are involved in every health authority throughout Italy.

One mechanism through which users' dissatisfaction can be voiced actively is a formal complaints procedure. In some European countries, including the United Kingdom, there is evidence of a rapid increase in the numbers of complaints over recent years. It is difficult to identify whether this is due to a real increase in grievances, a rise in users' expectations, or the fact that it is now easier to voice a complaint.

Most countries do have formal systems for channelling complaints, although the array of channels can be bewildering for the potential complainant. In the United Kingdom, the complaints system has recently been reviewed *(108)*. Complainants can pursue their grievances through an internal system and, if still not satisfied, they may ask for the complaint to be dealt with by a panel chaired by a lay person. It is the health authority or trust, however, that decides whether or not a panel is convened *(109,110)*.

One of the issues associated with complaints systems is that the agencies dealing with complaints are able to make decisions only about disciplinary measures, since financial compensation tends to be dealt with by the courts, particularly when there is disagreement between the parties. Finland attempted to deal with this problem in 1987 by passing legislation. A Patient Injuries Board was set up within the Ministry of Social Welfare and Health. The Board's task is to recommend whether compensation should be paid and, if requested, the Board must also give its opinion on the amount of compensation payable. Sweden has had a no-fault structure for several decades, administered by its National Board of Health and Welfare and funded by a small contribution per head paid by the county councils to a central fund.

Several complaints mechanisms exist in Poland. The complaints system, involving the state bureaucracy and rooted in administrative law, is largely discredited. Complaints procedures for patients also exist in the system of professional self-regulating associations, and patients may complain through the ombudsman for "patients' rights".

CHOICE OF INSURER AND/OR PROVIDER

The question of choice in health care is a complex one. In varying mixes, countries in Europe allow patients to select their providers, i.e. their general practitioner (GP), specialist, hospital and/or hospital doctor. In a limited number of countries, subscribers may choose their insurer, although in the northern European sickness fund countries this option has traditionally been available only to those on high incomes. Furthermore, in some countries some patients with a specific range of conditions (typically chronic or involving elective procedures) are able to influence clinical decisions concerning their course of treatment *(61)*.

With regard to choice of provider, most tax-based and sickness fund countries allow individuals to choose their GP *(6,111)*. This choice is typically for a fixed period (three months in Germany, one year in Denmark) and only a few countries require formal approval of these choices by a public regulatory authority. Finland is among the few countries in western Europe that still assigns individuals to GPs, in the belief that comprehensive holistic care can be more effectively provided if everyone in a particular neighbourhood is treated by the same physician or group of physicians. Finns who can afford to pay a private physician, however, are able to opt out of the public system of assigning GPs.

Choice of specialist and/or hospital for elective procedures remains controversial. There is no clear consensus among countries as to whether patients should be allowed to refer themselves to specialist care or whether, conversely, GPs should serve as gatekeepers, referring patients to specialists *(6,111)*. For further discussion, see the section on PHC in Chapter 6 (pages 236–239).

Examples of both approaches can be found in tax-based as well as sickness-fund-based health systems. Swedish patients can refer themselves to specialists, while those in Finland and the United Kingdom cannot. German sickness fund patients can refer themselves, while Dutch patients cannot. In Denmark, about 2.5% of the population choose Group 2 insurance, which allows direct access to a specialist but requires them to pay an additional fee *(112)*. A further complication is that in some tax-based systems, patients can choose to pay out of pocket (in Finland, for example, to pay the difference between the social insurance allowances and the actual cost) to visit a private specialist.

Choice of hospital follows a similar pattern to that of specialist referral. Since 1991 in Sweden and since 1993 in Denmark, patients have been allowed to choose their hospitals for elective procedures. This was designed to reduce waiting times and to stimulate hospital productivity, as well as to allow patients more control over their treatment in a publicly operated health system. Conversely, in the United Kingdom, the growth of contracting has served to restrict patient choice to those hospitals that have contracts with a patient's fundholding GP or health authority. While interim evaluations suggest that greater choice has been more successful than restricted choice in achieving these goals *(113)*, overall conclusions await an adequate comparative assessment.

The choice of insurer is also controversial; a detailed analysis is presented in Chapter 4. It is sufficient to note here that only one country in the European Region (Israel) currently provides universal insurance that allows patients to choose among competing private companies. When the Dutch attempted to introduce multiple competing insurers, they found that it created insuperable obstacles to maintaining social solidarity *(61,67,114)*. Competitive insurance has also proved to be a very expensive approach that offers few benefits in terms of additional services.

Patients only occasionally have an influence on clinical treatment decisions *(6)*. Some countries may, for example, consult elderly patients as to whether they wish to be placed in a nursing home or remain in their own home with home care services.

EVALUATION: THE IMPACT OF POLICY CHANGES

Evidence to date about the impact of these changes on levels of public participation and choice is largely derived from studies in the United Kingdom. Survey evidence (115,116) suggests that the impact has been mixed. For example, Bruster et al. (115), in their national study of patients' views on hospital care, show that the standards set out in the Patient's Charter were not being met in a number of areas: explanation of treatment, access to health records, choice about taking part in student training and guaranteed admission to hospital within two years of being placed on a waiting list.

Evidence from the British social attitudes survey (116) shows that the reforms seem to have reduced the demand for health spending and have helped restore confidence in the performance of the service. The public is not convinced, however, that its views do count regarding how the service is run. In 1987, nearly two thirds thought that if a hospital had to choose between making life easier for patients or easier for doctors, the hospital would opt to make life easier for patients. In 1993, only just over half thought hospitals would make that choice, while just over one in four believed that they would definitely or probably have a say in which hospital they would go to if they needed an operation. It has also been suggested (117) that the limit on waiting list times may be focusing on the less important aspects of waiting. Cartwright & Windsor (117) found that patients were more dissatisfied with the delay between referral by their GP and being seen at an outpatient department than with the decision to put them on a waiting list.

The evidence about the impact of fundholding on patient choice is limited, and thus difficult to judge (118). The hopes that the introduction of fundholding would lead to money following patients, and that fundholders would enhance patient choice by "shopping around" for health care, have not yet materialized, since fundholders tend to support their local hospitals. A recent Audit Commission report (119) found that patients of fundholding practices had better access to hospital care, owing to shorter waiting lists. An earlier study had found, however, that fundholding GPs were no more likely to take account of patients' preferences than those from non-fundholding practices (120).

There are other areas where United Kingdom policies have attempted to extend choice, and where the reforms have sought to encourage patients to act like consumers and shop around for their health care, but several commentators (e.g. Leavy, (121)) are sceptical about this. They question patients' motivation for acting as consumers and doubt their enthusiasm for shopping around. For those with chronic conditions, for instance, a relationship of trust and confidence, built up during the course of an illness, could provide a powerful incentive to stay put. A recent study found that the new system had led to no increase in the rate of movement of patients between GPs (122).

Similarly, while the increase in the proportion of the population covered by private health insurance in the United Kingdom has stabilized, it still remains largely the preserve of the well-off. The evidence suggests that the use of private health insurance only marginally increases "consumer choice" (123). Those who had used private health care stressed the quality of the facilities, the personal care, and the convenience of being able to choose when to be treated, but there was little evidence of shopping around between the private and public sectors. Subscribers had limited knowledge of treatment costs, and felt that they lacked the competence to evaluate the skills of different consultants in order to make an informed choice. Rather than shopping around for the best value, they depended on their NHS GP to decide whether they should opt for private treatment and, if so, which consultant they should see. This suggests that patients may well remain dependent on medical professionals, and that the issue is how to regulate this dependence *(124)*.

As to the effects of the new attempts by purchasing authorities to consult local people, there is a voluminous literature on the methods adopted *(109,110,125)*, ranging from surveys and rapid appraisal techniques to neighbourhood forums and user groups. The evidence available to evaluate these consultation methods is scarce, and it is difficult to know whether they are genuine attempts to take public views into consideration or token strategies that reflect managerial manipulation *(126)*. There is also the question of the internal organizational structure of health authorities, and the extent that the public's views, once elicited, actually influence decision-making.

With regard to the explicit rationing of services, purchasers have sometimes invited the public to prioritize their preferences *(127)*. This is a role that the public seems reluctant to perform *(128)*, claiming that it is mainly the responsibility of the medical profession. The methodology adopted in many of these studies has been criticized both for ethical reasons and for not accurately representing all sections of the community.

CONCLUSION

This brief review, based on selected countries' experiences, shows the similarities and differences in policies adopted and some evidence of effectiveness. Some countries, such as the United Kingdom, have taken the moral persuasion approach, while others, such as Finland, have adopted more interventionist government legislation aimed at enhancing patients' rights and public participation. In Italy, the policy was generated from a social movement rather than by a top-down prescriptive approach. There is still limited evidence available from which to make comparative judgements on the most effective mechanisms for representing users' views about health care.

The evolving role of public health

The health care reform debate often focuses largely on questions associated with the supply of services, seeking ways to organize, finance and deliver health care in the most cost-effective manner. Less attention has been paid to key aspects of the demand side, in particular how the need for health care might be reduced by improving the wider determinants of the population's health *(129)*. This is despite the fact that most European countries have formally adopted policies on both health care reform and public health, exemplified by the health for all strategy *(130)*.

Two important issues emerge. The first concerns the importance of ensuring that health sector reforms contribute to improvements in the health of the population. The second is the extent to which a strong public health infrastructure, with the appropriate skills, can contribute to the design and implementation of health sector reforms.

If the ultimate goal of health sector reform is to maximize the population's health, reforming health services must be part of a broader package that recognizes the impact of the wider social, physical and economic environments on health status *(131)* and vice versa *(132)*. The major determinants of health lie in these areas and they offer the greatest scope for health gain. Indeed, the main health challenges facing Europe call for policies that embrace a wide range of issues, including income distribution, employment, education, transport and agriculture.

In the second case, a strong public health infrastructure, with the ability to assess health care needs and to identify, develop and implement appropriate services in response to them, is an important factor in the success of reform programmes. This is increasingly important as reforms focus on the effectiveness of care.

The capacity needed for countries to develop a modern public health infrastructure requires technical skills to assess the need for health and health care, the ability to develop effective and achievable policies, and mechanisms to facilitate intersectoral action and achieve healthy public policies. Despite an increasing awareness of the role of public health, this issue is still not sufficiently addressed in some reform programmes.

This section considers these issues mainly from the perspective of health care sector reform. It includes a discussion on the definition of public health and on the intersectoral scope of public health. While recognizing that the public health function incorporates a wide range of bodies in different sectors, the section focuses on those components of the public health infrastructure that live within the health care sector.

DEFINING PUBLIC HEALTH

At the outset, it is necessary to define what is meant by public health, as it has had various definitions over the years and in different places. For example, in a recent exercise in Hungary, seven different words were identified to describe particular aspects of public health *(133)*, with meanings ranging from traditional hygiene to what is loosely translated as social medicine. In Hungary, as in some other countries, some terms that can be translated as public health, such as the German *Volksgesundheit*, have historical connotations that make them politically unacceptable.

Over 40 years ago, in 1952, a WHO Expert Committee on Public Health Administration *(134)*, based on a 1923 definition from Winslow *(135)*, stated that public health is:

> the science and art of preventing disease, prolonging life, and promoting mental and physical health and efficiency through organized community efforts for the sanitation of the environment, the control of communicable infections, the education of the individual in personal hygiene, the organization of medical and nursing services for the early

diagnosis and preventive treatment of disease, and the development of social machinery to ensure to every individual a standard of living adequate for the maintenance of health, so organizing these benefits as to enable every citizen to realize his birthright of health and longevity.

The influence of this definition can be seen in two widely used definitions: the first from the American Institute of Medicine, "organized community efforts aimed at the prevention of disease and promotion of health" *(136)*, and the second from the report of the Acheson Committee on the future of public health in England *(137)*, "the science and art of preventing disease, prolonging life and promoting health through organized efforts of society".

These definitions are extremely broad and do not refer explicitly to the curative sector as such. In practice, in many countries, public health services have been kept quite separate from the curative sector. It is, however, increasingly recognized that the two sectors must work together for their mutual benefit. The curative sector should not respond passively to those who seek care, but should also engage in preventive activities. Public health can contribute to the organization of health services by offering a population perspective, and by helping to develop policies that improve service effectiveness.

These concepts are central to the "new public health movement", which stresses that public health encompasses a broad range of activities, including medical care, that contribute to the protection, promotion and improvement of the health of a given population (Barnard, K., unpublished data, 1995). A detailed definition by Frenk *(138)* declares:

> The new public health addresses the systematic efforts to identify health needs and to organize comprehensive health services with a well-defined population base. It thus includes the process of information required for characterizing the conditions of the population and the mobilization of resources necessary for responding to such conditions. In this regard, the essence of public health is the health of the public. Therefore it includes the organization of personnel and facilities for providing all the health services required for health promotion, disease prevention, diagnosis and treatment of illnesses, and physical, social, and vocational rehabilitation.

INTERSECTORAL SCOPE OF PUBLIC HEALTH

The leading determinants of health act at several levels. In the first instance, there are differences in genetic factors, with some individuals being more susceptible to disease than others. Understanding of the contribution of genetics is expanding rapidly, drawing on a combination of epidemiological studies such as those of twins, family trees and adopted children, as well as new laboratory techniques that make it possible to identify both the genes and the associated proteins involved in disease. In a few cases, typically involving a single gene or chromosomal abnormality, they can be shown to cause disease. More commonly, they are simply an indicator of a predisposition to disease that will manifest itself only in the presence of other factors.

A second set of factors relates to lifestyle and environment; these include tobacco and alcohol consumption, diet and the causes of accidents. They can be shown to be closely linked to specific diseases, although even here evidence of the nature of relationships, such as the role of micronutrients in cardiovascular and cerebrovascular diseases, is emerging only slowly. Finally, there is a range of factors that have a more diffuse impact, influencing the rates of cardiovascular diseases, cancer, accidents and mental health. These include inequalities in income, sense of personal autonomy, and social support. The evidence for the importance of these factors is increasingly compelling *(34,139)*. While the mechanisms through which they act are still in need of clarification, there is growing evidence of the importance of links between psychological factors and the immune system.

These different factors can also interact, as illustrated by the case of smoking. A smoker with a genetically determined high level of blood cholesterol will be at greater risk of a heart attack than someone without it. Furthermore, an individual with a relatively low income will be both more likely to smoke and, for a given level of tobacco consumption, will be more likely to develop lung cancer.

Although the nature of the links between deprivation and ill health is only now beginning to be fully understood, the basic premise has been recognized for many years. Commentators such as Virchow called for changes in social policy in the mid-nineteenth century *(140)*. The practice of recording occupations in censuses and on death certificates in countries such as the United Kingdom has encouraged a steady increase in research on the association between deprivation and health. The Black report, published in 1980 *(141)*, demonstrated beyond reasonable doubt an association between social deprivation and ill health.

Increasing awareness of the complexity of the determinants of health has led to a new approach to health promotion, based on a multifactorial concept of health. This was set out clearly in the seminal 1974 Canadian government report, *A new perspective on the health of Canadians (42)*. This study, often referred to as the Lalonde report in honour of the study's chairman, introduced the "health field" concept, in which health is viewed as a product of lifestyle, environment, human biology and health care. This approach also constitutes the basis of the European health for all strategy adopted by WHO ten years later in 1984 *(142)*, and of the Ottawa Charter for Health Promotion in 1986 *(143)*, which set out five action areas:

- building healthy public policy
- creating supportive environments
- strengthening community action
- developing personal skills
- reorientating health services.

These principles reinforce the role of public health in enabling individuals and communities to increase control over the determinants of health *(143)*. The need for intersectoral action is a central theme of this approach. If factors such as poverty, nutrition and tobacco consumption are some of the major determinants of disease, then a wide range of agencies must be involved. These include central and local government, nongovernmental organizations and community groups, as well as private organizations.

Intersectoral programmes can be conducted through formal or informal means, involving public and private organizations, individuals acting alone or together, and organizations within and outside the health sector. In addition, many policies undertaken to achieve objectives not specifically related to health, such as community development or redistribution of wealth, may have important consequences for health.

One of the best known examples of this intersectoral approach is the WHO Healthy Cities project (144), which includes some 650 cities throughout Europe and more than 1000 worldwide. Within this movement, local governments and a wide range of statutory and voluntary agencies and organizations have come together to develop and implement healthy local policies. Areas of action include health promotion, ecological management, social support for vulnerable groups, and programmes addressing equity, community empowerment and integrated planning for health. These and other community-oriented programmes, such as the North Karelia Project (145), which addressed the high level of heart disease in Finland, have been shown to be effective in bringing about change in behaviour and thereby improving health.

At national level, several European countries have produced, or are in the process of producing, health strategies influenced by this intersectoral approach. The health of the nation strategy in the United Kingdom (146) is one example, but similar strategies are emerging in France, Luxembourg, the Netherlands, Switzerland and Turkey. Some CEE and CIS countries, such as the Czech Republic, Estonia, Lithuania, Poland and Slovenia, are also developing strategies embodying the principles of intersectoral action and health promotion. Various countries, including Bulgaria, Denmark, Finland, Hungary, Ireland and the United Kingdom (147), have established interministerial or interdepartmental committees to coordinate health policies. These provide a formal mechanism for placing health on the policy agenda although, inevitably, they cannot guarantee that it will remain there.

REFORMING PUBLIC HEALTH SERVICES

The various elements included in the term "public health services" vary widely in Europe. In the CEE and CIS countries, and in parts of southern Europe, the term has had a very narrow focus, covering only a few specific determinants of health such as environmental hazards and communicable diseases. In other countries, it has developed a broader role, monitoring the overall health of the population.

There is little official international guidance on what constitutes public health services. In the United Kingdom, the Acheson report (137) offers some assistance, defining public health medicine as:

> that branch of medicine which specializes in public health. Its chief responsibilities are the surveillance of the health of a population, the identification of its health needs, the fostering of policies which promote health, and the evaluation of health services.

This provides a good – if broad – working definition, although it must be recognized that public health services go well beyond public health medicine. Indeed, although the rate of progress varies between countries, there is a general trend towards a more multidisciplinary model of public health services in which senior positions are also held by sociologists, nonmedical epidemiologists, policy analysts and economists.

Given the differing views about what public health services are, a realistic approach is to examine the major functions common to most systems, recognizing that they often reflect different underlying beliefs and are organized in a variety of ways. These are considered here under five major headings *(148)*: communicable disease control and environmental health; provision of services for specific groups; health promotion; the commissioning, planning and evaluation of health services; and public health research.

Communicable disease control and environmental health

These two topics are considered together because, historically, communicable disease control and environmental health have been seen as the core roles of public health. In many countries, public health still focuses on these two traditional functions. Recently, the advent of new infections, such as those caused by antibiotic-resistent bacteria, has re-emphasized the importance of this role. Indeed, HIV infection and AIDS have been seen by some as galvanizing societies in a way not seen since the Black Death in the Middle Ages. In France and Switzerland, HIV has been responsible for a substantial strengthening of the public health function at national level. Despite the long tradition of public health involvement in communicable disease control, however, there are considerable national differences in implementation.

At a structural level, countries differ in whether responsibility for operational activities is located in local government, as in Germany and Scandinavia; in the health service, as in Italy and in the CEE countries; or split between the two, as in the United Kingdom, where public health medicine is part of the health service but environmental health is a local government responsibility. In practice, there is little evidence to suggest that one approach is better than another. What seems more important is that, wherever the service is located, there should be strong formal or informal links with other bodies involved, whether in the health system or in other public agencies, and that there should also be close links between practitioners and policy-makers.

There are also considerable differences between the methods used in the surveillance and investigation of outbreaks. These differences are arguably more important than structural considerations. For example, only a few countries have well developed surveillance systems with rapid transmission of information from hospital laboratories *(149)*. In the CEE countries and in some countries in southern Europe, investigation of outbreaks is based on microbiological methods, and this rather narrow approach often fails to identify avoidable risk factors. It is often ineffective where organisms with special culture requirements are involved, and where epidemiological clues that might indicate the need to look for them are absent. In contrast, western European countries, while recognizing that laboratory work is essential, place more emphasis on a coordinated approach, which includes epidemiological investigation based on case–control studies and mechanisms for developing policy to eliminate identified risk factors for infection.

Although communicable disease control is seen by many as somewhat peripheral to health care reform, each can have an impact on the other. Any failure of communicable disease control may have considerable economic consequences for health services, both in the direct cost of treating infected patients (150) and in the indirect costs to society of outbreaks; the closure of food factories, for example, can have consequences for national economic growth (151). Health sector reform can also affect existing systems for communicable disease surveillance and control. Many countries, especially those with large numbers of independent providers, have not developed integrated, comprehensive surveillance systems. This failure can mean that outbreaks go unrecognized. Health sector reform that leads to the fragmentation of laboratory networks may risk compromising existing surveillance activities (152).

Differences also can be seen in the approach to environmental health. Some systems, such as the sanitary and epidemiological (sanepid) stations in the CEE countries, only partially cover pollution. These should develop more sophisticated multidisciplinary approaches, recognizing the need for skills such as geography, economics, policy analysis and mathematical modelling, and they should move away from the existing model of medical dominance. The optimum model is one in which environmental control is based on a combination of exposure and health status monitoring, with the skills to integrate the two and to design and implement appropriate policy responses that encompass economic, educational and regulatory responses. No European country achieves this ideal but some, such as the Netherlands, have made more progress than others.

The wide variations in the quality of policies on communicable disease control and environmental health are a matter for concern. The EU is supporting projects to develop agreed definitions to be used in surveillance and to develop rapid communication networks. This is partly in response to the recognized threats from increasing population mobility, as well as the emergence of new diseases such as HIV infection and AIDS and transmissible spongiform encephalopathies. Governments also need to take action to ensure that effective surveillance and outbreak control networks are in place.

Provision of services for specific groups

The second area in which public health has been involved is the provision of services for specific groups, such as children (including school health), the elderly, people with learning impairments, and those with diseases such as tuberculosis. Traditionally, this role developed from the inability to design financial or other incentives that would persuade independent physicians to look after such groups. As a consequence, the state took responsibility for them. In countries with social insurance systems, health service benefits were initially limited to those in employment – mostly men – leaving the public health system to provide services for the unemployed and for mothers and children. Even where the government was responsible for all health services, however, as in the Beveridge model in the United Kingdom or the

Semashko model in the USSR, the two systems have remained separate. In a few countries, such as Belgium and the Netherlands, some of these services are provided by nongovernmental organizations.

Public health services are increasingly being integrated with mainstream health services. This reflects the recognition that the presence of two separate vertical systems frequently duplicated existing services, and often provided lower-quality care (153). There has also been a general move towards developing integrated models of PHC in which families have a single point of contact with the health services (see Box 11). As a result, public health is withdrawing from its role in the direct management of services for groups with special needs. In Germany, for example, there has been a steady transfer of responsibility for preventive medicine services since the early 1970s, from the public health service to sickness funds (154).

Box 11. Provision of preventive services in PHC in the United Kingdom

In the United Kingdom, child health surveillance and immunization have largely become the responsibility of GPs. High levels of immunization uptake have been achieved by the judicious use of contractual payments to GPs if they attain certain targets. Monitoring is carried out by public health staff based in health authorities, who can provide advice and support if targets are not met. The needs of the elderly and those with learning difficulties are cared for by specialists working across what is termed the "primary–secondary interface". This is intended to overcome the marginalization of these vulnerable groups from the mainstream health services.

In countries where public health still manages services for special groups in separate vertical programmes, there is a case for integrating these activities with the mainstream health services. It is not sufficient, however, to abolish the vertical systems still common in CEE and CIS countries and assume that the services they provide will be taken over by the mainstream services. In many countries, these programmes were established because of the failure of other providers to meet the needs of disadvantaged groups. Furthermore, adequate replacement will be difficult where strong PHC networks have not been developed.

Integration should be undertaken in a framework of explicit and measurable objectives, with effective monitoring and feedback systems, and with those responsible for implementing change given the scope to use a range of mechanisms. In some cases, it will be necessary to work within a contractual relationship between purchasers and providers. A complex combination of levers will need to be developed, including not only financial incentives but also capital controls and other forms of regulation. One caveat is that there may be a case for retaining some parallel services, such as family planning programmes targeted at teenagers and clinics for sexually transmitted diseases, in countries where cultural attitudes might inhibit people from seeking care from their GPs.

As with communicable disease control, any move towards greater pluralism carries risks. In countries where integrated services have developed, the introduction of competing providers may lead to a breakdown of carefully cultivated relationships.

Health promotion

As noted earlier, the model of health promotion adopted in some countries is based on an intersectoral approach, drawing on professionals from a range of disciplines that includes epidemiology, social policy, psychology, marketing, anthropology and economics. In a few countries, however, activities are still based on an outdated medical model that consists of poorly coordinated programmes of preventive medicine and health education.

Health promotion activities have not been given a central place within the reformed health care sector. In the CEE and CIS countries, health promotion is a relatively new activity. One barrier to the development of a health promotion function stems from recent moves to introduce a health insurance system, in which coverage is not necessarily universal and may be defined by individual contributions. Other obstacles include a lack of understanding of what health promotion activities involve, the lack of a health promotion infrastructure, and resistance by traditional public health systems.

Several countries, however, have recognized the importance of developing a health promotion function within the health care system. In Bulgaria, for instance, the Ministry of Health has set up a National Health Promotion Centre, which is seen as playing a leading role in the implementation of the national health strategy. This Centre is beginning to address the development of capacity building in health promotion within the health care sector and beyond. In Estonia, following the adoption of an insurance-based health care system in 1994, the National Health Insurance Board agreed to contribute to public health activities through a levy of 0.5% of its total revenue. This has provided a firm source of funding for the development of health promotion activities. Legislation on the organization of health care has placed the responsibility for health care and public health management on county physicians. These, together with public health specialists, have undergone health promotion training and are beginning to establish health promotion activities at county and local levels *(155)*.

As these examples show, the development of health promotion in some CEE countries has evolved according to local circumstances, interest and expertise. Successful health promotion seems to depend on a national commitment through legislation and national health policy. A national health promotion centre, with adequate funding to lead the development of competence building in health promotion, is also crucial. Any reorganization of the health care system must ensure that health promotion is built in at delivery level. In this sense, a defined role for health promotion within PHC is essential.

In western European countries, the impact of reforms on the health promotion function within the health care system has been varied. In some countries with social insurance, such as France and Germany, sickness funds have taken responsibility for some health promotion activities, which have been introduced in the reimbursement scheme for PHC practitioners. Box 12 illustrates the impact of the health sector reforms in the United Kingdom on health promotion activities.

Box 12. Health sector reforms and health promotion activities in the United Kingdom

In the United Kingdom, the health care reforms have provided some opportunities for health promotion in the commissioning of health care services, as well as in the delivery of health promotion services. The opportunity for strategic influence has also been strengthened by the health of the nation strategy, and the leading role given to the NHS in its implementation. Integration of the national health targets within the regulatory system has led to local purchasing plans addressing the national targets along with locally identified health priorities. Also, the GPs' contract has a specific requirement for GPs to give health promotion advice to patients. This is a significant development that is refined annually.

The purchasing of health promotion services through contracts has led to the evaluation of health promotion interventions in both clinical and cost–effectiveness terms. The issue of evaluating health promotion has also raised questions of how the health promotion process is understood within the health care system, and to what extent evaluation criteria should adopt additional success criteria such as equity.

In general, the concern for cost-containment of hospital services has shifted the emphasis to PHC. The extent to which countries have implemented policies to strengthen PHC services varies. This renewed focus on PHC, however, provides opportunities for health promotion and disease prevention.

In the long term, the need to reduce health care costs and demand will inevitably focus more attention on health gain and the effectiveness of clinical and health promotion interventions. The difficulties in measuring health promotion in terms that compare with clinical effectiveness has meant that health promotion has not played a central role in health sector reform. Until there are convincing ways of evaluating health promotion interventions that satisfy the needs of managers, clinicians and health promoters, the full potential of health promotion will not be recognized. Opportunities for increased health promotion work within PHC have also not been fully exploited.

Health promotion requires recognition at a strategic level. An effective infrastructure is also needed that can support health promoters at local and national levels. Those working in health promotion need to bridge the gap between health services and the other relevant sectors. They should assess, on the basis of sound epidemiological evidence, the major health challenges facing their populations, develop prioritized programmes for action, and implement policies that draw on the methods available to bring about change in knowledge, attitudes and practice.

The commissioning, planning and evaluation of health services

Public health professionals are increasingly involved in the overall direction of health services through planning or commissioning. This has arisen, in part, from the growing importance of health services research, which has revealed evidence of both underuse of effective and overuse of ineffective interventions, of variations in intervention rates and outcomes, and of unequal access to care affecting some of the most vulnerable groups. Issues relating to effectiveness are discussed in more detail in Chapter 6. The introduction of reforms based on separating the purchaser and provider functions, and on regulated competition between public and private providers, i.e. "planned markets" *(6)* or "quasi-markets" *(64)*, has further increased the need for these skills. As discussed earlier, planned markets seek to use market-based incentives to achieve socially desirable goals, but they must operate in a tightly regulated structure if they are to avoid the adverse consequences of market failure. Such a system requires bodies that serve three functions: insurance (matching income and expenditure), agency (providing information to support choice, and acting as a "prudent" buyer) and guarantee of access *(156)*.

Public health professionals in many countries have been able to adopt these roles, aided by the blurring of the distinction between prevention and cure in areas such as cancer screening and genetics, as well as by an improved understanding of the complementary nature of individual and population-based interventions *(157)*. For example, in several Scandinavian countries, there is input from public health professionals at both county and national levels.

In the United Kingdom, public health is a key element of the health authority purchasing structure. In the British model, health authorities are responsible for assessing the health needs of their populations, deciding priorities for meeting those needs, placing contracts accordingly, evaluating the performance of those contracts and taking other action to promote health and prevent disease. Public health is expected to play a central role in this process, including population-based epidemiological studies to identify needs and evaluate effectiveness. It also includes implementing strategies to increase access to care by those who encounter barriers, such as disabled people and members of ethnic minorities. There is an emerging trend towards employing public health staff in provider units. There may be a case for having public health skills available at this level, but there are also concerns about the lack of a population-based focus.

Other countries are also moving in a similar direction. In France, the Schéma régionale d'organisation sanitaire is developing mechanisms to coordinate regional priorities with the plans of health care providers, although this is proving difficult in a pluralist system *(158)*. In Germany, the sickness funds' research institutes are also beginning to develop this role but, to date, their focus has been more narrow, i.e. on cost-containment and in particular on controlling pharmaceutical expenditure *(159)*. This role has yet to develop in other countries, but in some, such as Belgium, it has been advocated by health policy analysts as a way of overcoming the identified problems of market failure *(160)*. It is likely that the absence of these skills played a part in the health care inflation experienced by the Czech Republic between 1992 and 1993 *(161)*.

Public health research

The final role of public health is to undertake research. Modern health services are driven by advances in biomedical research, and it is essential that public health research keeps pace. The direction it takes will be influenced by the concept of public health adopted in each country. In its broadest sense, public health research includes the use of epidemiological methods to describe a population's health needs, and to identify health hazards and the social determinants of disease. It also involves supporting the development of policies to tackle these hazards and determinants, including the evaluation of specific interventions. In practice, relatively few countries undertake such research and, when they do, it is rarely part of a well considered strategy designed to meet the health needs of the populations concerned.

Existing patterns in public health services

The preceding sections have examined the roles adopted by public health services and explored how they might develop in response to the challenge of changes in both health and health care. The following section moves away from this functional analysis to examine how, in practice, public health services are organized and what evidence exists to support the different approaches.

There is considerable diversity in the way that European countries have developed their public health services. Categorization of national public health infrastructures is complex, due partly to the difficulty of developing an unambiguous definition of what should be categorized as public health in each country, and partly to the lack of published information. In general, however, public health appears to be more developed in the Scandinavian countries, Ireland, the Netherlands, Switzerland and the United Kingdom. In some other countries, such as Italy and Spain, there are considerable variations, with some regions making a strong public health contribution. Although there are differences in structures and processes, all of these countries have modern communicable disease surveillance and control systems and well developed health promotion programmes, as well as mechanisms for building public health into the organization of the health services. Several countries are undertaking initiatives that will strengthen their public health function, either through major training programmes or by restructuring services; these include Denmark, France, Germany, Hungary and Poland. Others, such as Austria, Greece and Portugal, have done less, although services are well developed in some areas.

In the CIS countries, there has been little enthusiasm for reforming the sanepid system with its focus on traditional hygiene and narrow, laboratory-based approach *(162–164)*. As government budgets have shrunk, however, funding of these services has also fallen. Given the current challenges caused by social fragmentation, this budget shortfall has caused breakdowns even in areas where the sanepid services previously enjoyed success, such as communicable disease control. In the CEE countries, the picture is more complex. Hungary has undertaken an extensive restructuring of the former sanepid system to include health promotion as well as noncommunicable disease epidemiology, although the process of change has been difficult *(164)*. Some changes have taken place in Romania, leading to a reintegration of components of the service. Other countries, such as Bulgaria, the Czech Republic and Slovakia placed less emphasis on reforming the sanepid system.

The role of the state in public health services

As noted earlier, the characteristics of health systems are the result of a mix of economic, social, political and historical factors outside the system itself. Diversity may not matter if different approaches are equally effective, but this is not often the case. There are areas in which countries have different levels of success in developing and implementing health policies, indicated by, for example, the large variations in smoking rates and numbers of deaths from road traffic accidents.

One factor that does appear to play an important role is the way in which the state is involved in overall health policy. This includes the level of decentralization, the extent of national or local government intervention in health policy, and the degree of development of a public health infrastructure. Another key factor is the presence of a public health input at decision-making level.

The importance of public health input in decision-making is illustrated by the introduction of breast cancer screening programmes and of health promotion in connection with HIV infection and AIDS (see Boxes 13 and 14). Countries that introduced policies at an early stage were those where there was a public health presence at the relevant decision-making tier. In addition, it appears to have been easier to implement a programme where there was an integrated model of health services, as in the Scandinavian countries or the United Kingdom. Policies on sudden infant death syndrome also illustrate the importance of a strong public health function, although in some countries non-governmental organizations and clinicians also played an important role *(167)*.

Developing public health services

The development of the public health function in Europe is patchy. It is well developed in a few countries, with a large body of trained professional staff armed with

---

Box 13. Breast cancer screening

Breast cancer is the leading cause of death in women aged between 35 and 64 in western Europe. There is now clear evidence from several randomized controlled trials that screening by mammography is effective in reducing death rates. Screening is widely available on request, but is most effective when undertaken in the context of large-scale population-based programmes with dedicated facilities and robust quality control mechanisms. Such programmes have been introduced in only a few countries. They include Germany, Luxembourg, the Netherlands and the United Kingdom, with regional programmes in Belgium, Finland, France, Ireland, Italy, Portugal, Spain and Sweden. Differences in the strength of the public health component have contributed to this variation, either directly (such as through comprehensive review of the options) or indirectly (where the absence of population registers that could be used to identify the population at risk created obstacles).

Sources: Shapiro *(165)*; Tabar et al. *(166)*.

Box 14. Health promotion in HIV infection and AIDS

The case of HIV infection and AIDS offers an opportunity to study the relationship between public health policies and outcomes. A detailed study of national responses to HIV infection and AIDS, while noting the considerable methodological challenges involved, has shown how some countries, such as Norway and Switzerland, were able to mount effective and sustained campaigns early on while others, such as Finland, France and Portugal, acted relatively late. The different speed of response was not related to the prevalence of infection, but various factors were identified as having an impact. These included the presence (as in the Netherlands and Norway) or absence (as in Belgium and France) of a public health infrastructure on which to base interventions.

Source: Wellings *(21).*

the necessary skills to assess needs, advise on interventions and evaluate their implementation. At the other extreme, public health is marginalized, limited to relatively ineffective laboratory-based surveillance of communicable diseases, and responsible for providing often second-class services for disadvantaged groups.

There is a case for developing a new model of public health services, which would include an improved approach to communicable diseases and environmental health, withdrawal from the delivery of health services as they are integrated into the mainstream services, an intersectoral and multidisciplinary approach to health promotion and greater involvement in planning, commissioning and evaluating health services. Whether these roles should be integrated, or whether they should be distributed throughout a variety of structures, will depend on the context; an effective coordination mechanism is more important. There is a particularly urgent need to increase the availability of public health skills in those countries that are introducing market-based health sector reforms.

Reform of the public health function will succeed only if there are enough professionals available, and if they are given the appropriate skills. Investment in training and employing public health professionals with the relevant skills, however, varies considerably between countries *(168)*. There has been a substantial improvement in this area recently, as some countries have established new training programmes. Investment in training must be matched by a properly funded career structure, in which health care professionals receive levels of remuneration broadly similar to those of their colleagues in the curative services.

3 Confronting Resource Scarcity

As the resources available for paying for health care become more constrained and the pressures on health expenditure increase, national decision-makers have to develop strategies to deal with resource scarcity. There are two basic and often complementary options. First, countries may increase the resources for health care, either by shifting funds from other areas of public sector expenditure or by increasing taxation or social insurance contributions. The issue of the "right" level of funding is being widely discussed in the current reform debate. Several formulae have been suggested, including incremental funding adjusted by additional needs due to demographic, technological and policy changes, funding according to "affordability" by linking health expenditure to growth in GDP, or the use of international comparisons to look at the level of resources that other economically similar countries commit to health care *(169)*. None of these approaches has been found completely satisfactory. In practice, the appropriate level of funding depends on the value given to health and health care, both in itself and in relation to other areas of public spending. In short, the answer is not based on mathematical formulae but on political preference.

Second, countries can control health care expenditure by pursuing reform strategies that influence either supply or demand. This chapter will first provide an overview of the main cost-containment strategies available (some of which are assessed in detail in subsequent chapters). Two widely discussed cost-containment strategies that act on the demand for services – cost sharing and priority setting – are then reviewed.

Containing costs more effectively

The desire to control health care costs has been a key stimulus for the health care reforms of the 1980s and 1990s. Cost-containment strategies attempt to achieve such control by restricting health care spending to predefined limits. Cost-containment is frequently confused with spending cuts or with improved efficiency, but it should be distinguished from both. Cuts in expenditure may be used to achieve cost-containment, yet in certain situations it is possible for cost-containment to be associated with increased spending, as long as this is within predefined limits. Thus, cost-containment aims to control spending, not necessarily to cut it. Similarly, efficiency measures can be looked on as attempts to achieve cost-containment. While improved efficiency can lower costs for a given level of health services output, cost-containment does not necessarily involve greater efficiency. It is possible for cost-containment to lower costs and, at the same time, give rise to greater inefficiency.

There has been a degree of convergence in the measures countries have taken to control the costs of health care. The methods employed differ according to the way in which countries' health care systems are organized and financed. Where the government or the main health insurers own the health care facilities and employ salaried health professionals, change has been more rapid than where health care providers are contracted by government or insurers. Most cost-containment measures act only on publicly financed health care expenditures. Since some of these measures shift a proportion of health care costs on to the patient, it is possible for the total (public and private) health care spending of a country to remain unaffected by such reforms, or even to rise if additional private spending exceeds public savings. This section reviews cost-containment measures according to whether they seek to have an impact on the supply or the demand for health care services.[5]

DEMAND-ORIENTED MEASURES

The main measure seeking to influence demand levels is *cost sharing*. This option is reviewed in more detail below. Other approaches include no-claim bonuses in social insurance systems; introducing incentives for private spending, such as income tax concessions, for those who use private services; the right to opt out of the statutory system; and removing services from the public package of care. All these measures seek to reduce demand for publicly financed services by shifting a proportion of health care costs on to the individual.

Opting out involves the choice, usually offered to those with a high income or to the self-employed, of not being covered by compulsory health insurance. It is not a policy measure available in tax-based health care systems, where there is universal coverage of the population. Those who opt out may insure themselves privately, or may remain uninsured. This measure transfers total responsibility for health care financing on to individuals, and since opting out is usually confined to the better-off, it also weakens social solidarity by depriving the social insurance system of an important source of revenue. This option is available in Germany and the Netherlands, although in the latter proposed reforms are being planned to eliminate it. In addition, some CEE and CIS countries are considering this option. A different approach to opting out, applying to national health service systems, has been considered in the reform processes in Italy, New Zealand, Portugal and, more recently, Spain. This offers citizens the right to opt out of their national health services and take private insurance instead. In these cases, the national health service would allocate a capitation-based contribution to the insurer chosen by the individual. So far, this option has not been adopted in any of these countries, owing to its negative impact on solidarity.

No-claim bonuses are lower premium contributions to social insurance schemes, offered to individuals who limit their use of the public health care system. They are designed to increase cost consciousness, and are employed only in insurance-based systems. Since 1991 in Germany, people who do not use the health care system, apart from normal health check-ups in the course of the year, are eligible for a no-claim bonus

---

[5] This section is based on a review of cost-containment measures in western European countries published elsewhere (*170,171*). While few of these measures apply to current circumstances in the CEE and CIS countries, they can be expected to become relevant as these health systems develop. Some have already become relevant to CEE countries such as the Czech Republic, which experienced a cost explosion shortly after it introduced a social insurance scheme in 1992.

of one month's contribution to health insurance. Some CEE and CIS countries, such as the Russian Federation, are either considering or implementing no-claim bonuses.

Reappraisals of the benefits that should be included in the package of services funded by the public budget or social insurance system may lead to *reductions in services* in an effort to secure cost savings. Services may also be *rationed* through waiting times, or supplemented privately by the patient, through either out-of-pocket payments or private insurance. Such measures are intended to reduce the demand for publicly financed services by shifting financial responsibility on to patients.

A full review of rationing and priority setting can be found later in this chapter (pages 101–113).

SUPPLY-ORIENTED MEASURES

Costs can also be contained by influencing the supply of health services. A wide range of reform strategies can be included in this category, such as: introducing competition between public providers; setting global expenditure ceilings or global budgets for providers; reducing the production of doctors and/or the number of hospital beds; controlling the cost of the human resources (e.g. salaries) or supplies (e.g. pharmaceuticals) used to provide care; introducing more effective delivery patterns, such as substituting outpatient and primary care for more expensive inpatient services; regulating the use of technologies; influencing the use of resources authorized by physicians; and changing the methods of remunerating professionals. These strategies have met with different degrees of success in containing costs.

Expenditure ceilings have been introduced in many western European countries. The most commonly used method of control, as in Ireland, Italy and Spain, is a budget ceiling for all spending or for large parts of it (for instance, budgets for total payments made to physicians), reinforced by controls on staffing. Several countries, including Belgium, Germany, Ireland, Italy, Portugal, Spain and the United Kingdom, have used expenditure ceilings, often stated in advance in cash terms, as the main weapon to control costs. In Denmark and Sweden, there are negotiated limits for local government spending. Belgium and Germany have separate budgets for the main expenditure components, but in the latter health promotion and certain types of care outside hospital are not limited by budgets. In Belgium, Germany and the Netherlands, budgets have been introduced in individual hospitals irrespective of their ownership, even when they receive their income from several different insurers. Budgets for hospitals have accelerated the reduction in length of stay, and budgets for doctors' earnings in Germany have reduced the rate of spending growth. Performance-related payment systems for providers are reviewed in Chapter 5.

Restrictions on the numbers of medical students and physicians seek to control the supply of services, and attempt to deal with the oversupply of physicians. During the 1980s, France placed restrictions on the number of graduating physicians by sharply curtailing the number of students continuing from the first to the second year of medical school. The United Kingdom has limited entrance to medical schools by anticipating the future need for physicians. Since 1986 in Germany, physicians' associations and sickness funds have been authorized to deny access to new physicians if an area already contains more than a 50% excess of physicians in certain specialties. Measures have also been introduced to encourage early retirement. From 1989, the conditions for admitting physicians into practice with sickness funds have been tightened, while efforts are being made to reduce entrants to medical schools. Several CEE and CIS countries have begun efforts to reduce the number of medical students as a means of eventually reducing the oversupply of physicians.

Many countries in western Europe are making efforts *to reduce the number of hospital beds* in order to make savings. In some cases this is achieved through financial incentives. In Belgium, investment that results in a reduction of 25% or more in the number of beds allows regional governments to reduce their contribution from 60% to 30%, with the sickness funds paying the difference. As a consequence, regional governments give priority to construction projects that will result in fewer beds. In some western European countries, new capital developments in the public sector (and sometimes in the private sector) have to be authorized by national, regional or local planning bodies. Belgium, Ireland and the United Kingdom have taken extensive action to close hospitals or convert them to other uses. There are currently plans to close 22 000 public hospital beds in France and 3800 in the Netherlands. In Germany, legislation passed in December 1992 makes hospital closures easier. In Spain, smaller acute hospitals have been converted for use by the chronically sick or by convalescing patients, while others have been closed. The overprovision of hospital beds is a particular problem in the CEE and CIS countries; Hungary has announced a programme for closing 10 000 hospital beds, while other countries are also considering initiatives that will gradually reduce their bed numbers. The role of controls on capital investment is reviewed in Chapter 5.

Strategies that encourage bed reduction are closely related to the development of *substitution policies*. These refer to regrouping resources across care settings to exploit the best available solutions. Substitution frequently takes the form of replacing relatively more expensive inpatient care with less costly outpatient or primary care. Substitution policies can take numerous forms, such as developing day surgery, expanding home care instead of inpatient care, and strengthening PHC. Day hospitals and day surgery are well developed in Denmark, Ireland and the United Kingdom, and they are rapidly increasing in the Netherlands and Sweden. The restructuring of hospital services and substitution policies across care settings are dealt with in more detail in Chapter 6.

Countries are adopting a variety of measures in their attempts *to control expensive medical equipment*. Measures include increasing regulation, concentrating facilities, preventing uncontrolled growth and avoiding duplication. Introducing only those new technologies that have proved to be effective in improving treatment is a more fundamental approach. The economic burden that new technologies represent, together with issues of safety, ethics and social impact, suggest that careful evaluation is needed before their widespread acceptance in clinical practice is allowed. There is growing interest in setting up research bodies to undertake technology assessment. Chapter 6 deals with the assessment of health care technologies in the context of improving outcomes and quality of care.

The use of resources authorized by physicians is monitored in several European countries, including France, Germany and the Netherlands. France has recently introduced a system of "medical references", which specify the use of medical procedures, medical examinations, clinical tests or drug prescriptions related to a specific health condition. Physicians can be sanctioned if they do not follow these medical references. Prescribing patterns are under review in many western European countries. In some cases, monitoring is accompanied by sanctions and by financial penalties for high authorizers. An alternative way to control physicians' prescribing behaviour is to promote the use of generic drugs or to allow generic substitution, as in Germany, the Netherlands and the United Kingdom. Another development involves giving physicians responsibility for budgets in clinical departments, as in Germany and the United Kingdom, or at the PHC level, as in the fundholding initiative in the United Kingdom. Finally, an effective way of influencing physicians' behaviour is to change the method by which they are reimbursed for their work. Chapter 5 includes a review of the impact of alternative approaches to paying health professionals.

Overall, experience to date indicates that setting budgets for the health system or for each main subsector, based on targets and on limiting workforce members, appears to be the most effective means of containing costs. Reform strategies should not be exclusively evaluated in terms of their success in containing costs, however, but on a wider range of social objectives. Moreover, as noted above, success in containing costs does not necessarily imply greater efficiency. It is entirely possible for cost-containment initiatives to reduce total costs and increase inefficiency at the same time. Consequently, following the discussion of cost sharing and priority setting in the next two sections, this analysis then takes a twin approach: assessing health reform strategies in terms of their impact on specific objectives (including equity, efficiency and health gain) and in terms of the funding, allocation and delivery of services (see Chapters 4, 5 and 6, respectively).

An appropriate role for cost sharing

Cost sharing refers to any direct payment made by health service users to the providers. Because such payments directly affect the general population, the magnitude and extent of cost sharing often become a volatile political issue in national policy debates. The implications of cost sharing for health policy objectives, however, are not self-evident. This section describes the cost-sharing practices of countries in the European Region, and attempts to assess their consequences for sectoral objectives of efficiency, equity and health status.

To evaluate the efficiency and health effects of cost sharing, the main issues addressed here include the impact of cost sharing on total utilization levels, "appropriate" versus "inappropriate" utilization, total and government health spending, and health status. In addition, cost sharing's potential for generating supplementary revenues for the health system is assessed. To evaluate effects on efficiency and equity, any differential effects of cost sharing on each of these issues are examined across demographic groups, specific health services, payers or financing systems, and the type of cost sharing mechanism. Any assessment of these issues requires an understanding of what drives the demand for care and, more specifically, what drives the demand for particular types of health care service. Moreover, it is important to understand the main factors that contribute to health care costs, and how these are affected by cost-sharing policies.

THE CONCEPTUAL FRAMEWORK
Definitions

Patient cost sharing refers to a group of specific policy tools that act on the demand side of the market for health care services. These tools are usually applied in the context of (public or private) insurance or a national health system. The three main forms or mechanisms of patient cost sharing are the following *(172)*:

- *deductible*: the out-of-pocket amount that must be paid before the benefits of the insurance programme become active (e.g. the patient pays the first US $50 of the costs of a hospital stay, or pays the first US $200 of the year's outpatient care costs);
- *co-payment*: a flat amount that the beneficiary must pay for each service used (e.g. the patient pays US $5 per drug prescribed, or US $10 for each visit to the doctor); and
- *co-insurance*: the percentage of the total charge for a service that must be paid by the beneficiary (e.g. the patient pays 20% of the total charge for inpatient care).

Other policies are often associated with these forms of cost sharing, and they can also affect the level of out-of-pocket spending made by patients to providers. These include *(172)*:

- *benefit maximum*: a defined limit on the amount that will be reimbursed by the insurer for a specific period, over and above which the patient is entirely liable for payment (e.g. the patient pays all expenses in a year after US $100 000 in benefits has been reimbursed by the insurer, or the patient pays all lifetime expenses after US $1 million has been paid by the insurer);
- *out-of-pocket maximum*: a defined limit on the total amount of out-of-pocket spending for which an insured person or household will be liable for a defined period, over and above which all expenses are paid by the insurer (e.g. the insurer pays all expenses in a year after the patient has spent US $1000 on a combination of deductibles and co-insurance);
- *extra billing*: charges by the provider that are higher than the maximum reimbursement levels set by insurers, leaving patients liable to pay the difference (e.g. the patient must pay US $15 in addition to the US $10 co-payment, because the maximum reimbursement for a visit to the doctor is US $100 but the doctor charged US $115);

- *pharmaceutical reference pricing*: a price list established by the insurer for therapeutically comparable drugs that establishes a maximum reimbursement level per item prescribed, leaving patients financially responsible if more expensive items are chosen (e.g. the reference price for an antibiotic is US $60, and either the patient or the prescriber chooses a brand with a retail price of US $70, leaving the patient to pay US $10 out of pocket); and
- *coverage exclusions*: services or methods of using services that are not covered in the benefit package of public or private insurance plans, leaving individuals liable for their full costs or the costs over and above what is covered (e.g. drugs not included in the national formulary or considered to be of questionable therapeutic value, or the use of a hospital emergency department for non-urgent care instead of a defined PHC provider and referral channels).

These various cost-sharing options are viewed by most economists as potential policy tools. That is, they can constitute options for progressing towards the achievement of specific objectives. For many western European countries, the main objective of cost sharing is to reduce demand for services in order to contain the costs facing comprehensive social insurance or national health service systems. For many CEE and CIS countries, the main objective is to raise additional revenues to help sustain the functioning of health services, but overgeneralizing about the motivations and objectives of groups of countries in any part of the Region should be approached with caution. Some western European countries have viewed resource mobilization as an objective of their cost sharing policies, while some CEE and CIS countries see these measures as tools for demand management.

Cost sharing in theory

Economists are divided as to whether cost sharing can be an effective tool for improving efficiency and containing costs. There is more general agreement, however, that unless it is accompanied by compensatory measures for those on low incomes, cost sharing will be inequitable in terms of both the financing of and access to care. In countries that do not have functioning comprehensive health care systems, the rationale for cost sharing may be less one of demand management than of revenue raising for the purpose of sustaining and expanding service provision. For some of these countries, this may also reflect a history of informal payments (the "grey market") for services and supplies.

In neoclassical economic theory, the fundamental rationale for the use of cost sharing is to ration demand in the presence of public or private insurance. As reflected in Fig. 14, the socially optimal level of consumption would occur at point A, where the marginal cost (reflected in the supply curve) of producing services equals the marginal benefit (reflected in the demand curve) of consuming them. At this point, Q_1 of services is consumed at a price of P_1, which is equal to the marginal cost of supply at that quantity of output. With insurance, price is less than marginal cost, and so the level of consumption this implies occurs at a point where the cost to society of producing the services is greater than the value of their consumption.[6] If

---

[6] "Moral hazard" is the term used to describe the cause of the additional use of health care arising from insurance coverage (*173*).

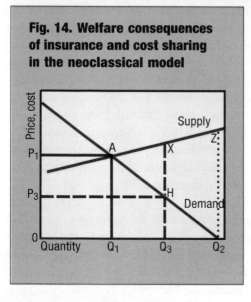

Fig. 14. Welfare consequences of insurance and cost sharing in the neoclassical model

insurance fully protects consumers from the price of health services, the quantity of services demanded will be that that would exist at a zero price (Q_2). At this point, marginal cost (corresponding to point Z on the supply curve) is far greater than marginal benefit (which is essentially zero). Standard neoclassical economic theory implies that this would result in a loss of welfare to society equal to the area contained by the triangle AZQ_2. This is why some economists contend that the demand for care exceeds socially desirable levels when services are fully covered by insurance. Cost-sharing measures introduce prices back into the medical market (P_3) in an attempt to limit the excessive demand[7] and consequent welfare loss believed to exist as a result of insurance. With cost sharing at price P_3 in Fig. 14, the quantity demanded is Q_3, and thus the welfare loss is reduced to the area of triangle AXH.

Some economists and others have questioned whether the above conclusion about the welfare loss from complete insurance coverage (and the implied welfare gain from cost sharing) derived from neoclassical economic theory is valid in practice. The theoretical rationale for cost sharing has been refined based on an analysis of health services from the perspective of welfare economics. Health services are not monolithic; they comprise various goods and services with different economic characteristics. One dimension where health services vary as an "economic good" is the extent to which the benefits of consumption are limited to the individual who receives the service *(174,175)*. Many health services are viewed by economists as purely*private* goods. From this perspective, the health benefits of consumption of these services are viewed narrowly, and seen as accruing solely to the individual receiving a service. In other words, those who do not receive the service are *excluded* from the associated benefits. An example of this would be an aspirin bought to treat a headache. For this type of product, welfare economics implies that marginal cost pricing (as in the standard neoclassical model described above) yields an optimal allocation of resources *(176)*.

---

[7] Technically, "excessive demand" does not refer to demand for services that are medically unnecessary or potentially harmful. Indeed, the additional services consumed may yield positive health benefits. In economic terms, however, utilization is considered to be excessive if the marginal social cost of providing this additional service is greater than the marginal social benefit arising from the consumption of the service. In other words, the resources used to provide the additional unit of service, such as a visit to the doctor, could yield a greater benefit to society if they were used for some other purpose. Despite this, many researchers (including several economists) have tried to operationalize a definition of excessive demand by testing whether the utilization deterred by cost sharing was for "necessary" services or had harmful health effects. Although this definition of excessive demand differs from that used in economics, it has intuitive appeal. The implications of this approach are that, if cost-sharing mechanisms are successful at reducing demand with no effect on health status, one can conclude that economic efficiency has been improved. The policy will lead to some costs being shifted to users, but overall costs would be reduced while benefits remain unchanged.

Alternatively, some health services are purely *public* goods, their benefits accruing to all members of society. If the service is provided, no one can be excluded from the associated benefits. Examples of public goods would include some environmental health interventions, such as controlling air quality and water pollution. Charging "users" for these services is not feasible because nonpayers would get the same benefits as those who pay, so there would be no incentive for any individual to pay.[8]

Finally, many health services are characterized by neoclassical economists as mixed goods: the individual receives the benefits of consumption, but others not directly involved in the transaction between provider and consumer benefit as well.[9] An example is the treatment of a communicable disease such as tuberculosis or syphilis. Such treatment protects not only the person who is treated but also those whom he or she would have infected had no treatment been available. Social benefits exceed private benefits for these types of service, so marginal cost pricing will result in a lower level of consumption than is socially optimal. For these goods, economists accept that a subsidy is desirable to raise private demand to the level that will equate social benefits with social costs, and thus maximize presumed (if narrowly economically defined) welfare (see *Jimenez (176)* for a full discussion). In this instance, the economic implications for cost-sharing policy are mixed. This subsidy may entail varying degrees of out-of-pocket payments by consumers, ranging from zero to a substantial percentage of marginal costs.

The market for health care services is imperfect, because the unregulated activities of producers and consumers do not result in a socially desirable quantity, mix and distribution of services. As suggested by the above discussion, one reason for this is the diversity of specific services in terms of capturing the benefits of consumption. There is an additional element of what economists term "market failure" that is relevant to a discussion of the effects of cost sharing. This is "information failure", which manifests itself in the health care market by consumers' reliance or dependence on providers for information about the services they "need". This asymmetry in information may lead to "supplier-induced demand", i.e. demand that would not have occurred had the consumer's agent, the provider, not encouraged the consumer to demand the services *(177)*. According to neoclassical economic theory, the assumption of supplier-induced demand implies that the preferences of providers determine at least some of the demand for health care services. The existence, precise definition, effects and appropriate policy response to supplier-induced demand is a topic of considerable interest and debate among health economists (see Labelle et al. *(178)* and Pauly *(179)* for a review and discussion of the issues).

Although some economists remain unconvinced that there is enough empirical evidence to demonstrate conclusively that supplier-induced demand exists *(179)*, most accept that providers do use their power to affect consumers' demand for care through their agency function *(180,181)*. If supplier-induced demand exists, the use of the standard supply–demand paradigm to measure welfare loss may be inappropriate,

---

[8] This is called the "free-rider" problem.

[9] The benefits that accrue to nonmarket participants are called "externalities".

since one of the underlying assumptions of that model is that supply and demand are independently determined. Given the asymmetry of information between the provider and consumer, and the agency role played by the provider, therefore, the debate among economists is whether the demand curve really is an appropriate tool for measuring consumer welfare. Some argue that the demand curve should not be used because of these information problems *(181–183)*; others say that there will never be perfect information, and that an estimated demand curve always incorporates existing levels of information. The demand curve can therefore still be used to measure the welfare consequences of insurance and cost sharing, because it reflects consumers' decisions based on the information they have at any point in time *(173,179,184)*.

Understanding the debate about supplier-induced demand is relevant to an assessment of the likely effects of cost sharing, which is a demand-side policy tool. Supplier-induced demand is not inherently bad. Providing lay people with information about their medical needs is a very important function of physicians, and providing medical training to the entire population would not be an economically efficient use of resources, even if it were feasible. If the model on which the analysis indicating that cost sharing reduces society's welfare loss is flawed, however, then the use of cost sharing for this purpose is called into question. Consequently, some believe that the scope for achieving efficiency gains from cost sharing are very limited, owing to the diversity of health services and the potential for supplier-induced demand *(181,185)*.

Many believe that supplier-induced demand compromises the usefulness of cost sharing. They reason that, if cost sharing initially reduces consumer demand for care, provider incomes will be threatened (in health systems where some or all providers are paid according to the volume of services). To the extent that they can induce demand for additional services, providers could compensate for a reduction in consumer-driven demand in order to maintain their level of income (see Fahs *(186)* for a description of this aspect of supplier-induced demand). This "supply response" will negate the demand-dampening effects of patient charges, which will therefore be an ineffective policy tool, along with other measures that act on the consumer side of the market. Others believe that there is scope for an appropriate demand-side policy response to the potentially harmful effects of asymmetry of information between providers and consumers. This is not to provide more complete insurance coverage (i.e. reduce cost sharing) but instead to arm consumers with more information *(173)*.

As indicated above, health care services include a mix of goods and services, with diverse market characteristics in terms of capturing the benefits of consumption. For each specific service, the key issue to consider is the extent to which demand is driven by consumers or by providers. Given consumers' reliance on their providers/agents for information that affects their demand for certain services, the theoretical basis for applying cost sharing as a demand-rationing tool to services that are largely provider determined (such as referral services) is weak *(181)*.

Some researchers and policy analysts have argued that there is an inherent conflict in using a tool that raises revenues as a tool to contain costs. This argument, put forcefully by Canadian health economists(*185,187*), rejects the use of cost sharing as a cost-containment measure. Owing to the assumption that the supplier induces demand, and that spending (by insurers and patients) is always equal to revenues (of providers), imposing or increasing cost sharing will not reduce costs but simply cause them to be shifted from those paying premiums (including taxpayers in a tax-based financing system) to those unfortunate enough to fall sick and require medical care. Furthermore, based on the experience of Canada and the United States, these economists argue that, in systems in which providers are reimbursed on a per-case basis, providers will respond to any general reduction in consumer-driven demand by increasing the volume and/or intensity (number of items of service provided per contact with the health system) of services, in order to maintain their income levels. From this perspective, if it is true that provider-driven utilization is a main cause of high health costs, then incentives and/or regulations affecting the supply side of the market are likely to be much more powerful tools for cost-containment. Moreover, these economists argue that systems utilizing per-case reimbursement will always generate provider-led cost increases. They also note that cost sharing increases health sector costs by increasing the complexity of financial administration.

Cost sharing raises obvious concerns about equity, in terms both of financing and of access to care. It can cause inequity in financing because of the potential for the burden of cost sharing to fall on households with low incomes. It can cause inequity in the consumption of health services by reducing access for the elderly, the young and the chronically sick. This differential impact of patient charges reflects the economic reality that price is more of a deterrent to use when it consumes a greater percentage of a household's available funds. Reductions in utilization or delays in seeking treatment can lead to lower health status, to the same degree that use of health services would have had beneficial health effects.

COST-SHARING PRACTICES IN EUROPE

The countries of the European Region employ a variety of approaches to cost sharing. The context for cost sharing, the objectives of these policies, and the way cost sharing is implemented in practice in the countries of western Europe tend to differ from those in the CEE and CIS countries.

The likely effects of cost-sharing policies are determined by a combination of conditions. These conditions also strongly affect the main objectives that countries assign (implicitly or explicitly) to cost sharing as part of their national health policies and systems. Where health services are operating at low levels of quality or are inaccessible to a significant proportion of the population, the revenue-raising objective tends to dominate other aims of cost sharing. These structural conditions set the context for overall policies on health financing, including decisions on sources of funding, risk sharing, provider payment options, and methods of ensuring access to care for the poorest members of society. These general policies, in turn, have implications for the likely consequences of cost sharing. In systems using fee-for-service or per-case reimbursement of providers, there is likely to be a greater reliance on cost sharing as a demand-side instrument to achieve policy aims, than in systems where doctors and hospitals are paid prospectively, since prospective systems (salaries, budgets or capitation, for example) build in cost-containment objectives on the supply side. Since cost sharing is only one feature of broader provider payment policies, it is essential to understand the motivation for these broader policies.

Cost sharing in western European countries

For the most part, western European countries have focused their cost-containment efforts on the supply side of the health care market, both through budgetary controls (especially for hospital care) and, in some countries, by requiring PHC practitioners to act as gatekeepers to referral-level care. Thus, most of these countries place little emphasis on cost sharing as a tool for either raising revenue for or containing the costs of services provided by doctors and hospitals. On the other hand, cost sharing for pharmaceuticals is widespread. Although the objectives of such policies are rarely stated explicitly, their main purpose appears to be to shift much of the cost of drugs to the users.

About half of the western European countries use some form of cost sharing for first-contact care, and about half also apply cost sharing to inpatient and specialty outpatient care (Table 7). The most common forms of direct cost sharing are co-payments and co-insurance; only in Switzerland is much use made of deductibles. Virtually all countries in western Europe use some form of out-of-pocket maximum to limit the liability of individuals or households for medical care costs, and none employs service or benefit maximums. Hence income protection is a strong feature of these systems.

Extra billing by physicians is not legal in most western European countries. Belgium, France and the Group 2 programme in Denmark[10] are exceptions to this.

Pharmaceutical reference pricing has been introduced in Denmark, Germany, the Netherlands, Norway and Sweden. In Germany, health care reform legislation in 1989 established a maximum reimbursement level (the reference price) for each drug, with consumers liable to pay the difference between the retail price and the reference price. In a way, reference pricing is a special case of coverage exclusion. Under this system, the health system's (or insurer's) expenditure per item is explicitly limited, but consumers are free to choose between the available products on the market. In Germany, reference prices are roughly the average price of similar types of drug (i.e. drugs with similar active ingredients, with therapeutically comparable active ingredients and with comparable therapeutic effects). By mid-1993, reference prices had been established for about half of the prescription drugs on the German market. The government's ultimate objective is to bring 70% of these drugs into the reference price system *(190)*.

The role that countries allow for voluntary (non-profit or for-profit) health insurance has implications for the effects of cost sharing. In most countries of western Europe, such insurance is either not allowed (e.g. Belgium and Norway) or can only be used to purchase private services not included in the standard benefit package of the national health service or social insurance system (e.g. Austria, Italy and the

---

[10] In this programme, patients have completely free choice of provider, but physicians are allowed to charge rates above the defined reimbursement levels. Less than 4% of the population opted for this programme in 1991.

Table 7. Patient cost sharing in western European health care systems

Country (source)	Type of provider		
	First contact	Referral	Pharmaceuticals
Austria (2)	Eighty percent of the population has none; the rest has co-insurance or is exempt due to low income.	Mix of co-payment and co-insurance (with exemptions). Out-of-pocket liability limited to first 28 days in hospital.	Co-payment for prescribed drugs. Non-prescription drugs are excluded.
Belgium (51,171,188)	Narrow range of co-payments or co-insurance (less for low-income persons). Extra billing allowed.	Variable co-payments according to fee schedule; benefit reduced after 90 days (lower co-payment for those on low income).	Co-payment or co-insurance with rates ranging, by type of drug, from 0% to 85%; drugs not on positive list are excluded from coverage.
Denmark (2)	None.	None.	Variable co-insurance rate (0–50%) applied to reference price. Drugs not on formulary excluded from coverage.
Finland (2)	None. Choice of annual prepayment or co-payment, or co-payment with out-of-pocket maximum; varies by municipality.	Maximum payment levels per hospital day and per specialist visit.	Co-insurance.
France (189)	Co-insurance; extra billing allowed for defined categories of physician.	Co-insurance for per diem rate plus co-payment to cover meals. No out-of-pocket liability after 30 days.	Most subject to co-insurance; no coverage for items not on national list of approved drugs.
Germany (172,190)	None.	Flat co-payment for up to 14 days per year; thereafter no out-of-pocket liability.	Variable co-payment; reference pricing; no coverage for items on negative list.

Table 7 (contd)

Country (source)	Type of provider		
	First contact	Referral	Pharmaceuticals
Greece (2)	None, although extra billing is common among private physicians.	None for inpatient hospital care. Some funds have co-insurance for diagnostic services.	Co-insurance.
Iceland (2)	Co-payment, with higher rate for visits outside of normal working hours. Higher co-payment for home visits. Out-of-pocket maximum.	None for inpatient hospital care. Mix of co-payment and co-insurance for specialist and hospital outpatient care. Co-payment for diagnostic services. Out-of-pocket maximum.	Mix of deductible per "day" of prescription, plus co-insurance, up to a defined out-of-pocket maximum. Some items entirely free and others excluded from coverage.
Ireland (171,188,191)	None for "Category I" population (37% in 1987). Full charges for others, unless they buy insurance. Insured persons face an annual deductible, which also serves as an out-of-pocket maximum.	None for "Category I" population in public hospitals. For the rest, co-payment for first hospital outpatient visit per episode and co-payment per diem for the first ten days of public hospital care per year. Insurance buys free care in public and private hospitals.	None for "Category I" population. Others face a monthly deductible, which also serves as an out-of-pocket maximum for the month. Items on the negative list of drugs are excluded from coverage.
Italy (2,171)	None.	None for inpatient care. Cost sharing introduced in 1990 in public hospitals for diagnostic procedures, specialist visits and spa treatment.	Deductible only for essential drugs. Most other drugs have a deductible plus co-insurance. Some drugs excluded from coverage.
Luxembourg (171)	Co-insurance.	Per diem co-payment indexed to inflation.	Co-insurance for outpatient drugs, except for "special diseases". Inpatient drugs are free.

Country			
Netherlands (172)	None for publicly insured; varies for privately insured.	None for publicly insured; varies for privately insured.	Reference price system; no coverage for excluded items.
Norway (2)	Cost sharing, with annual out-of-pocket maximum for all services.	None for inpatient care. Cost sharing for diagnostic services.	Reference price system for essential drugs.
Portugal (2,171)	Cost sharing.	Cost sharing.	Two co-insurance rates according to type of drug. Also, some items are free, but others are excluded from coverage.
Spain (171)	None.	None.	Co-insurance. Items not on approved list are excluded from coverage.
Sweden (172,192)	Co-payment, with annual out-of-pocket maximum for all services except inpatient care.	Co-payment per diem for inpatient care. Co-payments for therapeutic referrals.	Co-payment for first item prescribed; greatly reduced co-payment for additional items. Reference pricing for items with generic equivalents.
Switzerland (2)	Annual deductible plus co-insurance.	Co-payment per diem for hospital care.	Cost sharing varies among insurers. Items on negative list are excluded from coverage.
Turkey (2)	Mostly private providers who charge on a fee-for-service basis.	Social insurance schemes cover all charges; uninsured face user fees.	All social insurance schemes have co-insurance for outpatient drugs.
United Kingdom (172)	None.	None, except for amenity hospital beds.	Co-payments, but 83% of prescriptions are exempt. Items on negative list are excluded from NHS coverage.

United Kingdom). In Denmark and France, however, individuals are allowed to purchase insurance that covers the cost-sharing obligations of the national insurance system.

Virtually all western European countries reduce or eliminate cost-sharing obligations for low-income and chronically sick people. In Belgium, for example, people from low-income households receive complete or partial exemption from cost sharing. Charges are reduced or, for some services, nonexistent for the low-income "inactive" population comprising widows, orphans, pensioners and sometimes children *(51,171)*. In Austria, people requiring social services or with incomes below a defined level (17% of the population in 1990 *(2)*) are exempt from pharmaceutical cost sharing. In addition, charges often do not apply to preventive visits or for treatment of specified chronic or communicable diseases. In France, for example, exemptions apply to patients with any one of 30 diseases defined as serious, debilitating or chronic *(189)*. In Finland and Iceland, many preventive care visits are not subject to cost sharing *(2)*. In Ireland, everyone qualifies for free treatment of communicable and certain chronic diseases; infant screening, child health examinations, and prescribed medicines for certain chronic illnesses are also free *(2)*.

In most countries, policies are determined centrally, either by the national health service or on behalf of the social insurance schemes. In countries with multiple compulsory social insurance institutions, cost-sharing obligations may vary across schemes, as in Austria *(2)*. In Finland *(2)* and Sweden *(172)*, where the political systems are highly decentralized, decisions on cost sharing are made by local (municipal or county) authorities but within nationally legislated maximums.

Greece and Turkey are exceptions to the general picture of countries that provide universal access to well functioning health systems. In Greece, social insurance cover is universal, but the great geographical disparities in the distribution of providers mean that many citizens do not have ready access to services. Moreover, the practice of illegal extra billing ("envelope payments") by staff in hospitals and elsewhere is common, reflecting the low levels of pay for health professionals. In Turkey, only 60–65% of the population is covered by social insurance schemes. Everyone is entitled to use government health facilities, but user charges apply to a wide range of services. In both of these countries, therefore, official and unofficial charges are widespread and exist mainly for the purpose of raising additional revenues to fund health service provision.

Cost sharing in the CEE and CIS countries
The raising of revenue has been a principal concern of health policy in most CEE and CIS countries. Although insurance and general taxation are better methods of raising resources than direct charges to patients, the falling levels of employment experienced by most countries in recent years have reduced the scope for mandatory contributions to social insurance, since these are usually financed by the contributions of employers and employees. Similarly, there are limits to the amounts of revenue that can be generated through general taxes. Thus many (though not all) CEE and CIS countries are using direct charges to patients, primarily as a means of

providing additional resources to sustain the health services. At the same time, the available evidence suggests that providers are increasing relying on informal payments from patients.[11]

Table 8 sets out the cost-sharing policies of those countries for which information could be obtained, and includes a column that identifies the presence (and, if possible, the extent) of informal payments.[12]

It is apparent from Table 8 that informal payment for services is common in the CCE and CIS countries, reflecting the continuing low levels of remuneration. In Bulgaria, systematic underfunding of public sector services has led to widespread reliance on illegal payments and voluntary donations. Payments are often made by patients for drugs and medical supplies, food, clinical tests and other services *(193)*. In Hungary, the payment of "gratitude money" to health service providers has become widespread as their salary levels have dropped in real terms *(196)*. The low level of salaries for medical personnel in Poland contributes to the continuation of informal payments.

Household survey data from Kazakstan reveal that patients, during their stay in hospital, often have to supply goods and services "in kind" that are supposed to be provided by the government health services. A study of one Kazak *oblast* found that between one quarter and one third of hospital inpatients had to provide their own linen, food and laundry services. In Kyrgyzstan, evidence from household surveys conducted in 1993 and 1994 suggests that the use of both official and unofficial charges has grown *(197)*.

In the Czech Republic, macroeconomic performance has improved more rapidly than in many neighbouring countries. A universal compulsory insurance programme was introduced at the beginning of 1992, but this was soon followed by a cost explosion, largely because of the incentives of a fee-for-service reimbursement system. Supply-side and demand-side reforms have been introduced (or are planned) in an attempt to contain costs. This policy package includes low levels of cost sharing (limited by an out-of-pocket maximum), ostensibly to complement other cost-control policies *(195)*. Thus the main purpose of cost-sharing policy in the Czech Republic appears to be cost-containment rather than resource mobilization.

The rapid introduction of market mechanisms into the health systems of the CEE and CIS countries raises concerns about the ability of poorer citizens to meet the formal and informal charges required for access to health services. Moreover, the economic decline associated with the transitional period has led to a growth in the percentage of the population that is poor. In Hungary, for example, economic growth has declined during the 1990s; there has been a rapid increase in unemployment, and demographic changes have led to an increase in the number of pensioners. One consequence of these changes has been the economic polarization of the population.

---

[11] These non-sanctioned transactions are called by a variety of names, including "side payments", "black money", "under-the-table payments" and "gratitude money".

[12] A questionnaire was mailed to knowledgeable persons in the CEE and CIS countries in an attempt to obtain consistent information on both formal and informal cost sharing practices. Unless otherwise indicated in Table 8, responses to this questionnaire are the source of the information.

Table 8. Patient cost sharing in selected CEE and CIS countries

Country (source)	Type of provider		Pharmaceuticals	Informal payments
	First contact	Referral		
Bulgaria (193)	None in public sector; full payment in private sector (no insurance coverage).	None, but private donations are common.	Patients often pay for drugs that are officially free.	Widely used.
Croatia (194)	Low levels of co-insurance, but likely to increase.	Low levels of co-insurance, but likely to increase.	Low levels of co-insurance, but likely to increase.	
Czech Republic (195)	Modest cost sharing for specific PHC services, with out-of-pocket maximum. Private doctors can charge extra.	Plan to introduce cost sharing with out-of-pocket maximum.	Cost sharing; positive list of reimbursable drugs.	Yes.
Estonia	Modest cost sharing.	None for inpatient care; modest levels for specialist outpatient care.	High co-insurance with exemptions and reductions for specific groups.	Yes.
Hungary (196)	No formal charges.	Modest cost sharing for inpatient care.	Cost sharing with exemptions.	Widely used.
Kyrgyzstan (197)	Twenty-five percent pay official charges; the rest are exempt or not charged.	Twenty-five percent pay official admission charges; the rest are exempt or not charged. Families often provide food.	Most patients pay for drugs; prices vary widely.	Yes, and growing.

Latvia	Modest cost sharing.	Modest cost sharing for inpatient and outpatient care, with exemptions for specific groups.	Cost sharing.	Yes.
Lithuania	None or modest.	None or modest.	High co-insurance.	Yes.
Poland	None.	None.	Moderate co-insurance for domestically produced drugs; full payment for imported drugs.	Yes, and growing.
Romania	None.	None.	Cost sharing, but exemptions or reductions for specific groups.	Widely used.
Slovakia	None.	None.	Co-insurance rate varies according to category of drug.	Yes.
Slovenia	None.	None for inpatient care. None for specialist outpatient care unless use	Cost sharing.	Yes.

Those on higher incomes are more able to pay, more likely to be insured and less likely to be deterred from using health services than those on lower incomes. To provide some protection for disadvantaged people, certain pharmaceutical items are exempt from official charges. These include drugs for specified chronic conditions and communicable diseases, plus prescribed drugs for the "socially needy", whose status has been verified and who consequently hold a public health provision identity card *(196)*.

THE EFFECTS OF COST SHARING
Total health expenditure

Evidence suggests that cost sharing reduces utilization but does not contain costs. Overall costs are not contained because cost sharing is a set of demand-side policies, and costs are primarily driven by supply-side factors. Intercountry comparisons indicate that the United States has lower rates of contact with physicians and bed-days per head of population than many other countries, including Canada, France, Germany, Japan and the United Kingdom, but costs in the United States are much higher relative to GDP than in these other countries. This strongly suggests that it is the intensity of care provided per contact in the United States that is responsible for this apparent paradox *(198)*. The United States has the highest out-of-pocket expenses, mostly to meet cost-sharing obligations; it also has the highest overall costs. Other countries have lower cost-sharing and higher utilization rates, but lower costs. This does not mean that cost sharing causes higher costs; it means that measures other than cost sharing (supply-side measures such as budgetary controls) are much more effective mechanisms for cost-containment.

The Rand Study *(199,200)* suggests that cost sharing is associated with a decrease in total health spending, but the design of the experiment does not really permit strong conclusions to be drawn about the consequences for total expenditure of the broad implementation of cost sharing within a retrospective reimbursement system. The reason is that providers may compensate for a reduction in consumer-initiated demand by inducing increases in service volume or intensity. Table 9, which shows intercountry data *(198)* on contacts with physicians, hospital days and health expenditure as a percentage of GDP, suggests that consumer-initiated demand is not the major factor driving health care costs. Rather, it appears to be the intensity of services provided. Since intensity is largely provider initiated, there is little scope for cost sharing to make much of an impact on the overall level of spending.

Pharmaceuticals

In Sweden, the introduction of the reference price system led to a rapid decline in pharmaceutical prices. The generic market share for items covered by the reference price system increased from 35% to 49% during the first six months of 1993. The estimated annual saving resulting from this change was about 5% of the total pharmaceutical costs. The annual increase in total spending on drugs, however, continued at its previous rate, as additional costs were shifted to patients *(192)*.

Table 9. Health care utilization and expenditure in selected countries, around 1990

Country	Contacts with physicians per head	Bed-days per head	Expenditure as a percentage of GDP
Canada	6.9	1.5	9.5
France	7.2	1.5	8.8
Germany	11.5	2.3	8.3
Japan	12.9	–	6.7
United Kingdom	5.7	0.9	6.2
United States	5.5	0.9	12.2

Source: Rasell (198).

In the Czech Republic, pharmaceutical costs were completely covered until 1992, when cost sharing was introduced. This had very little effect on overall drug spending, however, which still accounts for about 30% of total health spending (195). By 1994 in Hungary, cost sharing accounted for about 25% of medications. Out-of-pocket spending on drugs grew more than fourfold between 1991 and 1994, but consumption has fallen as a result of the dramatic increase in drug prices. A 1995 survey indicated that 20% of prescriptions went unfilled because patients were unable to pay (196).

Equity in financing

Has cost sharing led to a relatively greater burden of health care financing falling on lower-income households? Based on data from the 1980s, Switzerland and the United States were found to have the most regressive health financing systems out of ten OECD countries studied (201). This finding was attributed to their heavy reliance on both private health insurance and private out-of-pocket payments. The latter were found to be very regressive in these two countries because, in most instances, cost-sharing obligations apply irrespective of the patient's income.

The equity consequences of cost sharing in France are unclear, because there is no direct relationship between income and complementary insurance coverage. Employees in small firms and young people, as well as the unemployed, are less likely to have complementary insurance. This suggests that voluntary complementary insurance that covers the cost-sharing obligations of a national insurance system can lead to a disproportionate financial burden (and probably inequitable access as well) for those unable to purchase that coverage.

Evidence from Kyrgyzstan suggests that the mix of formal and informal charges to users of health services increased inequities in financing. The out-of-pocket costs of a single episode of illness could impose a substantial financial burden on many households. In 20% of cases, the total costs of an episode for an individual exceeded the monthly income of his or her entire household. Almost 50% of inpatients reported severe difficulties in finding the money to pay for their stay, and one third of them borrowed money to pay for their hospital charges. Capital items were often sold (farm animals in rural areas, consumer goods in urban areas) to raise the necessary money. Overall, there is evidence that the incidence of out-of-pocket payments for health is inequitable, i.e. it creates more of a burden for poorer households and individuals *(197)*.

CONCLUSION

Cost sharing does not provide a very powerful policy tool, either for improving efficiency or for containing health sector costs. Because of the importance of providers in influencing the main drivers of health sector costs, policies that address the supply side of the market are likely to be much more powerful than those that act solely on the demand side. Cost sharing will reduce consumer initiated utilization, but such reductions will not be effective for cost-containment. This is because the main influence on health care costs is service intensity, which is provider driven.

The appropriateness and likely effects of cost sharing depend on the services to which it is applied, and on the broader context of the provider payment system. The use of cost sharing as a tool to limit demand is relevant only when applied to first-contact services. For (provider-initiated) referral services, cost sharing has little impact on utilization and is thus of little relevance in terms of efficiency. In systems in which providers are reimbursed retrospectively, reductions in consumer-initiated utilization caused by cost sharing will encourage providers to increase the volume of services per patient contact (i.e. service intensity) in order to maintain their incomes. In such systems, therefore, cost sharing does little to restrain cost growth because the available evidence suggests that providers can – and do – respond to a drop in consumer-initiated utilization by stimulating an increase in the use of diagnostic and therapeutic services. In systems where providers are prepaid, there are no obvious incentives for this response, but the effects of cost sharing are still likely to be marginal because supply-side incentives are enough to restrain growth in expenditure.

Without compensatory administrative procedures, cost sharing causes inequity in the financing and receipt of health services. Unless cost sharing is related to income, co-payments and co-insurance will impose a greater burden on the budgets of low-income households. Without specific measures to exempt low-income groups from out-of-pocket charges, access to care will depend on income levels. Evidence consistently shows that direct charges deter poorer people from using services to a greater degree than they deter the better-off. These limitations on access may result in adverse health effects for poorer and sicker groups of the population. To protect equity, therefore, measures are needed to compensate for the consequences of cost sharing on poorer members of society.

As a means of mobilizing revenue for the health services, direct charges to patients are not likely to generate substantial amounts without causing adverse consequences in terms of equity.

Priority setting in health care

Making choices about the allocation of resources between competing demands has always existed in health care systems. The choices made reflect the relative priorities attached to different services or types of patient; most often these choices were made implicitly by health care professionals. Rationing[13] of services to individuals also existed, achieved indirectly through waiting lists or by introducing cost-sharing arrangements. What is new is the growing interest of both politicians and citizens in this process, and the consequent demand for explicitness and transparency.

The priority-setting debate has become more significant as fundamental questions have been raised about the future scope of publicly funded health services. This is most evident in those systems that have sought to define core services or a basic care package, but it has also emerged as a point of discussion in other systems. At a time when the future of the welfare state as a whole is coming under scrutiny, the ability of governments to support universal and comprehensive health services is a subject of debate. Some economists argue that there should be a move away from government to individual responsibility and a retreat from state-financed health systems. This view has been strongly contested by other analysts, and the need to ration health services by excluding services from public funding is by no means universally accepted.

Some have argued that rationing would not be necessary if additional funding were made available and/or if resources were used more efficiently. Indeed, as discussed above, countries could change public expenditure priorities to shift more resources to health care, increase revenue collection through taxation or social insurance, or shift costs to the private sector. Also, as shown in the following chapters, there is ample scope for achieving greater operating efficiencies by funding only those interventions that are appropriate and by adopting more cost-effective patterns of resource allocation and delivery. The search for cost-effective patterns of care should be the first objective of policy-makers, since it may forestall or reduce the need to ration individual access to necessary services.

Against this background, this section explores in more detail the issues involved in priority setting and rationing. It deals first with the main strategies for setting priorities, and then reviews experience in the European Region. Finally, a number of emerging lessons are summarized.

APPROACHES TO PRIORITY SETTING

Health care priority setting has attracted interest from researchers from quite different disciplinary backgrounds. Apart from economics, the most significant contributions have come from political science, philosophy and epidemiology. In the case of epidemiology, two themes are important. First, by analysing patterns of mortality and morbidity, epidemiology helps decision-making by identifying the main causes

---

[13] Throughout this review, the terms "rationing" and "priority setting" are used interchangeably. Both are used to describe the process by which choices in health care are made, particularly in circumstances where the demand for health care exceeds the resources available. Rationing emphasizes reductions in packages of care, resulting from setting priorities between competing demands.

of death and disability and the burden of disease. Second, the contribution of economics enables comparisons to be made of the cost–effectiveness of different procedures.

Political scientists and policy analysts have often been critical of the work of epidemiologists and economists, arguing that priority setting cannot be reduced to a technical exercise since in essence it involves a debate about values. Political scientists therefore see techniques as only one element of the decision-making process, and not necessarily the most important. Klein *(202)*, for example, emphasizes the importance of the process by which decisions are made and the role of different groups in this process. Political scientists also maintain that techniques can be misleading if the basis on which they are constructed is not understood. According to this school of thought, the aim should be to muddle through elegantly *(203)* and to ensure that the debate about priorities is open and fair. In highlighting the role of values in priority setting, political scientists enter the territory of philosophers, in particular drawing attention to the moral basis of decision-making and to the ethical principles that underpin choices in health care. This includes different concepts of justice, for instance, utilitarian and "needs-based" approaches *(204,205)*. Like political scientists, philosophers are often critical of economists, arguing that their work is based on questionable moral assumptions and fails to recognize that, in a democratic society, every individual has the same value and rights *(206)*.

There is also a growing body of empirical work describing experience in those systems that have given particular attention to priority setting. Studies that draw on empirical research to conceptualize approaches to priority setting are of particular relevance here.

Klein *(207)* has argued that there are different levels of priority setting in health care. At the macro level there is the priority attached to health care in relation to other competing claims on resources. Next, there are choices involved in allocating the health care budget between different geographical areas and services. At another level, decisions have to be taken about allocating resources to particular forms of treatment within service areas, e.g. the priority to be given to heart transplants versus open-heart surgery. There are also decisions to be made about which patient to treat first if treatment cannot be administered immediately. Finally, priorities have to be set for individual patients, particularly in the case of innovative or expensive procedures, when it may be necessary to decide whether a treatment should be provided at all and, if so, for how long.

This categorization offers a useful framework for analysing priority-setting processes in health care. While decisions at the micro level are influenced by those at the macro level, discussions about priority setting often fail to distinguish between different levels and result in a lack of clarity about the nature of the choices being made and the responsibility for those choices. The responsibility of politicians at the macro level is paralleled by the responsibility of clinicians at the micro level. At intermediate levels of priority setting, a range of political, clinical and managerial influences operate and these vary between systems. The manner in which decisions on priorities are made is not always easy to comprehend, because of the lack of transparency in the processes involved.

Another approach is summarized in Fig. 15, which shows in simplified form the forces that guide priority setting: government, providers, the public and patients, as well as evidence on health needs and on the cost and effectiveness of available interventions *(208)*. The roles and relative importance of these factors will vary between different health systems. In planned systems, the influence of politicians and the government is particularly important, both in determining priorities at the macro level and in shaping the way in which decisions are taken at lower levels. In contrast, in competitive systems, patients and clinicians have a significant influence on decision-making and the role of the government is commensurately weaker.

There are several methodological approaches to measuring the need for services, as well as the cost and effectiveness of available health care interventions. As discussed in Chapter 2, methods based on the burden of disease combine a series of epidemiological and economic techniques to measure the impact of disease on mortality and morbidity, as well as to quantify the cost and effectiveness of available interventions *(27)*. Some techniques employed are years of life lost, avoidable mortality and the quality-adjusted life-year (QALY). The latter relies on a scale of individual preferences for different levels of disability or impairment to adjust life-years resulting from different interventions. Data from a range of studies can then be combined with information about the cost of these interventions to produce cost-per-QALY league tables. An example from the United Kingdom is given in Table 10 *(209)*. This technique in turn led to the development of the disability-adjusted life-year (DALY) *(22)*, first used extensively in the World Bank's 1993 *World development report (28)*. Data on DALYs gained from particular interventions are combined with the

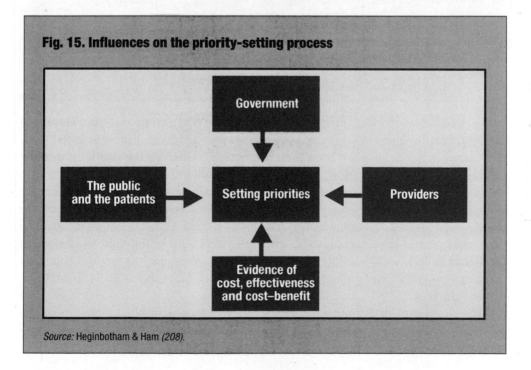

Fig. 15. Influences on the priority-setting process

Government → Setting priorities ← Providers

The public and the patients → Setting priorities

Evidence of cost, effectiveness and cost–benefit → Setting priorities

Source: Heginbotham & Ham *(208)*.

Table 10. Cost per QALY of some NHS interventions, August 1990

Treatment	Cost per QALY (£)
Cholesterol testing and diet therapy (ages 40–69)	220
Neurosurgery for head injury	240
Advice to stop smoking from GP	270
Neurosurgery for subarachnoid haemorrhage	490
Antihypertensive treatment to prevent stroke (ages 45–64)	940
Pacemaker implantation	1 100
Valve replacement for aortic stenosis	1 140
Hip replacement	1 180
Cholesterol testing and treatment	1 480
Coronary artery bypass graft (left main vessel disease, severe angina)	2 090
Kidney transplant	4 710
Breast cancer screening	5 780
Heart transplant	7 840
Cholesterol testing and incremental treatment (ages 25–39)	14 150
Home haemodialysis	17 260
Coronary artery bypass graft (one vessel disease, moderate angina)	18 830
Continuous outpatient peritoneal dialysis	19 870
Hospital haemodialysis	21 970
Erythropoietin treatment for anaemia (dialysis patients, assuming 10% reduction in mortality)	54 380
Neurosurgery for malignant intracranial tumour	107 780
Erythropoietin treatment for anaemia (dialysis patients, assuming no reduction in mortality)	126 290

Source: Maynard (209).

cost of these interventions to produce a cost per DALY, which economists then employ to assess alternative interventions or to define a basic package of health care benefits.

Various approaches have been used to attempt to involve the public in priority setting (see Box 15). There is, however, considerable disagreement as to whether these involve participation or simply cooption. Much depends on whether the purpose is to use the public's views to shape decision-making, or only to inform the public about the need to make choices. Evidence from the United Kingdom suggests that most people are reluctant to be involved in priority setting and would prefer decisions to be left to the medical profession (210). None the less, several countries have made significant efforts to involve the public, and this seems likely to continue in the future.

The domain of health priorities inevitably overlaps with other elements of the health system. Fig. 16 maps the process of setting priorities, indicates the main elements involved, and highlights the process's dynamic nature.

Box 15. Public involvement in priority setting

Public involvement in rationing has taken a number of forms. In the Netherlands, an extensive period of public consultation followed publication of the Dunning committee's report *(58)*. About 60 organizations were involved in discussions on choices in health care. These started in 1991 and ended in 1995. An evaluation of the process concluded that the public discussions reached about one third of the population. As a consequence, there were changes in public opinion. For example, in 1990, 55% of the population believed that all treatments must be available irrespective of cost, whereas in 1994 this had fallen to 44%. Less positively, the results of the exercise were not used by the Dutch government in its decision-making process on choices in health care.

In Sweden, the work of the Parliamentary Priorities Commission *(211)* was guided by a number of surveys of the public and of health care professionals. The survey of the public was carried out by questionnaire in January 1994, and involved a random sample of 1500 people. A 78% response rate was achieved. A majority of respondents felt that medical care should be mainly devoted to people with the severest illnesses. A majority of respondents also agreed with the Commission's recommendation that terminal care should be given the same high priority as emergency health care. Services that the public felt might be restricted included cosmetic surgery, removing harmless birthmarks, smoking cessation programmes and *in vitro* fertilization. Overall, the questionnaire survey strongly endorsed the principles set out in the Commission's first report.

In the United Kingdom, various approaches have been tried at local level *(212)*. These include public meetings, postal questionnaire surveys, Delphi techniques, consultation with the public and GPs in small areas or localities, the use of consensus conferences, consultation with community health councils, market research, rapid appraisal and focus group discussions. Focus groups have been found to be particularly effective *(213,214)*.

In Oregon in the United States, the methods used included public hearings, community meetings and telephone surveys. An organization known as Oregon Health Decisions was commissioned to help with this work. Focus groups involved participants drawn from different sections of the community in discussing some of the choices that had to be made. Oregon Health Decisions concluded that this was a particularly effective way of extracting information from the community about values. Because of the small numbers involved, however, it was less effective as a method of engaging the community at large.

In the health sector, priorities cannot be set in a vacuum. They need to be congruent with societal values and principles, and with health policy objectives. The institutional and legal framework of the health system provides the limits in which priorities can be set and implemented. Current priorities are strongly influenced by a number of factors, including budgetary limitations, demand for services and political pressures. Among the criteria commonly used to select priority interventions in public institutions are the ability significantly to reduce the burden of disease, to be reasonably cost-effective and to satisfy population preferences. Not all technically defined priorities can be implemented in the short or medium term. They need to comply

Fig. 16. The dynamics of setting health priorities

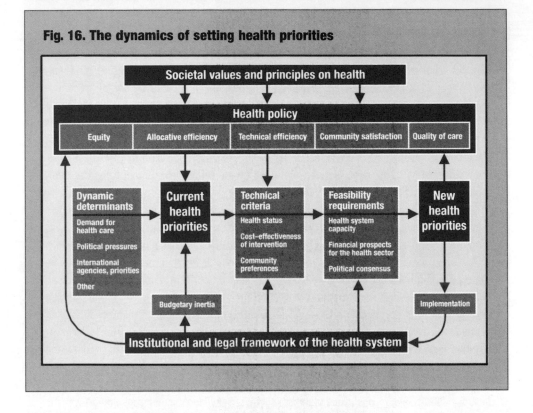

with three critical feasibility requirements: that they be deliverable with reasonable quality by the current health system; that they be available to all, or almost all, within the projected budget; and that they reflect reasonable political agreement on their appropriateness. If new health priorities are set, they will need to be implemented. Mechanisms to change the current allocation of resources will be needed, as well as changes in the rules that govern the relationships between the actors in the health system.

TRENDS AND DEVELOPMENTS
Priority setting in western Europe
In recent years, several countries in the European Region and elsewhere have taken initiatives to examine priority setting on a more systematic and explicit basis. The countries in western Europe to have done so include the Netherlands, Norway, Spain and Sweden. Overall, however, there have not been any substantial reductions in coverage or in the packages of benefits offered by their statutory systems.

The government of the Netherlands appointed the Dunning committee in 1990 to "examine how to put limits on new medical technologies and how to deal with problems caused by scarcity of care, rationing of care, and the necessity of selection of patients for care" (58). In its report, the committee reached the view that it was necessary to make explicit choices about care, such as excluding some treatments from funding. It suggested that the best way would be to apply four criteria to determine whether a health care intervention should be included in the basic package. These criteria, illustrated in Fig. 17, included asking whether the care was necessary from the community's point of view, whether it was effective and efficient, and whether it should not be left to personal responsibility. If services passed these tests, then they would be included in the care package; if they did not, they would be left to individuals to purchase from their own resources.

Using this framework, the Dunning committee argued that dental care for adults, homeopathic medicine and *in vitro* fertilization could be left out of the care package. It also emphasized that the government should legislate to protect the quality of care for vulnerable groups such as the mentally and physically disabled. Beyond these proposals, the committee argued that priorities should be set by assessing the effectiveness of health care technologies, and by devising explicit criteria for determining access to waiting lists and from waiting lists into hospital. It also called on the health care professions to take the lead in drawing up guidelines for service provision. Although initial reaction to the report was cautious, it was accepted by the Dutch government and action has been taken on most of its recommendations. In the Netherlands, the key to further progress is seen to be influencing physicians' decisions to promote more effective clinical practices (Mulder, J., unpublished data, 1995).

Priority setting in Sweden has been strongly influenced by work originally undertaken in Norway. In both countries – as in the Netherlands – the desire to reduce waiting lists was one of the factors that led policy-makers to take action. In Sweden, a Parliamentary Priorities Commission was set up by the Government in 1992 and produced its final report in 1995 *(211)*. The Commission concluded that priority setting should be based on a sound and explicit ethical platform. To this end, it proposed three principles as the starting point:

1. *human dignity*: all human beings have equal dignity and the same rights, regardless of their personal characteristics and their functions in the community;
2. *need and solidarity*: resources should be committed to those fields where needs are greatest, and special attention should be paid to the needs of those groups unaware of their human dignity or who have less chance than others of making their voices heard or exercising their rights; and
3. *cost–efficiency*: when choosing between different options, one should aim for a reasonable relationship between cost and effect (this principle should be applied only when comparing methods for treating the same disease).

These principles are listed in order of rank, and in practice this means that the cost–efficiency principle is given relatively low priority. The Commission also emphasized that certain criteria were not acceptable as a basis for prioritization. These included advanced age, self-inflicted injuries and social position. On this basis, the Commission outlined a number of priority categories. The highest priority was attached to treating life-threatening acute conditions, chronic diseases and severe mental disorders, followed by prevention and rehabilitation; the lowest priority was

Fig. 17. A method to determine the basic package of care

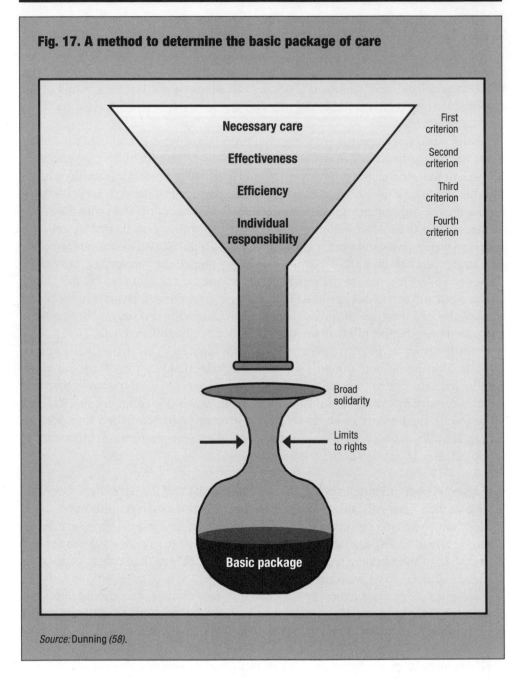

Source: Dunning (58).

given to mild disorders and illnesses where self-care was sufficient. Unlike the Dunning committee, the Swedish Commission did not make specific proposals for excluding services, but recommended instead that its framework should be used as a basis for guiding decisions on priorities. Another feature of the Swedish approach worth noting was the effort put into consulting the public.

In the United Kingdom, there has been no national initiative of the type found in the Netherlands and Sweden. Nevertheless, the recent NHS reforms, which separated the responsibility for purchasing and providing health care (together with a number of well publicized cases of patients being denied care), have given rise to a great deal of interest and activity in relation to priority setting. Health authorities have been at the forefront of efforts to develop more systematic approaches to priority setting, and a number of studies have reviewed their experience (212,215,216). Increasingly, health authorities are arriving at decisions after consulting key stakeholders in their areas, including local people and GPs. They are also undertaking epidemiologically based health needs assessments to aid decision-making. In a few cases, this has resulted in decisions to exclude services from funding, but most health authorities have made only incremental changes to their plans and have shifted priorities only at the margins.

One effect of separating the responsibilities of purchaser and provider has been to encourage health authorities to question established spending patterns and adopt a more critical attitude to providers' demands. The Department of Health has launched a number of initiatives designed to promote evidence-based medicine through its research and development programme (217). These include the establishment of a Centre for Reviews and Dissemination, which publishes reports that review the effectiveness of different services, and the Cochrane Centre (218). A key objective has been to ensure that clinical decisions are based on research findings. Health authorities have been asked to develop the use of guidelines and clinical protocols, and to introduce clinical audit as a means of reviewing professional practices and promoting high standards. At national level, the Department publishes annual guidance on planning and priorities, and this provides the framework within which health authorities are expected to operate. The guidance contains a large number of priorities, however, and little effort has been made to identify those that really matter.

The British government's view is that priority setting should initially be approached by increasing efficiency, before any services are excluded from the remit of the NHS (219). In practice, some services have been excluded or are limited in availability as a result of financial pressures, and more seem likely to follow (220,221). The government has resisted calls for a national debate on priority setting or, as in other countries, for setting up a committee to review the way forward.

Outside the European Region, there have been a number of examples of systematic approaches to priority setting, notably those adopted by the Core Services Committee in New Zealand and the State of Oregon in the United States. These are summarized in Box 16.

Priority setting in the CEE and CIS countries

The justification for and importance of setting heath priorities depend greatly on the policy context. Some commentators have argued that the policy context in the CEE and particularly the CIS countries makes priority setting a necessary step towards ensuring an efficient use of public funds for health. They contend that the average expenditure per head in the CIS countries is insufficient to pay the generous health

Box 16. Examples of priority setting outside Europe

In Oregon, a State Health Commission was appointed in 1989 to make recommendations to the state legislature on how Medicaid coverage could be expanded and how priorities could be set in the Medicaid programme. The Commission tried out a number of methods, beginning with an approach based on economic evaluation. This produced such anomalous results that it was abandoned, and the Commission resorted to a judgemental approach supported by a number of exercises in public consultation. The resulting list of almost 700 condition–treatment pairs was presented to the legislature, and after amendments had been made to satisfy the federal government and to avoid infringing disability legislation, the Oregon Plan was implemented in 1994. At the time of writing, 565 treatments are funded under the Plan and population coverage has been extended in line with the expectations of the Plan's architects. The Oregon list, however, has not yet been extended beyond the Medicaid programme to form the basis of health insurance throughout the state. The attempt to involve the public in priority setting through public hearings and community meetings was a key element of the Oregon approach. In practice, concerns were expressed at the lack of representativeness of those attending the meetings, which were dominated by health care providers *(222,223)*.

In New Zealand, the Government appointed a Core Services Committee in 1992 to advise on the services that should be included in the publicly funded health system. The Committee decided that it would not be appropriate to draw up a list of Oregon-style services. Instead, it argued that the current services were those that should be provided, and it set in train a process for determining priorities in specific areas of provision. This was done through a range of methods, including consensus conferences, reviews of published research and international evidence, expert evaluation of contemporary practice, closed workshops, contested public hearings and public consultation. In most cases, the aim was to draw up guidelines on the service concerned, and these would then be offered as advice to the Minister of Health. The Committee's view was that whole categories of care should not be excluded because this might discriminate against those who could benefit from receiving such care. One of the purposes of the guidelines was to identify those most likely to benefit from receiving a service, thereby targeting resources where they could achieve the most health gain. By the middle of 1995, 18 areas had been systematically reviewed. In the next stage of its work, the Committee will examine the question of priorities between services or treatment areas *(224,225)*.

care coverage provided by the previous system, and that many cost-effective interventions are currently neglected, underfunded or of a low standard. If health status is to be improved, such interventions should be granted greater priority.

Initial exclusions have focused on relatively uncontroversial, nonessential services such as cosmetic surgery and some prosthetic devices (e.g Croatia and The Former Yugoslav Republic of Macedonia) or health sanatoria (e.g. the Czech Republic and Slovakia). Continued economic contraction and/or unanticipated cost escalation in health services are now leading some countries to consider more profound reductions in benefits. The Former Yugoslav Republic of Macedonia, for example, is defining a guaranteed basic package of benefits that is more in line with available resources. In Georgia, the state minimum package includes only 10–15% of all necessary clinical care.

Burden-of-disease and DALY methodologies have been used in studies to guide priority setting in several CEE and CIS countries. Most of these studies, however, have been confined to measuring the burden of disease in terms of mortality, morbidity and disability. Little work has been done to assess the cost–effectiveness of health interventions, and no work has been done on identifying social preferences for health outcomes.

THE EMERGING LESSONS

The debate about priority setting raises uncomfortable questions about the scope of publicly funded health service provision. The review of experience indicates that no country has so far retreated from the commitment to play a major part in funding and regulating health services. Rather, the aim has been to increase the efficiency with which resources are used and to make changes to services in an incremental manner. Different countries have approached priority setting in different ways, and various methods have been pursued. Much of the work that has been done is at an early stage of development, and therefore its impact remains uncertain. Nevertheless, certain patterns have emerged.

Priority setting is inherently complex, and is not amenable to a "quick fix" approach. As the above discussion suggests, a strategic approach is needed that involves action on the different levels of decision-making. Some of this activity will be at the political level, in terms of setting priorities for the system as a whole. Some will be at the clinical level, ensuring that decisions about which patients to treat and in what order of priority are based on the results of research. A continuing effort is required at all levels if decisions are to be soundly based and defensible. This is best illustrated by experience in the Netherlands, where the national debate on the care package was combined with investment in technology assessment, the development of practice guidelines and the establishment of criteria to govern waiting lists.

There is also considerable variety in the national frameworks that guide priority setting and on the strategies that have been pursued. There is a key distinction to be made here between rationing services by exclusion and rationing by guidelines (226). Oregon has chosen to ration by exclusion, specifically services for poorer women and children. In contrast, the New Zealand Core Services Committee rejected exclusions and concentrated instead on drawing up guidelines for specific services. The Netherlands sought to combine these two approaches, by excluding some services from the care package while attaching priority to the development of guidelines by professional associations.

In all systems, there is concern to combine the use of priority-setting techniques with public debate about the choices that should be made. While some systems emphasize formulaic approaches more than others, there is general recognition that priority setting cannot be reduced to a technical exercise. This particularly applies to the use of some economic approaches such as QALYs and DALYs, whose educational value is widely acknowledged but only as one element in the priority-setting process. Technical methods need to be reviewed in a thorough public debate about the choices to be made. Methodologies for involving the public in the priority-setting process are at various stages of development; they have significant problems and little is known about their relative effectiveness. None the less, there is wide-spread consensus about the importance of continuing to develop ways of engaging the public in decisions about priorities.

The need for public involvement is closely linked to another aspect of the pro-cess: the need to legitimize rationing decisions. This cannot be done by arguing that these decisions are correct, since there can be no right answer to questions about health care priorities. Such decisions are essentially value judgements, which will vary between individuals, groups and societies. Legitimacy, therefore, is derived from the decision-making process. This process is more likely to be seen as legiti-mate if it is open, and if it enables different interests to contribute. The approaches taken in the Netherlands and Sweden illustrate how two European countries have sought to address these issues at national level, while developments in the United Kingdom have placed greater emphasis on the need to establish effective decision-making processes at local level. Notwithstanding these differences, there is a com-mon concern to move away from implicit to explicit rationing, and to develop greater public accountability for specific rationing decisions.

In making choices in health care, policy-makers have to balance a range of objectives. Decision-making involves trade-offs between these objectives, as a bal-ance is sought between universal coverage, comprehensiveness, equity, efficiency, choice, cost-containment and other goals. As the Dunning committee in the Nether-lands noted, health care choices have to balance the aim of achieving basic care for all with the need to contain costs. In the Netherlands, the degree of comprehensive-ness has been sacrificed to some degree in the pursuit of cost-containment. The same applies in the United Kingdom, where the effect of government policies limiting the growth of spending on the NHS has been to limit the provision of certain low-priority services such as infertility treatment.

Another important objective is equity. In the Netherlands and Sweden, equity or solidarity is explicitly mentioned as one of the key principles that should guide priority setting. In both countries, particular priority has been attached to care for vulnerable groups. For instance, the Parliamentary Priorities Commission in Sweden emphasized the need to ensure that cost–efficiency in resource use was not pursued at the expense of equity. All this illustrates the trade-offs inherent in priority setting. While the aim of achieving greater efficiency in the use of resources is widely acknowledged, it is just one objective among many and has to be balanced against other considerations.

There can be a gap between the conclusions reached by national committees and what happens in practice. The Dunning committee report illustrates how the work of an expert committee can act as a force for debate and change. Establishing a national framework, however, is only one step in the process. The framework has to be translated into action and, most importantly, it has to influence clinical decisions. If, as international experience suggests, ensuring that physicians use resources effec-tively and appropriately is central to priority setting, then strategies for improving clinical decision-making are at least as important as broad statements of national principles. In practice, it is not a question of seeking to change clinical decisions or of developing a national framework, but of how the two can best go hand in hand.

Feasibility is a further aspect. Even when technical priorities are clearly defined, it is not always possible to implement them in the short or medium term. They need to comply with three feasibility requirements as set out above on page 106. Changes must also be introduced into the financing and provision of health care to account for shifts in priorities, such as the introduction of regulations, modifications in provider payments, the review of clinical protocols to diagnose and treat some conditions, or changes in programming and budgeting.

Finally, each country needs to find its own solution to the priority-setting dilemma, reflecting its own starting point, spending levels and expectations. Policy-makers have a number of options available:

- allowing priority setting to remain implicit, with clinicians deciding on the best use of resources;
- using waiting lists to regulate access to services for non-life-threatening conditions;
- introducing cost-sharing arrangements for services seen as low priorities, with exemptions for low-income groups where appropriate;
- limiting the availability of some services through positive or negative lists, as for pharmaceuticals;
- concentrating resources on services of proved effectiveness;
- introducing the assessment and regulation of technologies;
- developing evidence-based guidelines to determine access to services;
- commissioning research to guide decision-making on priorities;
- providing information to users, to encourage an appropriate use of services;
- defining a process for determining priorities, either through the health ministry or through an expert group;
- drawing up a set of principles and priority categories to guide debate on priority setting;
- transferring responsibility for certain health services to the private sector; and/or
- defining a list of services to be funded.

Also, key priority-setting decisions should be reviewed regularly, owing to the dynamic nature of health care systems and services.

Ultimately, it is the responsibility of elected public officials to use their best judgement in determining priorities. Their decisions will be shaped by the availability of resources, information on the health needs of the population, evidence on the cost and effectiveness of available interventions, population preferences, an assessment of what is politically feasible and, of course, the values they bring to bear. The one clear message from international experience is that health care rationing cannot be divorced from values.

4 Funding Systems Equitably

The effort to balance equitable funding of health services with scarce resources is a major challenge to national policy-makers. This chapter reviews two aspects of that dilemma. It first discusses funding trends across the European Region. It then assesses the compatibility of solidaristic funding mechanisms with multiple competitive third-party insurers.

Trends in health care funding

There are four key sources of funds for health care: taxation, contributions to social insurance schemes, voluntary subscriptions to private insurance schemes and out-of-pocket payments. These four sources can be classified as compulsory or statutory systems (social health insurance and taxation) or as voluntary systems (voluntary insurance and out-of-pocket payments).

Many health care systems in the European Region rely on a mix of all four sources. Nevertheless, it is possible to distinguish five categories of country in the Region, grouped according to the predominant type of statutory financing arrangement that characterizes their health care systems, or the predominant type of statutory financing they wish to develop. The five groups are (Table 11):

1. health care systems that are based on the Bismarck model (i.e. that are predominantly insurance-based) with well established financing systems;
2. health care systems that are based on the Bismarck model, but are at present in a state of transition;
3. health care systems that are based on the Beveridge model (i.e. that are predominantly tax-based) with well established financing systems;
4. health care systems that have relatively recently begun to change from being predominantly insurance-based to being predominantly tax-based, and hence are in a state of transition; and
5. health care systems that have historically been based on the Semashko model and that are planning or have implemented, in whole or in part, a shift to an insurance-based system.

Although this classification centres on the predominant type of statutory financing arrangement, there is no "pure" system: tax-based financing systems typically also include elements of social insurance, and insurance-based systems often include strong elements of tax-based financing. Moreover, whether tax-based or insurance-based, virtually all health care systems in the Region either include or have plans to include some elements of the two types of voluntary financing.

Table 11 gives a rough categorization of prevalent tendencies in financing health care systems in the European Region. It does not, however, reflect the

Table 11. Countries of the European Region grouped according to the actual or planned method of financing

Insurance-based system	Tax-based system	From central control to an insurance-based system (5)	
		CEE countries	CIS countries
Well established (1)	**Well established (3)**		
Austria	Denmark	Albania	Armenia
Belgium	Finland	Bosnia and	Azerbaijan
France	Iceland	Herzegovina	Belarus
Germany	Ireland	Bulgaria	Georgia
Luxembourg	Norway	Croatia	Kazakstan
Netherlands	Sweden	Czech Republic	Kyrgyzstan
Switzerland	United Kingdom	Estonia	Republic of Moldova
		Hungary	Russian Federation
		Latvia	Tajikistan
		Lithuania	Turkmenistan
		Poland	Ukraine
In transition (2)	**In transition (4)**	Romania	Uzbekistan
Former German	Greece	Slovakia	
Democratic	Italy	Slovenia	
Republic[a]	Portugal	The Former Yugoslav	
Israel	Spain	Republic of	
Turkey		Macedonia	

[a] Strictly speaking, the territory formerly occupied by the German Democratic Republic should be grouped with the CEE countries, as it is in a process of transition from central control to insurance-based financing. Because of its accession to the Federal Republic of Germany and the resulting integration of the two health care systems, however, it is considered here as an insurance-based system in transition.

essential time element. Most of the countries in group 1 adopted their systems long ago, some even in the last century. In group 2, the insurance-based systems are at present in transition. The health care systems of all the countries in group 3 initially had social insurance systems, which were transformed into national health (tax-based) systems in recent decades. The countries in group 4 have more recently embarked on a process of transformation from insurance-based to tax-based financing. Thus groups 2 and 4, listing countries currently in transition, are distinguished from groups 1 and 3, respectively, only by time. Finally, group 5 consists of the CEE and CIS countries, which recently transformed their state financing systems into predominantly insurance-based systems or plan to do so in the near future.

INSURANCE-BASED FINANCING
Well established systems

Social insurance evolved from risk spreading by groups of individuals, who voluntarily pooled money in order to have some financial security in the event of hardship. The earliest voluntary associations paid cash benefits to their members during periods of unemployment or interruption of income, to compensate them for lost income or for the costs of medical care. The development of social insurance from these early mutual-aid societies entailed the use of four mechanisms to ensure affordable cover for the majority of unskilled workers for whom the insurance was initially intended *(227)*:

- spreading the risk broadly by making social insurance compulsory;
- requiring employers to pay for part of members' contributions;
- providing insurance through public or quasi-public non-profit institutions; and
- devising a mechanism for redistributing income from the higher to the lower paid.

The first compulsory sickness insurance legislation was passed in Germany in 1883, and made workers' membership of the previously voluntary funds compulsory. Accident, old-age, long-term disability, survivors' and unemployment insurance legislation was subsequently enacted in the years up to 1927. Virtually all other European countries followed in Germany's footsteps, and by 1930 social insurance was widespread throughout Europe *(227)*. In all cases, the evolution of social insurance involved the inclusion of more groups in insurance schemes, thus gradually increasing coverage of the population.

Although they were inspired by the same underlying principles, and aimed to achieve similar ends, social insurance systems in Europe differ significantly from each other. Many of the differences derive from the uniqueness of each country's social, economic, institutional and ideological structures, within which social insurance financing gradually evolved over many years.

The major source of funds for health care in this group of countries is social insurance. In all cases, funds collected through contributions to social insurance are earmarked for health care purposes. For example, in the early 1990s financing through statutory health insurance accounted for 70% of total health care financing in France and 60% in Germany and the Netherlands *(188)*.

In virtually all countries, social insurance funds are subsidized by the state, though the extent of such subsidies varies widely between countries (Table 12).

Funds from the state budget are used in part to subsidize the social insurance system. In addition, state funds are generally used for such items as public health, and medical teaching and research. Hence financing through the state budget from general taxation makes up a substantial proportion of total health care financing. For example, in the early 1990s the contributions of budget financing to total health care financing were 39% in Belgium, 21% in Germany, 37.9% in Luxembourg and 33.9% in Switzerland *(2,188)*.

Table 12. Premiums and government subsidies in some social insurance systems, early 1990s

Country	Premiums (%)	Government subsidies (%)
Austria	88.0	12.0
Belgium	58.0	42.0
Switzerland	73.9	14.1

Source: OECD *(2,188).*

In all countries, compulsory health insurance is part of the social security system, which includes other items of social protection such as pensions and unemployment benefits. The precise conditions, however, are not the same everywhere. For example, in some countries, such as Belgium, France and Germany, health insurance law is part of the social security code that covers other items such as pensions and work disability. In other countries, such as the Netherlands and Switzerland, health insurance law is separate from other social security items *(228).*

In all countries, health insurance funds are independent bodies, with their own management, budget and legal status. This ensures their independence from the government and from the government budget. In France, according to administrative law, they are private organizations charged with the provision of a public service, but because of their close supervision by the government they are in effect nongovernmental quasi-public organizations *(189).* Similarly, in Germany, they are private non-profit entities or what are termed "public law corporations". In Switzerland, they are non-profit "mutual insurance companies" (i.e. private commercial insurance firms) conforming to statutory conditions *(228).* In all countries, health insurance funds, though independent, are subject to close regulation by the government.

There are wide variations in the number of health insurance or sickness funds in countries, ranging from as few as 6 in Belgium to 11 in Luxembourg, about 16 in France, 24 in Austria, 53 in the Netherlands, some 200 in Switzerland and about 1100 in Germany *(2,188).* In most cases, current numbers represent a significant reduction, as many mergers and alliances have taken place over the years. In Germany, for example, at the time of the first health insurance legislation in 1883 there were about 22 000 sickness funds in existence *(229).* One important reason for the mergers has been the concomitant increase in membership, as a means of spreading risk over a relatively larger population.

In some countries, such as France and Luxembourg, funds are organized mainly according to occupational groups. They were organized mainly geographically in the Netherlands, until recently, and according to religious or political affiliations in Belgium. In Austria, Germany and Switzerland, sickness funds are organized according to several principles. In Austria and Germany, for example, funds may be organized on the basis of occupation, region or locality, or business enterprise *(2,188)*.

Membership of statutory insurance funds is compulsory for virtually the entire population in Austria, Belgium, France and Luxembourg. In Switzerland it is voluntary, with the exception of four cantons and some municipalities that have made it compulsory, and some cantons that have made it compulsory for certain groups (such as the elderly, children and those on low incomes). In Germany and the Netherlands, membership is compulsory only for people below a certain income level. In Germany, people above this income level can choose to be insured with the statutory system or with a private insurer, while in the Netherlands (in the case of coverage for acute care) they may choose a private insurer or remain uninsured *(2,188)*.

No system financed predominantly by social insurance has completely universal coverage, since cover follows entitlement based on some criterion relating to insurance contributions. Most countries cover some 99% of the population, however, either through statutory insurance alone or through a combination of statutory and private insurance. It is possible to distinguish four patterns of coverage.

The first pattern is exemplified by those countries in which nearly the entire population is covered by compulsory statutory insurance and where cover is comprehensive, such as Austria, France and Luxembourg.

The second pattern is exemplified by those countries in which nearly the entire population is covered by compulsory statutory insurance but where some people receive only partial coverage, such as Belgium and the Netherlands. In Belgium, about 15% of the population (the self-employed) is covered only for major risks, while comprehensive cover – for major and minor risks[14] – is reserved for the remainder of the population). In the Netherlands, comprehensive cover by statutory insurance is provided for about 60% of the population, the remainder being covered only for health care for chronic conditions.

The third pattern is exemplified by those countries, such as Switzerland, in which nearly the entire population is covered by statutory insurance but where membership is voluntary.

The fourth pattern is exemplified by those countries in which only a portion of the population is covered by statutory insurance, as in Germany where about 90% of the population is covered by the statutory system.

Within these limits, most countries have a legally specified package of benefits that applies uniformly to all sickness funds within a given insurance scheme. Some countries, however, have more than one insurance scheme, with benefits varying from one scheme to another. Austria, for example, has four schemes based on occupational categories, with different benefits and cost-sharing requirements. Some countries, such as the Netherlands, have separate schemes for public employees. In addition, sickness funds in virtually all the countries offer supplementary optional benefits, over and above those offered in the benefit package, which also vary from fund to fund.

---

[14] Major risks refer to inpatient care and special technical services; minor risks refer to such items as outpatient care, dental care and pharmaceuticals.

In all these countries, contributions paid into the sickness funds are related to income and at a flat rate, and shared between employers and employees. In Austria, Germany, Luxembourg and the Netherlands they are shared on a 50:50 basis, while in Belgium and France employers pay a higher proportion than employees. The contribution rates are negotiated on various levels, but usually with the central government taking final responsibility. In a number of countries, such as Austria, France, Germany and Switzerland, contribution rates are permitted to vary from fund to fund, frequently reflecting the differing risk profiles of their members. By contrast, Belgium and Luxembourg require identical contribution rates for all funds. Contribution rates (employer plus employee) are quite low in Austria, ranging from 5.6% to 8.5% of gross income, while they are fairly high in France, being 19.4% for the largest fund that insures the bulk of the French population. Most other countries have intermediate contribution rates *(2,188)*.

Individuals can choose their insurance fund in Belgium and Switzerland, and to a more limited extent in Germany, where free choice is available mainly to white-collar workers (about half of all members of Germany's statutory funds). In the remaining countries, the occupational or geographical organization of sickness funds precludes choice *(2,188)*.

As noted earlier, social insurance funds in all countries are closely regulated by the government. For several years, there has been a marked trend in virtually all countries towards increasing government regulation and control of health insurance financing. Health insurance is increasingly subject to legislation, regulation and the decisions of national governments. This applies equally to countries with a federal structure, such as Austria, Germany and Switzerland *(228)*. Factors behind this trend include the increasing government preoccupation with cost-containment issues and, to a lesser extent, issues of equity and solidarity. As government control increases, the traditional autonomy of health insurance funds tends to be correspondingly circumscribed.

Systems in transition

Two countries in the European Region, Israel and Turkey, currently have health insurance systems in a stage of transition, while in the eastern *Länder* of Germany the health care financing system is being transformed in accordance with the principles of the rest of the country.

Most of Israel's population is insured by four insurance organizations, membership of which is wholly voluntary *(229)*. Reform legislation passed in 1995 provides universal access to a specified benefit package, uniform premium contributions for all employers and employees, choice of sickness fund and the option of supplementary voluntary insurance *(230)*.

In Turkey, there are three insurance funds for blue-collar workers, the self-employed and pensioners, respectively; benefits vary from fund to fund, and coverage of the population is only partial *(229)*. Social insurance funds account for only one sixth of total health care spending, with tax revenues contributing about one third. A key objective of proposals to reform health care financing is to extend social insurance cover to the entire population. The reforms propose to provide a basic package of care, contributions related to ability to pay (being zero for the very poor), social insurance subsidized by the general budget and administration by a new quasi-governmental body *(2)*. Implementation of the reforms has yet to begin.

The German Democratic Republic had a tax-based health care system under strong central control. In the negotiations leading to accession to the Federal Republic of Germany, it was decided that the health care system of the eastern *Länder* would be put on the same organizational and financial basis as the rest of Germany as quickly as possible. On 1 January 1991, a network of sickness funds was established; the bulk of the population was compulsorily insured, and the contribution rate was set at 12.8% for at least one year, i.e. the average rate for the western *Länder (188)*.

TAX-BASED FINANCING
Well established systems
The countries whose health care systems are financed predominantly by general tax revenues comprise Ireland, the United Kingdom and the Nordic countries. Here, the earliest social protection systems for health care benefits made their appearance in the late nineteenth or early twentieth century, and took the form of social insurance schemes. As in the group 1 countries, these generally involved a multiplicity of sickness funds covering small portions of the total population (generally urban workers and their families), which were sometimes subsidized by the state. With the passage of time, efforts were made to increase population coverage, as in all countries that relied on social insurance. However, the following features distinguish this group of countries from those that still rely predominantly on social insurance:

- as coverage was extended to more of the population, the state assumed an increasing responsibility for financing through general tax revenues;
- coverage of the population was made universal (i.e. to include all residents in a country) so that contributions to an insurance fund ceased to be the factor determining entitlement to health care;
- the sickness funds tended to lose their separate identity and independence from the state; and
- the provision of health care services (operation of hospitals and other health care facilities, and employment of physicians and other health care personnel) increasingly became the responsibility of the public sector.

The process of transformation from social insurance to predominantly tax-based financing was completed for most of the countries in this group in the period shortly after the Second World War. Most of these countries still retain, although to varying degrees, an element of social insurance financing for health care.

The following are some of the key features of the financing systems of those countries that, some decades ago, completed the transition to predominantly tax-based financing:

- most of the costs of health care are provided from general taxation, which is raised at central, regional and/or local levels;

- unlike those raised through social insurance, these funds tend not to be earmarked (for example, in Denmark, Norway and the United Kingdom);
- in the United Kingdom in 1989, 79% of the cost of the NHS was financed by general tax revenues, with social insurance funds contributing 16% *(2,188)*; and
- in Finland since 1972, roughly 80% of costs have been financed by general tax revenues *(229)*.

In contrast to insurance-based systems, all residents or citizens of a country with tax-based health care financing are covered by the statutory system, and the range of services provided is comprehensive. In addition, all residents are eligible to receive the same range of services, unlike under social insurance systems. Ireland is an exception, as it has two categories of citizen linked to income level: only the poorest third of the population is eligible to receive all health care benefits without additional charges, while the remainder is subject to various out-of-pocket payments *(188)*.

Health care systems financed predominantly through taxation and providing universal and comprehensive coverage of the population on equal terms, tend to avoid some of the difficulties that could otherwise arise with respect to solidarity, as there is no room for risk selection.

Funds collected through social insurance are earmarked in accordance with the principles of social insurance financing, and used for different purposes in different countries. They are often used to finance other social security programmes, such as pensions and disability benefits, but a proportion of the funds collected through social insurance may be used for health care purposes. In the United Kingdom, the original intention was that the NHS was to be financed exclusively by tax revenues, but owing to limits imposed on such funding it has been forced to draw additional funds from social insurance *(228)*. In Sweden, social insurance pays for drugs and medical services in outpatient care, and in 1984 also paid a small part (8%) of hospital services *(229)*. In Finland, social insurance contributions are used mainly for private medical and occupational health services, drugs and auxiliary services *(2)*.

The initial division of social insurance contributions between employers and employees has been kept in some cases, as in the United Kingdom *(188)*. Other countries, such as Finland, Norway and Sweden, have eliminated the employee's contribution *(228)*. In Iceland, health insurance funds are publicly funded *(2)*.

As noted above, the health insurance funds lost their independent identity and became submerged in the public sector. In Denmark, for example, the hundreds of sickness funds that had existed since the end of the nineteenth century were abolished in 1973, and health insurance payments were assigned to Denmark's 280 municipalities *(229)*. In Norway in 1930, local benefit societies were converted into branch offices of the National Insurance Institute, a division of the Ministry of Social Affairs; in 1971, the collection and allocation of insurance funds were integrated with general income tax collection *(229)*. In 1989, health insurance funds were totally abolished in Iceland, and their role was taken over by the State Social Security Institution *(2)*.

There has been a pronounced trend towards devolving financial and corresponding service delivery responsibilities away from central government. Finland has progressed furthest in this respect, and since 1972 the basic administrative levels have been the municipalities; these have the authority to raise taxes and have legal responsibility for health service delivery *(2)*. Denmark and Sweden have also achieved a significant degree of decentralization. In Denmark, the counties are responsible for financing and delivery with respect to hospitals and health care reimbursement, while the municipalities have the responsibility for home nursing and for some preventive programmes *(2)*. In Sweden, the county councils finance most hospital services, including the payment of hospital doctors, through local income taxes *(2)*. In the United Kingdom, trends in decentralization are taking a somewhat different form since the recent separation of purchasers from providers, but here, too, the trend is towards allowing greater financial autonomy to local units. Only Iceland appears to be an exception, in that recent years have seen an increasing role for central government financing and a correspondingly decreasing role for local government *(2)*.

Central government still has a role, not only for financing public health, medical research and university teaching hospitals, but also as a source either of subsidies to the social insurance system (as in Sweden) or of grants and subsidies to local government units (as in Denmark, Finland and Norway) *(2,188)*.

Systems in transition

The countries in this group are in southern Europe. They have all embarked on a process of switching from predominantly social-insurance to predominantly tax-based financing, similar to that in for the group 3 countries. The main factor distinguishing them from the group 3 countries is time: they began the transition later (late 1970s to mid-1980s) and have not yet fully established their tax-based health systems.

The countries in this group were prompted to establish predominantly tax-based systems by the perceived need to extend coverage to sections of the population not previously covered, and by the desire to provide comprehensive services for the entire population. An additional consideration, in the cases of Greece and Italy, was the need to address fragmented financing and organizational structures.

Italy and Portugal were the first of these countries to establish national health services, in 1978 and 1979, respectively. Greece introduced similar legislation in 1983 and Spain followed in 1986, passing additional legislation in 1989 providing for a shift in financing towards general taxation. Numerous difficulties associated with efforts to reform financing mechanisms persist in all four countries, and financing at the present time remains mixed. In Greece, for example, where the 1983 legislation has only partially been implemented, hospitals are largely financed by tax revenues while outpatient care is still financed by the insurance funds. In Italy, social insurance contributions made up almost 40% of total public health care spending in 1990 *(2)*.

FROM CENTRAL CONTROL TO INSURANCE-BASED FINANCING
Reform of health care financing systems

The CEE and CIS countries have, almost without exception, declared their intention to change to an insurance-based system of financing, and some countries have taken major steps towards establishing such systems. The attraction of this type of financing is partly its dissimilarity to state financing under previous regimes. In addition, some CEE countries perceive this as a return to the health care arrangements prevailing before these regimes. Additional factors include greater choice for patients and personal entitlements through direct health care contributions, as well as higher levels of remuneration for physicians, changes that are supported by physicians' organizations. In addition, the CEE and CIS countries have been encouraged by those western European countries that themselves finance health care through some form of health insurance. Finally, a major consideration has been the hope that social insurance contributions will increase the total funds available for health care.

Most of the CEE and CIS countries have either passed or are in the process of preparing legislation to lay the basis for a transition to a system of social insurance financing. A number of them have begun the necessary preparations to make their social insurance systems operational; in others, contributions from employers and employees have already become one source of funding for health care.

Key characteristics of social insurance systems in the CEE and CIS countries

A number of characteristics of the newly established systems can already be identified from the experiences of those countries that have begun to set up health insurance.

EARMARKED FUNDS

In accordance with the principles of insurance financing, all monies accumulated by health insurance funds are earmarked for health care purposes in all countries planning or implementing statutory health insurance.

THE CONTINUING ROLE OF TAX-BASED FINANCING

In all these health insurance systems (actual or planned) there are provisions for supplementary budget financing, either in the form of contributions for non-paying sections of the population or for financing public health activities, medical education, medical research and large national research institutions.

INDEPENDENCE OF HEALTH INSURANCE FUNDS

While dependence on the state budget continues, the administrative body or bodies responsible for health insurance tend to be, to varying degrees, financially independent of the state budget and the finance ministry. In the early phases of implementation, financing comes from the state budget; at a later stage, it is separated from the state budget (for example, the Czech Republic, Hungary and Slovakia). This involves administrative separation, with the health insurance funds tending to become quasi-public entities.

GOVERNMENT CONTROL

The insurance companies or sickness funds are usually under some form of government control, with varying degrees of independence from the state *(231)*. In the

Czech Republic, for example, the National Health Insurance Company is a publicly sponsored private firm, as are the sickness funds *(232,233)*, which have a high degree of independence from state control. In Slovakia, by contrast, the health and finance ministries exercise relatively stronger control over the insurance companies.

NUMBERS OF INSURANCE FUNDS AND ORGANIZATIONAL STRUCTURE

Some countries have established, or are in the process of establishing, a plurality of insurance funds. A number of countries have established a central "national health insurance company" with local branches or specialized sickness funds (for example, the Czech Republic, Estonia, Hungary, Slovakia and Slovenia) *(155,231–234)*. The national level insurance company is a primary insurer covering, for example, 83% of the population in the Czech Republic *(233)* and 85% of the population in Slovakia *(234)*. At the same time, the national company has the responsibility for overseeing the local companies. Not all countries have a plurality of insurance funds; Albania's health insurance system, for instance, is run by a single social insurance fund *(235)*.

COMPULSORY INSURANCE

The insurance systems being developed stipulate that insurance is to be compulsory for those groups intended to be covered by the new system. In some isolated instances, more wealthy people may be permitted to opt out, as in Hungary *(236)*.

ENTITLEMENT

It is possible to discern a diverging pattern in health care reform documents. Some countries, such as the Russian Federation and Slovakia, are focusing on citizenship or residence as the basis of entitlement *(234,237)*, while a smaller group, including the Czech Republic and Hungary, is focusing on insurance contributions *(238)*. While most reform documents refer to the importance of maintaining universal or near-universal coverage, in practice some relatively small groups appear to be excluded, even in those countries that are trying to overcome the problems of achieving universality. In cases where entitlement is based on insurance contributions, the objective of universal coverage is more difficult to fulfil *(239)*. Estonia provides an example of a country that restricted population coverage in 1994; while in its earlier health care reform legislation entitlement was based on citizenship, a 1994 amendment made it dependent on contributions *(155)*.

THE BENEFITS PACKAGE

Countries introducing health insurance design a package of health care benefits that is stipulated in the appropriate legislation, and that applies equally to all insurance funds and to all those who are covered. There are often differences in the benefits offered by the different insurance funds over and above the basic package.

CONTRIBUTIONS

Contributions tend to be at a flat rate and related to income, and in most cases are shared between employer and employee. Nevertheless, there are very wide variations between countries both in contribution rates and in employer:employee ratios. Table 13 provides an indication of these rates and ratios in different countries.

CONTRIBUTIONS FOR NON-PAYING SECTORS OF THE POPULATION
These are typically the responsibility of government, which finances non-paying sectors of the population through budget revenues. In some cases, such as in Hungary, the unemployed and/or pensioners have their contributions paid by an unemployment fund or pension fund, respectively *(240)*.

CHOICE OF INSURANCE FUND
Most countries have either permitted or plan to allow the insured a choice of insurance fund, in order to foster competition between funds. In practice, however, the occupational or geographical composition of fund members may limit the actual degree of choice.

SOLIDARITY AND RISK ADJUSTMENT
Countries usually make efforts to adjust for unevenly distributed health risks *(155,233,234,237,241)*. The mechanism by which this is accomplished usually involves the transfer, in whole or in part, of health insurance funds to a central fund, which then redistributes these to the sickness funds according to specific criteria such as the size of the population and its age and sex distribution. In the Russian Federation, for example, according to the 1993 amendments to the 1991 health insurance legislation, special compulsory health insurance funds at the regional level were to be established to collect premiums for all residents of a region or of a large city. Health insurance companies would receive money from this regional fund. These payments were not to be based on the social position or income level of the insured, but on the age and sex structure of the insured group. At the beginning of 1994, there were 82 regional funds. A federal fund will redistribute premium revenues to ensure interregional equity *(237)*.

Table 13. Contribution rates and employer:employee ratios in selected CEE and CIS countries

Country	Contribution rate	Employer:employee ratio
Czech Republic	13.5	66:33
Estonia	13.0	100:1
Hungary	12.5	19.5:4
Slovakia	13.5	66:33
Slovenia	12.8	50:50
Russian Federation	3.6	100:1

Source: Chinitz *(240)*.

MOBILIZATION OF FUNDS FOR HEALTH CARE

Countries where health insurance has become a major source of funds for health care tend to show an increase in health care revenues, even though funding from the state budget has shown a net reduction. This is contrary to what was previously believed, namely, that rising unemployment and poor compliance would erode the revenue base. The proportion of GDP spent on health care has increased in these countries following their introduction of health insurance, and tends to be higher than in countries where health care is still financed from the state budget *(242)*.

Difficulties in switching to insurance-based financing

The CEE and CIS countries are attempting to set up health care financing systems in a relatively short period. Moreover, some are setting up health insurance systems under conditions that are not the most suited to rapid change: weak economies, unstable governments and inappropriate institutional infrastructures.

LOSS OF EXPENDITURE CONTROL

While the introduction of insurance appears to mobilize more funds for health care, it is not clear whether this is an effective use of resources. Health care financing under the former regimes was the responsibility of ministries of finance, which collected general revenues and allocated them for various purposes and thus exercised some form of spending control. Under health insurance financing, contributions are collected and distributed by various agencies that bypass the ministry of finance. Initially, ministries were pleased to be relieved of the fiscal responsibility for financing health care out of state budgets. In view of the deficits being accumulated by the health insurance funds (see below), which are subsidized by the state budget, however, government departments are still indirectly involved in financing health care but without the spending control they formerly enjoyed. This has led to significant tensions between the semi-autonomous social insurance funds and finance ministries in the Czech Republic, Hungary and Slovakia, where health spending increased significantly in the period immediately following the introduction of health insurance. Moreover, as noted above, any increase in the funds available for health care following the adoption of social insurance may be a reflection of inadequate long-term incentives for cost-containment *(240)*.

THE EMERGENCE OF STRUCTURAL DEFICITS

Health insurance schemes in the CEE and CIS countries aim to provide near-universal coverage, though to varying degrees. As noted earlier, governments achieve this by paying contributions for non-paying sections of the population from taxation, or through indirect contributions for pensioners and the unemployed from pension and unemployment funds. Since the cost of providing health care services for these sections of the population tends to be greater than the transfers received by the health insurance funds, many of these funds are experiencing persistant deficits. Examples include those in Croatia, the Czech Republic, Estonia, Hungary and Slovakia *(232,234,243,244)*. It was estimated that, in Hungary in 1996, the cost of health care benefits for the economically inactive population would be Ft 77.3 billion for pensioners, Ft 14.3 billion for the unemployed and Ft 22.8 billion for the remainder. The actual funds available will be Ft 65.7 billion in transfers to insurers to pay premiums for pensioners, Ft 7.3 billion for the unemployed and Ft 12 billion for the rest, resulting in a shortfall of about Ft 29 billion or 0.5% of GDP. This will be only partially offset by the contributions from the paying population. Efforts by governments to use deficit financing techniques to balance their budgets result in rapidly accumulating permanent deficits *(240)*.

DIFFICULTIES ENCOUNTERED IN RISK ADJUSTMENT

The aim of distributing funds equitably between insurance companies or sickness funds encounters difficulties similar to the structural deficits described above. In the Czech Republic, for example, a percentage of the premium income of all branch insurance companies (sickness funds), as well as the state contribution for target groups (the non-paying population) are transferred to a central fund, which then redistributes these funds to the insurance companies. There are problems, however, with the redistribution mechanism. The primary insurer, the National Health Insurance Company, has the highest proportion of pensioners and children and is not compensated sufficiently by the redistribution mechanism, while branch insurance companies (which are specialized sickness funds for employees of certain government agencies and economic sectors) receive premium revenues in excess of their spending on health care. This is due to the fact that the state contribution for special groups is significantly lower than the contributions made by paying individuals. While, in principle, anyone has the right to join a branch health insurance company, in practice they tend to discriminate in favour of people in good health and with high incomes. Their superior financial position allows them to provide more benefits to their subscribers, as well as to pay more to physicians and to purchase health care facilities *(232,233)*.

Similar problems have been encountered in Slovakia, which relies on a similar risk adjustment mechanism. The Slovak National Health Insurance Company, covering a great part of the economically inactive population (about 65% of the total) has been permanently in debt *(234)*.

INCREASING LABOUR COSTS

The shift from budget sources to health insurance results in increased labour costs. This has implications for international competitiveness as well as encouraging the non-reporting of economic activity, as both employers and employees seek ways to avoid the resulting heavy financial burden *(240)*.

THE INCREASING BURDEN OF CONTRIBUTIONS

Usually, health care is not the only service provided through social insurance; pensions and unemployment contributions are added to health contributions and these can sometimes reach considerable proportions. In Hungary, for example, the combined contribution rate is 60.8% of the net wage bill (including pensions, health care and unemployment), compared with an average of 31% in western European countries. Yet even this high contribution rate is not sufficient to cover the cost of health care without a significant transfer of resources from the state budget to the health insurance funds. Hungary is therefore now considering ways of shifting some of the redistributive elements of health care financing (pensions and unemployment) back to the state budget *(240)*.

COMPLIANCE PROBLEMS

As a result of the increasing burden of contribution payments, many state-owned enterprises and private employers are accumulating large arrears with their health insurance and other social insurance obligations *(240)*.

OTHER ISSUES

In seeking to organize and implement a shift to health insurance financing, many countries have discovered that the process is more difficult than they originally envisaged. The reasons include:

- the lack of adequate information technology;
- the lack of sufficient experience with information systems;
- the lack of technical expertise in insurance management and related areas;
- an insufficiently developed institutional infrastructure, including a well functioning banking system, capital markets, and contract and property law; and
- the absence of an appropriate government regulatory framework for operating newly established insurance institutions *(238)*.

Some of these institutional structures were not part of the previous socioeconomic framework, and will need to be developed in tandem with the development of health insurance systems.

THE ROLE OF PRIVATE HEALTH INSURANCE

Private insurance is currently available mainly in western European countries. A number of the CEE and CIS countries have declared their intention to allow private insurance at some future date, while some have already begun procedures for its establishment and operation.

The western European countries

In western Europe, private insurance serves two purposes. It provides voluntary, supplementary cover for certain sections of populations covered by a national health service or statutory insurance scheme. Private health insurance also provides voluntary cover for certain parts of the population in countries with statutory insurance systems, mainly those on a high income who have no other cover.

Voluntary health insurance for medical expenses is purchased for several different reasons. These partly depend on the country's predominant method of health care financing, and partly on arrangements peculiar to specific statutory financing systems.

Health care systems financed predominantly through taxation offer comprehensive cover for services, free at the point of entry. There is therefore relatively little scope for private insurance, which is, by and large, considered a luxury. Queues and rationing, which are associated with certain tax-financed health systems, however, encourage the demand for supplementary private health insurance for benefits such as shorter waiting times, choice of time of treatment, a wider choice of physician or hospital, and greater comfort. Examples of countries in this group are Italy, Spain and the United Kingdom *(245)*.

Health care systems financed predominantly through statutory health insurance are marked by the diversity of their arrangements. In Belgium and France, for example, while care is virtually universal, substantial payments are made at the point of delivery for which patients are only partially reimbursed. In France, reimbursement varies between 40% and 100%, while in Belgium it is set at a minimum of 75% *(245)*. In these countries, private insurance is taken out to reimburse the patient for the percentage of medical costs not funded by the statutory system, as well as for providing more comfortable accommodation.

In the cases discussed above, most private insurance policies are supplementary. By contrast, in Germany and the Netherlands, whose health care systems are also financed predominantly by social insurance, private insurance plays a role similar to statutory insurance for certain sections of the population. Coverage by the statutory system is not universal, owing to the arrangement that allows those with income above a certain level to opt out. In Germany, the better-off are offered the choice between statutory and private insurance. This involves about 20% of the population, half of whom choose to be insured privately *(246)*. In the Netherlands, those with income above a certain level have the option to become insured privately or remaining uninsured. About 40% of the population have been excluded from the statutory system *(188)*,[15] and the majority have taken out private cover *(245)*. This arrangement may be about to change, as proposed reforms make statutory insurance compulsory for all. In these two countries, therefore, private insurance either provides basic medical coverage to those excluded from the statutory system, or supplementary cover to those who already have statutory cover. In both Germany and the Netherlands, basic medical cover accounts for the bulk of insurance premiums, because it is more expensive than supplementary insurance.

The Swiss health care system, also predominantly based on social insurance financing, represents a somewhat different case in that, in contrast to all the countries mentioned above, statutory health insurance is optional. (Four cantons and certain municipalities make it compulsory, however, while some municipalities make it compulsory only for certain groups such as the elderly, children and those on low incomes.) None the less, almost 99% of the population is insured with the statutory system, and there is thus relatively less scope for private insurance for basic medical services. There is, however, greater scope for supplementary insurance coverage owing to a significant amount of cost sharing: Swiss households are responsible for

---

[15] This only applies to acute risks, as virtually the entire population is covered for chronic risks by the statutory health insurance system.

just under 30% of health care costs (not including insurance premiums paid by individuals) *(2)*.

The patterns discussed above are depicted in Fig. 18 and 19, which show the highly variable inroads made by private insurance in various western European countries. Health care systems relying predominantly on tax-based financing show the lowest reliance on private insurance financing, as shown by premium levels per head of population and penetration rates of private insurance (i.e. the percentage of the population taking out private insurance). This is a consequence of the comprehensive care provided by the national health services.

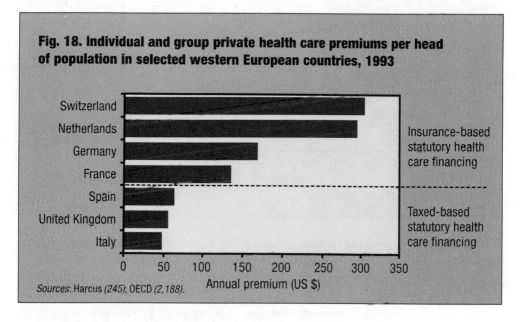

Fig. 18. Individual and group private health care premiums per head of population in selected western European countries, 1993

Sources: Harcus *(245)*; OECD *(2,188)*. Annual premium (US $)

Two countries in this group stand out: Denmark and Ireland. In Denmark, the bulk of private insurance reimbursement is for dental care and for drugs not covered by the publicly funded system. Ireland differs from other countries in the tax-based group, as it is the only one where benefits covered by the publicly funded system vary with income. There are two categories:[16] the poorest third of the population is entitled to comprehensive cover free of charge; the remainder is liable for certain out-of-pocket payments, either as co-payments or full payment for services not included in the benefits package *(188)*. There is therefore relatively more scope for private insurance penetration in Ireland.

As a group, the insurance-based countries show both higher private health care premiums per head and higher penetration rates. Penetration rates are very high in the Netherlands, because of the high percentage of people opting out of statutory insurance, and in France, because of the relatively low reimbursement rates. The Netherlands and Switzerland also have the highest levels of premiums per head. The

---

[16] There were three categories until 1991, when the two covering people on higher incomes were merged into a single category.

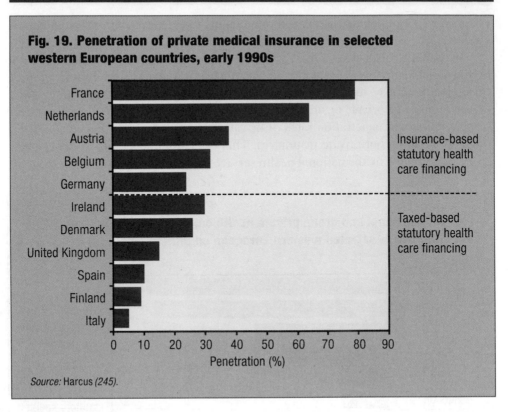

Fig. 19. Penetration of private medical insurance in selected western European countries, early 1990s

Source: Harcus *(245).*

intermediate level found in France – which at the same time has the highest penetration rate in Europe, 80% – is due to the fact that private health cover is almost exclusively supplementary, and therefore entails far lower premiums than cover for basic medical services.

In several countries of western Europe, funding from private insurance is increasing, although sometimes from a very low base. Growth rates could accelerate in coming years if governments attempt to curtail spending by shifting an increasing proportion of health care costs on to patients.

The CEE and CIS countries

The CEE and CIS countries had no private insurance during the Soviet era. Since then, as part of the processes of economic transformation, liberalization and health system reform, many countries have been debating the possibility of introducing private insurance, while others have begun procedures for its introduction. The policy rationale is to offer citizens the option of voluntary, supplementary insurance. In certain isolated instances, the possibility of allowing the better-off to opt out of the statutory insurance system and insure themselves exclusively with a private insurer has been considered. For the most part, however, private insurance is seen as a means of supplementing scarce resources for health care.

Slovakia has begun to offer voluntary insurance. This is offered: to people not covered by the compulsory insurance scheme, for services agreed in the private policy, and to people included in the compulsory scheme but desiring supplementary insurance. Cover by the statutory scheme is nearly universal, and therefore only small groups are excluded; these comprise people without permanent residence in Slovakia, those with permanent residence but employed by people who are insured in another country, and citizens who live abroad for more than six months of the year. As to supplementary insurance, the most important service so far offered involves reimbursement of health care costs incurred abroad. Both these types of insurance are offered by Slovakia's 11 statutory insurance companies, as well as by commercial (private) insurance companies (234).

Similar arrangements can be found in the Czech Republic, where voluntary insurance provides cover for foreign nationals not insured by the compulsory system, as well as supplementary insurance for services not offered by the compulsory system (233).

Voluntary insurance is available in the Russian Federation, and some citizens are making independent arrangements to supplement the benefits provided by the statutory system. Private companies have been set up, and these administer both compulsory and voluntary insurance (241).

In Latvia, private insurance companies provide voluntary insurance, and offer the same range of benefits as those offered by the statutory package as well as some additional services: dental care, rehabilitation treatment and pharmaceuticals. In addition, they provide access to advanced health care facilities with high levels of service and accommodation. By 31 January 1996, some 120 000 people were covered by these companies. This, however, is considered to be an interim arrangement during the transition from tax-based to predominantly insurance-based financing. It is expected that, once the social insurance system is in place, voluntary insurance will be utilized only to supplement the statutory package (247).

Where voluntary insurance is available in the CEE and CIS countries, it currently provides only a small proportion of total health care financing. It is, however, a source of financing that may grow significantly as institutional and regulatory frameworks are developed and the transition to new funding mechanisms progresses.

Solidarity and competition

Historically, the concept of "solidarity" has a variety of roots, among them Protestant as well as Catholic religious thinking on social justice, conservative reasoning about social order, Marxist–socialist ideas, and even the libertarian concept of a social contract (248,249). It was central to various pre-welfare-state arrangements such as friendly societies or company-based sickness funds, as well as to twentieth-century welfare states.

Solidarity is a rather vague term, however. Traditionally, the term was used for the "face-to-face" solidarity in small groups "keeping together", which became less important in the emerging welfare states. In a second meaning, solidarity has become a synonym for "risk pooling". This refers to all arrangements in which health care costs are not financed individually, and in which people who re-mained healthy through a given period financially support those who were sick and used the health care services.

In Europe, however, the term is predominantly reserved for health care systems that are designed to reduce health-related inequalities *(67)*. This has consequences for both the funding and the delivery of health care. According to this notion of solidarity, individual financial contributions should not depend on a person's previous health status, but should be related to his or her ability to pay. Services should not be delivered according to the ability to pay but according to "need" – although this is a vague and multidimensional term *(250)*. As a consequence, a health care system is judged to attain solidarity if it achieves some kind of *ex ante* redistribution between age groups, between income classes, between single people and families, and between good and bad health risks compared to a hypothetical, unregulated private health care market.

Whether a society can base health care funding on competition and maintain a high level of social solidarity at the same time is a challenging question.

PRIVATE INSURANCE

In many countries, including the United States, private health insurance schemes are operated in a manner that corrodes social solidarity. This is because the basis of payment from individual families to the health insurance company usually takes the form of risk-adjusted premiums reflecting the individual's health status. Under such a system, the chronically sick (if they manage to get access to health insurance at all) have to pay more for insurance than healthy people. This violates the principle of solidarity in both of the meanings described above: in risk pooling as well as in reduction of health-related inequalities.

In private health insurance markets, there is normally competition between health insurers. Even when premiums are adjusted for risk, competition between insurance companies still focuses on identifying the good risks and trying to attract those, rather than on simple price competition in the market. Through a process known as adverse selection, individuals who view themselves as good risks tend to opt out of insurance schemes that charge premiums high enough to cover the bad risks. As a result, premiums for the "self-confessed bad risks" who need to remain in the pool are driven up. Insurance companies that do not try to identify good risks and offer lower premiums may find themselves attracting bad risks, and are then liable to be driven out of the market *(251,252)*.

GENERAL TAXATION

The opposite extreme from competitive risk by means of adjusted premiums is health care funding through some form of general taxation. Solidarity, understood as risk pooling, is generally achieved through such a system. The amount of redistribution achieved depends largely on the progressiveness of the tax system. One recent study *(253)* demonstrated that funding from taxes is usually progressive, though the degree of progressiveness depends on the mix of specific taxes used to fund the health system. Thus, funding health care from this source can be viewed as contributing to social solidarity.

There is no market competition over health care funding in such an arrangement.[17] There can, however, be political–budgetary competition between health and other areas of government spending, and this may have implications for solidarity. Moreover, solidarity will be affected by the level of private health care financing that operates alongside, and is sometimes mixed with, public funding (67).

SOCIAL INSURANCE

Social insurance usually involves mandatory contributions by employers and employees, as well as by independent workers, pensioners and sometimes even the unemployed, that are used to fund social programmes such as health care, unemployment benefits and pensions. Sometimes a specific percentage of social insurance contributions is earmarked for health.

Unfortunately, social insurance systems do not usually contribute to solidarity in financial terms. Most social insurance systems fund health care in a regressive fashion (253), since contribution rates are usually calculated as a flat percentage of salaries or income and there is often a ceiling on the amount of income on which the social assessment is levied. In this situation, those earning above the ceiling pay a lower proportion of their incomes for social insurance and health care. Solidarity is also affected by rules governing those included or excluded from social insurance, or those who may opt out of it. If those with a high income are not included (or are able to opt out), they will not contribute to the system's funding, thus making it more regressive.

If a country has one social insurance agency that provides health care services, there is no competition. The same is true if there several agencies but individuals are not entitled to choose between them. Competition can be introduced into social insurance schemes, however, by allowing an individual to choose between them if they have an interest in attracting members. As in systems relying on private health insurance, there will be a "natural" conflict between solidarity and competition, in that social insurance schemes will try to attract good risks. Government regulation can attempt to set a framework for maintaining solidarity in such systems, and the extent to which solidarity will be eaten away by competition will depend heavily on this regulation (as well as on self-regulation, consumer education and scrutiny by the mass media).

OUT-OF-POCKET PAYMENTS

In most health systems in the western part of the Region, direct out-of-pocket payments by patients at the point of delivery make up a limited portion of overall health care funding. In terms of solidarity, out-of-pocket payments represent the most regressive form of payment for health care, since such payments constitute a greater share of income for the poor, who are also higher consumers of medical care. If regulatory guidelines exempt lower-income groups from co-payments, the

---

[17] As the British as well as some Scandinavian examples of "internal" markets have shown, there may be competition between providers for the money raised by general taxation (60).

consequences for social solidarity are less severe (see the section on cost sharing in Chapter 3, pages 83–100).

RECENT REFORMS IN THE CEE AND CIS COUNTRIES

As already noted, one central trend in the reforms in the CEE and CIS countries has been the desire to shift from funding health care through general tax revenues towards a significant reliance on national health insurance *(242)*. The former Yugoslavia had such a health insurance system before the transition, while Hungary (1991), the Russian Federation (1991), the Czech Republic (1992), Estonia (1992), Kyrgyzstan (1992), Latvia (1993), Slovakia (1993), Georgia (1995) and Kazakstan (1996) have all since adopted such systems. Even Albania, with an annual income per head of only US $340, has introduced a limited form of health insurance. Although the implementation of social insurance has already begun, a number of these countries still find it necessary to rely predominantly on general revenues to fund health services. Other countries, such as Belarus, Bulgaria, Lithuania, Poland and Romania, which currently rely on general revenues as the principal source of health care funding, are considering national health insurance laws.

While this trend is an expression of the countries' will to decentralize and liberalize their health care systems, in terms of solidarity the impact of the new source of funding is likely to be regressive. In practice, all CEE countries that have introduced national health insurance also continue to rely in part on general budgetary revenues. In the CIS, budgetary revenues continue to provide the majority of health care funds.

In the process of shifting from a tax-funded system to social insurance, discussions have often taken place on "opening" the system to allow some of the population to opt out of mandatory insurance. There was pressure from some newly self-employed health professionals to introduce more "freedom of choice" by giving the financially well-off the opportunity to insure privately or to pay their doctors out-of-pocket. To date, however, none of the CEE countries has "de-insured" any part of its population or turned to private health insurance as the main source of health care financing. Thus the potential problems for social solidarity that would result from abolishing or severely limiting mandatory arrangements have been avoided in the official sector.

There is, however, a growing informal sector. Since, in this sector, services are provided only for those who can afford them, the ability to pay is playing a more important role in health care than before. Although most CEE countries continue to offer a more or less comprehensive benefits package through their public health care systems (with only minor exclusions of coverage for nonessential activities),[18] overall solidarity in health financing has therefore been reduced. Another problem created by the informal sector in some systems is a loss of control over total spending, as well as "leakage" of health professionals' earnings from the income tax system.

---

[18] Examples are the exclusion of treatment at health sanatoria (the Czech Republic and Slovakia), plastic surgery (Croatia) and ambulance services (Hungary). Poland has also introduced a "negative list" of activities that are not covered through its national health service. Almost all the CEE countries have restricted the list of drugs and medical appliances that are fully or partially reimbursed through public funding.

It is too early to evaluate the impact of these reforms on equity, health gain, efficiency and quality of care. This is especially true since reforms in the health care sector are taking place within a dramatically changing social and economic context. Those changes – rising rates of unemployment and poverty, as well as structural changes in the economy – are also having a serious impact on health and health care systems.

RECENT REFORMS IN WESTERN EUROPE

Although most health politicians in western Europe would emphasize that health care systems still achieve a certain level of solidarity, the concept of a solidaristic health care system has been the target of increasing scepticism. Although conditions and debates vary between countries, the basic reasons for this scepticism are similar *(2)*:

- rising health care spending conflicts with strong pressures on governments not to increase taxes or quasi-taxes in a globally competitive environment;
- a powerful libertarian, neoclassical philosophy argues that health should be much more a private than a public good *(254)*; and
- rising health care spending is increasingly perceived to be the result of the collective, public organization of health systems – moral hazard and supplier-induced demand being prominent issues.

A shift in the age structure is expected to lead to an increase in spending on health care per head of population, yet most European governments have been cautious about introducing funding reforms that would directly damage solidarity. The eight-year story of health reform in the Netherlands reflects in key respects the reluctance of successive governments to embrace competitive financing if it would exact a cost in solidarity *(67,114)*. This tension also can be seen in the 1995 health insurance law in Israel, and in reforms currently under way in the German sickness fund system.

In Israel, the new law sought to rearrange previous financial flows in order to promote more equity. Assessed contributions by employers and employees are paid into a central fund. These funds, combined with direct government contributions, are distributed to the sickness funds on an age-adjusted capitation basis. The result is that the largest fund, which has a higher proportion of elderly and poor subscribers, now receives more revenue and the three small funds, with healthier subscribers, receive less. Moreover, funds are prohibited from selecting their members. The overall financial position of the large fund has been improved, while the small funds must now cover all types of subscriber with less revenue.

While it is too early to evaluate these changes, one outcome appears to have been a redistribution of the burden of health contributions. A recent survey revealed that very few of those with the lowest incomes report that their health payments have increased, while most of the wealthy report an increase *(255)*. This is an indication that the law is achieving one of its goals: increased equity in the burden of health care funding, based on principles of solidarity.

In Germany, a risk-adjustment formula was introduced in 1994 to take account of the income, age and sex of those insured and whether they received invalidity pensions. Funds that insure the young, wealthy and healthy must pay part of their revenues to sickness funds with "bad" risk structures. As a result, the differences in contribution rates between funds have fallen considerably. A second element of the reform was the introduction of a degree of "freedom of choice". Starting in 1996, more than 95% of the insured can choose membership in more than 15 large sickness funds, and may change insurers annually. There is mandatory open enrolment, intended to guarantee that these sickness funds cannot deny access to applicants.

The major political reason for introducing these measures was not to stimulate competition but, as in Israel, a concern for equity and solidarity *(256)*. None the less, giving everybody the right to choose health insurance inevitably leads to competition between sickness funds.

So far, German sickness funds have lacked the mechanisms for "real competition". Apart from activities in some minor areas, such as antismoking programmes, diet courses and administrative services, opportunities for competition were significantly reduced during the 1970s and 1980s because the government required all sickness funds to pursue common policies in their relations with providers *(257)*. Today, sickness funds are calling for deregulation of their relations with health care providers, in order to have more opportunities to compete with each other. Some of the sickness funds also want to be allowed to provide supplementary insurance. At present, it is unclear to what extent health politicians will satisfy these requests.

CONCLUSION

In Germany, Israel and the Netherlands, as well as in Belgium and Switzerland, politicians have sought to introduce competition between sickness funds while maintaining solidarity. The objectives were not the same everywhere – sometimes (most clearly in Israel, but also in Germany) equity and solidarity were the main concerns. In other places (most clearly in the Netherlands, but in Switzerland, too) the driving motivation was to use competition between health insurers as a mechanism for introducing market-oriented health care reform.

Yet competition between insurers (regardless of whether they are private or public) tends to erode solidarity in health care financing, since health insurers will inevitably engage in adverse risk selection. In all these countries, politicians have had to find solutions to this problem. One common answer has been mandatory open enrolment. Another, closely linked to financing, was introducing a risk-adjustment system for redistributing the health insurance systems' revenues to competing health insurers. Although technical procedures have differed between countries, the central idea is the same: the financial wellbeing of sickness funds should not depend on the "risk structure" of their members. Neither the income, gender or age of the insured nor the number of his or her children should have any impact on the ability of funds to compete against each other. The objective is that solidarity be maintained despite the fact that insurers are competing. Choice of health insurer shall be given to the population without disadvantaged individuals paying the bill.

There are few definitive data yet available to support empirical conclusions about the impact of these financial reforms on equity, health gain, efficiency and quality of care. Some tendencies can be described in general terms, however.

The risk adjustment formulae currently applied are far from perfect *(114)*. Differences in morbidity are in most cases measured only by age and sex, which are crude indicators at best. Thus differences in nominal premiums (as in the Netherlands and Switzerland) or in contribution rates (as in Germany) are partly due to uneven risk structures. This may be seen as a violation of equity. It is also a violation of the allocative signalling function of the level of premiums, in that individuals may choose not the most efficient health insurer but the one with the best risk structure. Thus allocative efficiency due to competition among insurers may be suffering. In the case of Germany and Switzerland, differences in contribution levels due to the uneven risk structures between sickness funds were larger before the new system was introduced. In these countries, therefore, equity and allocative efficiency were improved within the existing framework of competition.

Since different risk structures are not completely neutralized by the risk-adjustment system, health insurers still have incentives to "skim the cream". Consequently, they have begun to develop marketing strategies with which they try to attract good risks *(67)*. Within the limitations defined by public regulation, health insurers are also trying to tailor their benefit schemes and to negotiate contracts with providers that will be attractive to the wealthier (and healthier) people they prefer to insure. To the extent that these activities limit the benefits provided for vulnerable groups or for the chronically sick, competition will result in a reduction in health gain.

From the viewpoint of advocates of market-oriented health care, competition between health insurers makes sense only if insurers are freed from detailed hierarchical regulation of provider contracts. Yet health politicians in most of these countries are reluctant to reduce cost-containment regulations developed over the last 20 years. If health insurers are not given more freedom to behave as prudent, competitive buyers of health care, the potential benefits from competition (in efficiency terms, but also in terms of choice based on different contracts between purchasers and providers) may not be achieved. One advantage, however, would remain even then: if consumers could choose between several health insurers, insurers would be likely to show somewhat greater responsiveness towards their members than they would in the case of a monopoly.

Maintaining solidarity in health care funding while introducing competition between insurers is an ambitious and difficult undertaking. Owing to the forces unleashed by competitive markets, introducing competition without damaging solidarity cannot be achieved solely through deregulation. The solidarity safety net has to be designed very carefully, and this requires sophisticated supervision of health care markets. Moreover, several crucial questions have not yet been answered. It remains to be demonstrated whether competition among insurers leads to more efficient and effective health care, and whether newly implemented mechanisms that combine solidarity with competition will be successful in sustaining both policy objectives.

5 Allocating Resources Effectively

A number of countries in both the eastern and western parts of the Region have begun to move from integrated models of provision towards separating public, or quasi-public, third-party payers from health service providers. As direct managerial relationships between these actors weaken, resource allocation mechanisms become increasingly salient in enabling payers to achieve macro-level control of expenditure as well as improved institutional efficiency. Key strategies for allocating resources more effectively include contracting mechanisms, payment systems for professionals and institutions, purchasing mechanisms for pharmaceuticals, and allocation of capital for investing in health.

Buying better health: resource allocation, purchasing and contracting

In a number of countries in Europe, contracting is seen as an instrument for implementing health policy objectives. It is a coordinating mechanism that offers an alternative to the traditional command-and-control models of health care management. An essential element of contracting is that it facilitates a more market-oriented form of institutional resource allocation based on separating purchasers from providers. Contracting mechanisms bind third-party payers and providers to explicit commitments, and generate the economic motivation to fulfil those commitments.

In health systems based on social insurance, contracts between third-party payers and suppliers of health services have existed for many years. In Germany and the Netherlands, for instance, complex institutional structures have developed to represent health insurers and physicians in negotiating payment schedules. These contracting arrangements, however, primarily existed to stabilize the relationships between insurer and provider. In current reforms, particularly in tax-based health care systems, contracting has become a device for price and quality negotiations, as well as for ensuring provider compliance.

The introduction of contracting should not be seen as a development that is occurring only in health care. In practice, it is part of a wider process currently taking place in many sectors of public policy and society. The Dutch sociologist De Swaan has described this process in terms of a transition from a command society towards a negotiating society, in which contractual relations replace traditional hierarchical relations. In his view, there are two main explanations for this movement towards a more symmetrical balance of power in society. Rapid technological change and the growing need for more efficiency and innovation require a more efficient type of coordination than the rigid command-and-control model. The process of democratization and individualization in society points in the same direction. In De Swaan's view, the contract model has a greater potential for responsiveness to individual or small group needs than the command-and-control model *(258)*. These observations are also relevant in understanding the present process of change in health care systems.

CONCEPTUAL ISSUES

Proponents of contracting present four major reasons for introducing contractual relationships into tax-based, command-and-control health systems.

Encouraging the decentralization of management

A study in the NHS in the United Kingdom points out that contracting permits delegation of responsibility down the line of management, allowing lower-level managers more power to deploy resources to meet population needs *(259)*. Two major mechanisms can be used for decentralizing management through contracting: clear specification of commitments between contracting parties in terms of services to be provided, and reallocation of risk between purchasers and providers.

The first mechanism makes providers' commitments actual rather than merely formal. They are bound in terms of outcomes rather than performance inputs. These commitments are linked to the availability of financial resources, which is particularly important for the CEE and CIS countries where the health sector is greatly underfunded owing to the traditional allocation of funds to this sector by a "residual" method. The clear specification of commitments on both sides also makes decentralization of management an imperative of state policy rather than only the subjective choice of decision-makers.

Contracts also offer traditional risk-sharing arrangements. The responsibility of third-party payers for covering unpredicted expenditures gives way to contractual sharing of risks between purchasers and providers. The types of risk-sharing arrangement range from simplified contractual provisions in cost and volume contracts with hospitals (in the NHS reforms in the United Kingdom) to various PHC budget holding schemes (in the Russian Federation, the United Kingdom and some regions of Sweden). Their common feature is that providers become responsible to some degree for unplanned spending.

Improving the performance of providers

Clear-cut contractual provisions can overcome blurred responsibilities by giving payers levers with which to influence providers' behaviour. Hospitals and physicians become financially responsible for providing a specified volume, quality and mix of services at negotiated or regulated prices.

Contracting also incorporates the monitoring and evaluation of a set of performance indicators. For example, current contracts in the British NHS formalize this process by specifying targets and performance indicators. This enables purchasers to substantiate claims for better provider performance, and also to settle disputes. Here, the major limitation on implementation is the lack of adequate data.

Improving the planning of health care development

The rationale for using contracting as a planning tool is that it provides a direct link between planning and resource allocation. Providers are economically motivated to follow the planning strategy embodied in the contractual arrangements.

Contracting can be regarded as an alternative way to do some of the things that have traditionally been accomplished by planning. Purchasers engaging in health needs assessment and setting priorities pay selected providers to deliver services that will best meet the needs of resident populations. For example, plans for an interregional diagnostic centre may take a contractual form whereby the regions involved in the project are committed to sharing resources and expenses for running the new facility.

Moreover, contracting can encourage the development of information systems. Purchasers interested in the practice of good contracting require information about health status, health needs, health outcomes, the costs of services and the performance of providers, without which informed contracts cannot be drawn up.

Improving the management of care

One of the major objectives of contracting is to encourage a shift from inpatient to outpatient care, and also to more cost-effective medical interventions. This strategy is of particular importance for the CEE and CIS countries, where previous bureaucratic control led to severe distortions in the structure of health care provision. Inpatient costs in the Russian Federation, for example, amount to around 70% of health spending, against an OECD average of 44% for hospitals and 55% for hospitals plus long-term care.

CONTRACTING AND PUBLIC HEALTH
Contracting and equity

Contracts can support equity if, through needs assessment, they take explicit account of vulnerable and disadvantaged groups as well as underserved communities. From this perspective, purchasers represent the interests of their populations, allocating resources and purchasing services in accordance with the needs of their communities.

Contracting also brings dangers, however, that can undermine equity. For example, it has been argued that services that are less profitable, as opposed to less efficient, may be underemphasized or phased out *(55)*.

Contracting and community participation

Community participation in contracting can generate a democratization process in health services, increase the accountability of governments and the medical profession, and make health policy more relevant to the needs and priorities of society.

The contracting process can be divided into three stages: the pre-contracting stage, the actual contract or written agreement stage, and the post-contracting stage. The community can participate in all three of these stages.

Contracting and intersectorality

It can hardly be argued that intersectorality is present in contracting as currently practised, since contracting today focuses mainly on primary, secondary and tertiary curative care. Yet numerous aspects of curative care are linked with other activities in the community, such as education, employment and social protection mechanisms, to mention but a few. Contracting could therefore be used as a mechanism for involving the different interfaces of these activities in health care. In addition, there is potential for contracting to be introduced in areas other than health care, i.e. in community and environmental health services.

APPROACHES TO CONTRACTING

Two such approaches are possible. First, contracting can be seen as an instrument of health care planning and management in both competitive and noncompetitive environments. This implies that contracts can be an integral part of the planning process, irrespective of the role market mechanisms play in resource allocation. In other words, contracting is regarded as the formalization of the planning and management process, with the contracting parties making explicit commitments to objectives and targets.

In the second approach, contracting is viewed as a tool for making an informed choice of providers. This type of contracting is implemented in competitive environments, and is designed to encourage competitive tendering for packages of medical benefits and services.

The two approaches are not necessarily mutually exclusive. The requirements set by purchasers in the course of competitive tendering may include provisions designed to improve resource planning and the management of the health care structure.

Contracts define the relationships between different categories of participant in any health care system. Types of contract can vary widely. Contracting can be analysed according to four basic elements: who the contracting parties are, the legal status of health sector contracts, the particular type of contracting mechanism and the comprehensiveness of contracting (e.g. bilateral as against multilateral relationships).

Contractual parties

In the Beveridge model, the demand side is represented by public sector health authorities. A recent innovation in the Russian Federation, Sweden and the United Kingdom is that PHC providers also act as purchasers of care. The providers are on the supply side. The subject of the contracts might be not only inpatient or outpatient care but also public health, programmes for specific diseases or community care. In the Bismarck model, the scope for contracting by the government is much narrower, as statutory insurers act as the purchasers of care. Here, contracting is between insurers and employers or individual subscribers, and between insurers and providers. This might be supplemented by contracts between insurers and the government for providing subsidies, and between insurers and central insurance agencies.

In the Bismarck model, purchaser/provider relationships may be regulated by collective rather than by individual contracting, such as contracts between physicians' associations and insurers (or their associations). Sometimes, collective contracting is also used in countries with a predominant model of individual contracting. In the United States, so-called "umbrella contracting" has recently been used by informal associations of physicians. In this format, the physician authorizes a loose association of peers to negotiate service contracts with purchasers *(260)*. Similar contracting is taking place in the Russian Federation: agreements between a regional authority, insurance funds and associations of health providers serve as the basis for individual contracts.

There is a distinction between "hard" and "soft" contracting. In hard contracting, the contracting parties are relatively autonomous and press their interests actively and strongly. In soft contracting, contracts have a lower degree of formality, and the contracting parties have a closer identity of interests. The relationship between third-party payers and providers depends more strongly on cooperation, mutual support, trust and continuity in relations, as opposed to competition and opportunism *(6)*. Soft contracts are less likely to be legally binding. In the contractual relationships following the reforms of the British NHS, for example, contracts are not legal documents and the government did not intend that they should be legally enforceable. As such, they can also be described as "service agreements" and "understandings", and would not be defined as contracts in the legal sense.

Purchasers play different roles in contracting, depending on the legal status of providers. When contracting with independent or autonomous providers (e.g. hospital trusts), health authorities are acting as purchasers with all the rights and responsibilities that apply to the relationships between entities, each of which is voluntarily and deliberately engaging in an exchange. When contracting with state-owned providers, they are acting as "commissioners", as representatives of the government. In the former case there is a purchaser/provider split, and in the latter a commissioner/provider split.

The distinction between purchasing and commissioning can be related to the distinction noted above between hard and soft contracts. Purchaser/provider relationships can be based on either hard or soft contracts. Commissioner/provider relationships are more likely to be less formal, and to be based on trust, continuity and cooperation.

The content of contracts
Three types of contract are employed.

BLOCK CONTRACT
This can be compared to a budget for a defined service. The purchaser (or commissioner) agrees to pay a sum in exchange for access to a broadly defined range of services. Block contracts may additionally contain agreements concerning the maximum and minimum volume of the services to be provided and the assessment or monitoring of quality, although this area still remains underdeveloped owing to the lack of information on cost–effectiveness and health outcomes.

COST-AND-VOLUME CONTRACT
This represents a refinement of the block contract, in that payment for specific services is more explicitly related to the services to be offered. For example, it may entail an agreement for the purchaser (or commissioner) to pay a specified amount

for a specified number of patients to be treated in one specialty. In a further refinement, the payments may be differentiated in accordance with the service rendered (for example, high-, medium- and low-cost categories).

COST-PER-CASE CONTRACT
A single cost is set for each item of service. To date, limited use is made of this type of contract as it requires information on the cost of individual treatments at a level of detail and precision not currently available. Cost information systems are in the process of being developed, and are increasingly used to achieve more effective resource management.

THE IMPLEMENTATION OF CONTRACTING
Contracting practices in the European Region differ widely, reflecting the model of financing and organization of health care found in each country. Countries can be divided into four groups with regard to contracting: those following the Beveridge model, those following the Bismarck model, southern European countries with a mixed model, and the CEE and CIS countries. The rationale for forming a special group for the CEE and CIS countries is that these emerging health systems often do not fall into the traditional typologies. Rather, they are a transitional type of system.

Beveridge-style health systems
Health care reforms introducing contracting in the Beveridge group of countries seek to soften the command-and-control elements of this model. Contracting entails the introduction of a split within the public health sector between payers and providers. Among the countries in this group, three have directly introduced contracting.

FINLAND
Since the beginning of 1993, reforms of the state subsidy systems have created a commissioner/provider configuration. The financing and provision of health care in Finland are the responsibility of municipalities. As part of reforms that altered the system of state subsidies, the municipalities were given greater freedom to organize service provision and were permitted to take on a more active role vis-à-vis providers, although they retain responsibility for providing health (and social) services. As a result of the reforms, hospital financing has changed so that revenues depend on the services requested by the municipalities.

A key objective of these reforms is increasing municipal (local-level) flexibility in service provision, with a corresponding reduction in central government control. This goes hand-in-hand with efforts to strengthen municipalities' position vis-à-vis hospital providers. It is unclear at present whether these reforms will lead to a fully fledged purchaser/provider split.

SWEDEN
A number of counties have introduced purchasing and selling activities between a public agency at county or subcounty level and the county's hospitals. Other elements of

these reforms include: contracting relationships between counties and private providers, PHC providers in some counties acting as purchasers of inpatient care, and consumer choice of outpatient and inpatient care settings (6).

UNITED KINGDOM

The contracting parties on the purchasing side emerging from the purchaser/provider split include: local health authorities, which were previously involved with both the financing and management of hospital and community services; and fund-holding GPs, originally organized in large group practices with over 9000 patients, who have exercised the option to hold budgets for certain inpatient, elective and outpatient services. These two groups of purchaser contract with self-governing but publicly owned NHS hospital trusts, private hospitals and/or community services.

According to the classification of contracts described above, local health authorities act as commissioners rather than as purchasers; GP fundholders, on the other hand, act only in the capacity of purchasers.

Bismarck-style health systems

Contracting has been a part of the Bismarck-style, social-insurance-based health systems of continental Europe since their inception. Until recently, however, these contracts did not focus on price or efficiency; neither were they understood to be contestable. Rather, traditional social insurance contracting simply formalized a long-term payment arrangement. These contracts were typically negotiated between associations of sickness funds (payers) and associations of hospitals and/or physicians (providers), overseen and guided by national legislation.

Since the late 1980s, however, the Netherlands has attempted to introduce a more price-sensitive form of contracting, which would incorporate premium payments by individuals as well as contracts between the third-party payers (sickness funds) and provider institutions. Germany is scheduled to introduce a similar arrangement.

GERMANY

Contracting in Germany remains largely an exercise in formal relationships, although elements of financial efficiency are beginning to play a role. An effort was made to increase the discretionary power of insurers over providers following the 1989 health care reform legislation, when sickness funds were given the freedom to cancel contracts with inefficient hospitals. Nevertheless, the collective (as opposed to the selective) nature of contracting remains. Another relevant provision in this legislation was that hospitals were obliged to publish price lists.

Remuneration of physicians in the outpatient sector is based on a points system. Contracts concluded at national level between federal sickness fund associations and federal physicians' associations establish a fee schedule that includes about 2500 items of service, as well as a relative points scale. These agreements are revised only infrequently. Sickness fund associations at the *Land* level (the purchasers) negotiate with physicians' associations at the national level to pay a prospective lump sum, distributed to physicians in accordance with the nationally negotiated fee schedule and the volume of services provided. Physicians are reimbursed on a fee-for-service basis using the fee schedule, the relative points value scale, and a monetary value per point. Since the total amount to be transferred to the physicians' association is fixed in the agreement, the fee per point is inversely proportional to the volume of services provided collectively by the physicians.

Hospital remuneration is determined by contracting between hospital associations and sickness fund associations, and is based on an agreed average daily rate to be paid for each patient day. Volume is controlled through prospective global budgeting, which, from 1996, was also to be handled through a revenue pool at the *Land* level. Contracts can also include agreements on the quality of services.

Compared to contracting as currently practised in the United Kingdom, German purchasers are more limited, particularly regarding the specification of services.

NETHERLANDS

The 1987 Dekker committee *(261)* proposed using contracting as a tool to shift the balance of power away from providers to insurers. The sickness funds' relationship with providers (hospitals and physicians) was to be altered by abolishing the requirement that the funds should conclude contracts with all interested providers, and by granting them the freedom to contract selectively. In the new system, insurers would be able to exercise discretion with regard to the providers they contracted with. Such voluntary contracting would transform insurers from passive administrators and funders into more active purchasers and managers. While insurers have been granted freedom to contract selectively with physicians, this has yet to be implemented with respect to hospitals *(156)*.

The new scheme of contracting is designed to change the pattern of relationships between insurers and individual citizens. Insurers seek to expand their market share by offering additional medical benefits, such as annual check-ups, cross-border care in order to limit waiting time, and medical services in addition to the basic package. This is a new development, as until recently in the Netherlands (and in other Bismarck-style countries) the contracts were determined by government regulation, and citizens below the sickness fund income ceiling had little choice among insurers.

The southern European countries

Greece, Israel, Italy, Portugal, Spain and Turkey all have mixed systems that combine elements of both the Bismarck and the Beveridge models. Greece, Italy, Portugal and Spain are in transition from primarily insurance-based to primarily tax-based systems, and as such either have established or are in the process of establishing national health services. Although there are continuing reforms in some regions of Italy (Emilia Romagna and Veneto) and Spain (Catalonia and the Basque Country), in general these countries have not implemented contracting between payers (in this instance government or public bodies) and providers.[19]

---

[19] In Spain, reform proposals in 1991 included provisions for a purchaser/provider split that would lead to the development of contracting. The recommendations, however, have only been partially implemented.

Turkey differs in that it is in the process of extending insurance coverage to parts of the population not previously covered. Recent health care reform proposals include arrangements for purchaser/provider contracting. The proposals provide that insurance premiums (which are to be subsidized by tax revenues) collected from four insurance funds (three existing funds, plus a new one to be established) are to be transferred to provincial health directorates. These directorates will therefore be the payers and they will contract with selected hospital providers. The selected hospitals, for their part, are to be autonomously managed. These proposals have not yet been implemented.

The CEE and CIS countries

Health care systems in these countries were historically based on the Semashko model, a rigorously hierarchical, nationally controlled system in which all health personnel, including physicians, are state employees. A number of countries in this group have already begun the change over to an insurance-based system inspired by the Bismarck model, while others have expressed an interest in the possibility of doing so in the future. A few are attempting to introduce contracting between payers and providers in the context of newly established health insurance systems. Many of the issues surrounding the contractual arrangements between insurers and providers have yet to be worked out. Countries attempting to implement contracting through a purchaser/provider split include Bulgaria, the Czech Republic, Estonia, Georgia, Hungary, Romania and the Russian Federation.

RUSSIAN FEDERATION

In accordance with health insurance legislation passed in 1991, mandatory health insurance (MHI) has been introduced on a highly decentralized basis. Each of the 88 regions can build up its own system of MHI, though the major elements of the system are determined by federal legislation. These elements are: employers make income-related contributions to the MHI regional fund for their employees; local authorities make contributions to the fund for the nonworking population, and directly finance a number of health programmes and providers; the regional fund allocates resources to competing insurers based on a weighted capitation formula; and insurers (in some regions, the branches of the fund) pay health providers (262).

According to this pattern of financial flow, at least four areas of contractual relationship arise: between employers and insurers, between insurers and the MHI regional fund, between local government and insurer (or the fund), and between insurers and health providers. In some regions, regional or local health authorities contract directly with medical providers (195,239). These contracts are relatively rare, since most health authorities allocate resources directly. Thus the major purchaser is the insurer or the branch of the fund.

The types of contract with providers are similar to those used in the United Kingdom. The emphasis, however, is on different cost-per-case contracts for hospitals and capitation contracts for polyclinics. Quality control and consumer complaints settlements are also included in the contracts. Providers are committed to perform according to approved clinical standards, and they are subject to monitoring by insurers. There are specific provisions on the financial sanctions for violating standards, and on procedures for quality control. The scope for decentralizing hospital management, according to the contract, is no less than for the British hospital trusts.

In most of the regions, contracts provide for purchasers to be the major risk bearers. They are committed to pay for each case of inpatient care and in some regions, such as Moscow, for each service by polyclinics. To make this possible, risk arrangements are contracted between the regional fund and insurers, each party retaining reserves to pay for unpredicted expenditures. There is some evidence, however, of growing interest in risk management between insurers and providers. In the Kemerovo region, for example, polyclinics are close to becoming fundholders for all types of outpatient care and a specified portion of inpatient care, and they thereby share risks with the insurers as final purchasers.

The regional MHI scheme is regulated by the collective contract (agreement) between the regional government, the regional fund and medical associations. It specifies the general rules of funding and management of the MHI system, including the methods and rates of payment and the basic package of medical benefits. The major provisions of the collective agreement deal with the mechanisms of equalization of funding across insurers and, correspondingly, across subscribers. Thus the system is designed to introduce contractual relationships with providers, while seeking to maintain solidarity and equity.

KEY ISSUES CONCERNING CONTRACTING

The move to more sophisticated cost-and-volume and cost-per-case contracting models is limited by the fact that there is insufficient information to conduct an effective purchasing policy. The minimum information requirements for effective contracting cover patient flow data, cost and utilization information across specialties or diagnostic groups, and demographic and risk group information. Large investments need to be made in information systems, including the capacity to process bills. It is also important to disseminate information that will facilitate rational choice of providers. The resistance of health authorities and medical professions to collecting and disseminating health information, and as well as their tendency to manipulate the available information, must be overcome.

An associated issue is rising transaction costs, i.e. the costs associated with the continuing interaction of purchasers and providers (needs assessment, performance analyses, negotiating, monitoring, etc.). Substantial increases in quality and efficiency are required in order to justify these additional costs. To reduce transaction costs, some scholars encourage purchasers and providers to enter into long-term contractual relationships, rather than to view their task as one of making spot market deals (19,263).

Adopting a contract-based allocation system has a number of implications for human resources. Staff have to be trained and supported over the long term while they develop the sophisticated negotiating skills necessary for effective contracting. Even with these skills, purchasers typically encounter difficulties negotiating on an equal basis with providers, as the latter have long dominated most service delivery decisions. Conversely, providers are extremely wary about the redistribution of authority involved in contracting.

There are several additional issues involved in contracting in the Russian Federation and other CEE and CIS countries, the main one being the underfunding of the system. Public funding needs to be adequate and predictable in order to meet the bills of contracted providers. In transitional economies, this condition is rarely met. Health spending in the Russian Federation amounts to only 3–4% of gross national product (GNP). In addition, the state's commitment to provide services without (at least officially) instituting user charges is generous, even by the standards of more developed countries. Hence, political commitments may conflict with contractual arrangements.

The transition from directly allocated resources to contractual relationships with providers is not an easy process. One major reason for a slow pace of reform is unclear specification of the responsibilities of insurance funds and health authorities. Health authorities retain their responsibilities as direct providers of a high proportion of health care, and keep control over finances for noncontractual allocations to providers. For example, in most of the regions in the Russian Federation, the share of contracted health expenditure in 1995 varied from 20% to 30%.

The fragmentation of funding policy is a further constraint. This results in one payer – health insurers – acting as a purchasing agency, while a second – health authorities and local government – allocates additional health sector resources directly. Thus providers must respond to two different economic regimes: contractual with insurers and noncontractual with the health authorities and local government. This limits the scope for efficiency related to performance. There is growing concern about this dual structure and the mixed incentives it creates. In response, some health authorities and territorial health insurance funds have started working together to coordinate their purchasing policies.

One more constraint in CEE and CIS countries is the lack of skills to manage the contracting process. Contracts require skills not needed under direct public provision, such as negotiation, monitoring the performance of providers, and the ability to identify cost-effective medical interventions. Furthermore, contracting implies a high degree of decentralization in resource allocation, since bids are likely to involve local providers that are too numerous to be dealt with at central level, and are better known to local purchasers. The relevant skills must therefore be developed at the middle or lower levels of the system, where capacity may be particularly weak. In short, capacity building is a prerequisite of viable contracting.

CONCLUSION

The growing interest in contracting can be attributed to disillusionment with the traditional mechanisms of command-and-control resource allocation. Contracting can be implemented in both competitive and noncompetitive environments. In both cases, contracting can be regarded as a planning and management tool.

Hence contracting represents a new way to do many of the things that have traditionally preoccupied health care planning and management, in a way that can simultaneously address the difficulties inherent in traditional planning methods while achieving a number of public health objectives.

It is possible to identify four main trends in contracting across countries with different health models:

- from block contracts to cost-and-volume and cost-per-case contracts;
- from universal to individual contracting;
- from contracting with all providers to selective contracting; and
- from contracts with a few provisions (primarily on volume and quality) to more sophisticated contracts (with a number of provisions on cost containment, utilization management, quality assurance, risk sharing arrangements, etc.).

The actual implementation of a contracting process, however, does not necessarily match the theoretical expectations. Contracting presents many obstacles and issues, of which the most important are the lack of adequate information, the management skills of health purchasers and providers, high transaction costs and, in the CEE and CIS countries, the inadequacy of public funding.

Performance-related payment systems for providers

Policy-makers across the European Region require payment systems for professionals and institutions that both encourage access for patients to efficient and high-quality care and achieve efficiency and cost-containment objectives. This section reviews the impact of different systems for paying physicians and hospitals, and describes recent reforms of these mechanisms that have been adopted in different countries of the Region.

PAYING PHYSICIANS

Designing payment systems for physicians involves recognizing the particular objectives and constraints that motivate their behaviour. One key element is the uncertainty and asymmetry of information between doctor and patient, which is the source of the agency relationship between them. While this arrangement is intended first and foremost to protect the patient's interests, it can produce a supply-induced demand phenomenon by which doctors, acting as agents for the patients, increase the demand for their own services in order to maximize their personal incomes. (See the discussion on cost sharing in Chapter 3, pages 83–100.)

Towards an optimum payment system

An optimum payment system should achieve a variety of policy objectives, including: the efficient use of resources; accessibility; quality (including aspects such as comprehensive care and coordination between services); a global approach to health, including prevention; choice of doctor for the patient; professional freedom for the doctor; and straightforward implementation.

There are three main forms of payment for physicians – fee-for-service, salary and capitation *(264)* – together with allowances to reward good practice, which can be combined with any of the first three. When trying to set up a typology of payment systems that encompasses the organizational environment in which physicians practise, the following three questions need to be asked *(265)*.

WHAT IS PAID FOR?

Three different payment systems can be defined under this category. The first is (salary-based) remuneration for the actual resource, i.e. the time spent by the physician. Under this system, the physician works within a predefined schedule and combines different activities such as medical work, administrative tasks and teaching.

The second system is (fee-for-service) remuneration for the services that this resource produces. Such systems are organized around fee schedules that classify the activities of physicians with varying degrees of precision *(266)*. The Quebec fee schedule, for example, is very detailed and includes no fewer than 7000 procedures. By contrast, in France, the schedule is more opaque since it combines a type of medical activity identified by a letter (e.g. K for surgery) with a coefficient (e.g. 50 for minor surgery). In this group, two types of case can be distinguished according to whether fixed costs (e.g. capital equipment) are included. If they are included, the purchase of capital equipment may turn out to be an important determinant of the volume of services performed, for example in radiology.

The third system is (capitation) payment for the responsibility for the health of the patient. Two types can be distinguished here: responsibility for the health of a population covered for a certain period, or responsibility for the treatment of an episode of care, such as a lump sum for antenatal care. This second is half way between fee-for-service and capitation, and remains rather circumscribed.

WHO DETERMINES THE LEVEL OF REMUNERATION?

Three options can be identified here. The first, "free fee fixing" by physicians themselves is not common but is employed in France for Secteur II physicians.[20]

The second comprises negotiations between physicians' representatives and the third-party payer. Fee schedules may determine the level of fees that physicians can claim, but they have discretionary powers in applying the schedule. In a "closed" system, i.e. where limits on global expenditure are applied, the negotiations will determine total expenditure, while in an open-ended system quantity adjustments may take place and total expenditure will be known only retrospectively.

The third option is the determination of income level by a central agency. In this case, the income level and its evolution over time may depend on the number of years worked or may be related to actual performance.

WHO PAYS?

There are three alternatives, according to who pays the physician: the consumer, as in France, where the patient pays the whole bill and is later partly reimbursed by

---

[20] In France, a new option for outpatient physicians, Secteur II, was set up in 1980. In this system, physicians are free to set their own fees, but those who opt for this system face higher social insurance contributions than Secteur I physicians. About 25% of physicians (mainly specialists) have chosen Secteur II.

health insurance; the third-party payer, such as an insurance company; or the institution employing the physician.

Combining these yields 15 possible combinations (options) that allow a policy-maker to consider the environment (the relationship with the third-party payer and the patient) in which the physician practises. Beyond the typological value of this approach, it can help to predict the possible impact of different types of payment system. It suggests, for instance, that no fewer than seven different options, depending on who sets the fees and who pays, should be considered when analysing fee-for-service methods. Indeed, the likelihood of supply-induced demand will increase according to the degree of freedom in each setting. At one end of the spectrum, physicians have greater freedom under fee-for-service systems, in which they set their own fees and patients themselves pay. At the other end, fee-for-service systems will be more constrained if physicians are paid by their institution and their levels of income are determined by a central agency *(265)*.

Trends in the European Region

THE WESTERN EUROPEAN COUNTRIES

Table 14 summarizes current patterns of paying PHC physicians in a number of western European countries. It also shows the relationship between the type of payment and other key factors, including the annual number of visits to the doctor per head of population, the extent of cost sharing and whether the doctor carries out a gatekeeping function in relation to referrals.

Salary-based systems predominate among directly employed doctors. In insurance-based systems, PHC practitioners are independent contractors, mainly paid fee-for-service. This contrasts with the approaches adopted in national health service systems, which tend to employ PHC practitioners directly and pay them a salary. In the latter group, however, there are several countries, including Denmark, Italy and the United Kingdom, where PHC practitioners are self-employed and paid by capitation or by a mix of salary, capitation and fee-for-service.

While countries with a predominantly fee-for-service system never mix payments, those based on capitation either mix them according to the patient's economic status (Ireland and the Netherlands) or according to the service covered. For instance, in Denmark and the United Kingdom, GPs are paid fees for specified activities. Gatekeeping is associated with either capitation or salary, but never with fee-for-service. Another interesting observation is that countries with gatekeeping and either capitation or salary usually have low or zero out-of-pocket payments. Countries with fee-for-service, on the contrary, emphasize out-of-pocket payments to reduce moral hazard to patient and doctor. The French term for co-payment – *ticket modérateur* – which means moderating payment, is a good illustration of the policy assumptions underlying out-of-pocket payments. It should be noted that in France and other countries, however, out-of-pocket payments are totally refunded by private voluntary complementary insurance, thus negating any impact on moral hazard. Moreover, as discussed in detail in the section on cost sharing in Chapter 3 (pages 83–100), co-payments of all types have been demonstrated to be inequitable regulators of service demand.

Table 14. Principal methods of payment for PHC physicians in western European countries

Country	Type of payment	Annual visits per head, around 1992	Gatekeeping	Cost sharing
Indirect provision (contracted)				
Austria	Fee-for-service	5.1[a]	No	20% of population pays 10% or 20%
Belgium	Fee-for-service	8.0[a]	No	Self-employed pay full cost
Denmark	28% capitation (flat fee); 63% fee-for-service; 9% allowances	4.4[b]	Yes	None
France	Fee-for-service; salary in health centres	6.3[a]	No	25% including extra billing
Germany	Fee-for-service	12.8[c]	No	None
Ireland	Fee-for-service if higher income; capitation (age-differentiated fee) if lower income	6.6[d]	Yes	None if lower income
Italy	Capitation (age-differentiated fee)	11.0[d]	Yes	None
Luxembourg	Fee-for-service	–	No	5%
Netherlands	Fee-for-service if higher income; capitation (age-differentiated fee) if lower income	5.8[e]	Yes	None if lower income

Table 14 (contd)

Country	Type of payment	Annual visits per head, around 1992	Gatekeeping	Cost sharing
Switzerland	Fee-for-service	11.0[e]	No	10% of cost
United Kingdom	Capitation (age-differentiated fee); fee-for-service; allowances and target payments	5.8[c]	Yes	None
Direct provision (employed)				
Finland	Salary	3.3[b]	Yes	US $0.17
Greece	Salary	5.3[f]	No	None
Norway	35% salary; 65% fee-for-service	–	Yes	30% of costs for selected items
Portugal	Salary	3.1[a]	Yes	None
Spain	Salary; capitation (age differentiated fee)	6.2[g]	Yes	None
Sweden	Salary	3.0[a]	No	US $6–9

[a] 1993; [b] 1991; [c] 1992; [d] 1988; [e] 1994; [f] 1982; [g] 1989.

Sources: OECD *(2)*; Abel-Smith *(170)*.

THE CEE AND CIS COUNTRIES

While recent reforms of arrangements for paying physicians have resulted in only marginal adjustments in most western European countries, reforms in the CEE and CIS countries have involved more structural changes. Typically, there has been a move away from a model of salaried practitioners employed by the state towards contractual relationships, with self-employed practitioners paid by a mix of salary, capitation and fee-for-service methods.

The move towards social insurance systems in the CEE and CIS countries has had clear implications for the methods by which doctors are paid. While no connection necessarily exists between the type of health care funding system and the type of mechanism by which physicians are paid, countries tend to perceive the reform of their funding systems as an opportunity to reform provider payment mechanisms, with the aim of raising very low remuneration levels as well as improving efficiency.

In the initial phases of reform, most countries have continued to rely on salary-based payments, while the introduction of fee-for-service and/or capitation systems is so far limited to the small privatized health sector. As financial reforms progress, capitation and/or fee-for-service elements are progressively incorporated into the payment mechanisms. For example, Bulgaria, Lithuania, Poland and Romania rely on tax-based financing, but all four are moving towards introducing insurance systems. In these countries, physicians in the public health care system are still paid by salary, but all four countries are considering a transition to new forms of payment. In Romania, for example, under the family doctor system that is being developed, physicians' remuneration will mainly be based on capitation fees, with additions for some medical activities (chronic diseases, immunization, health promotion and health education). Reforms of the payment system have already been implemented in pilot districts. Similarly, Poland has set up a series of experimental schemes for paying family practitioners in order to evaluate different combinations, including salary and fee-for-service schemes, salary and capitation, and fundholding.

There appear to be two general trends among those CEE countries that have made a complete or partial switch over to health insurance financing. First, there are countries such as Croatia, Estonia and Hungary, which rely mainly on forms of salary or capitation for public and contracted PHC and specialist practitioners. A second group of countries, including the Czech Republic, Slovakia and Slovenia, relies on fee-for-service methods (Czech Republic) or on a mix of capitation and fee-for-service methods (Slovakia and Slovenia) for self-employed PHC practitioners and specialists.

In the Czech Republic, which has adopted the German points system (see page 161), PHC physicians and specialists under contract are reimbursed according to a list of services containing more than 4000 items. Each item has a fixed points value, with values assigned to some services and procedures that differ according to specialty and payer. This system was introduced in 1992, before adequate information systems had been developed to track costs, and before a process for negotiating prices had been set up. The result was that control of expenditure was lost within a few months of the initiation of the programme *(174)*. The Czech Republic is currently considering plans for replacing it by a combination of capitation and fee-for-service.

The expectations of physicians about target earnings are a key problem in CEE countries. The economic transition has substantially increased wages for well educated workers – except in the health sector. As discussed in Chapter 1, economic recession has led to lower health spending in several countries, as well as the erosion of real wages for health workers. Among other problems, low salaries have prevented the eradication of informal or "under-the-table" systems of payment. These are the equivalent of an informal fee-for-service system, and they have been prevalent in most CEE and CIS countries since the Soviet era. There are few data on the extent of this phenomenon, but it appears to provide a significant proportion of physicians' incomes in both outpatient and inpatient care. (Further details are provided in the section on cost sharing in Chapter 3; see pages 83–100.) Informal payments have implications for equity of access, since patients of low socioeconomic status are unable to pay PHC practitioners – the gatekeepers – for access to medical facilities and services. Ultimately, the challenge for policy-makers is how, in an environment of continuing budgetary crisis, to secure necessary funds to pay physicians at a level that is close to their expected target earnings.

Evaluating current payment systems

Assessing the usefulness of payment systems for physicians can best be accomplished by dividing them into two groups: retrospective and prospective. Indeed, the difference between capitation and fee-for-service payment is better understood with reference to time: payment for the resource (fee-for-service) is a retrospective type of payment, while payment for responsibility (capitation) is a prospective payment for the period covered by the agreement. Salary-based systems will be grouped with capitation, inasmuch as total remuneration is known in advance and several of the incentives influencing physicians are similar.

RETROSPECTIVE PAYMENT SYSTEMS

Providers themselves often describe the advantages of fee-for-service payment in terms of enhanced freedom and greater continuity of care. This has been documented in a number of studies. For instance, Hickson (267) compared the effect of randomly assigning 18 paediatric physicians to either fee-for-service payment or salaries. The results showed that the former had 22% more visits per patient enrolled with them than the salaried doctors. In terms of continuity of care, patients were more likely to be seen by their regular doctor if he or she was paid fees for services.

The disadvantages are that fee-for-service payments are open-ended systems that give providers a blank cheque to encourage demand if they so wish. A number of studies have documented differences in surgical rates between countries with different payment systems, such as Canada and the United Kingdom. Higher rates of surgery for common operations in Canada and the United States, compared with those in the United Kingdom, were due not so much to differences in the incidence and prevalence of disease as to factors such as the lack of agreement about indications for surgery, variations in the use and availability of technology, and the fee-for-service system in Canada and the United States (268,269).

Several studies have looked at the effect of an increase in the physician:population ratio on the level of fees and utilization rates, but these investigations present several methodological problems. More recent studies, based on natural experiments, have sought to reveal alternative evidence about physicians' discretionary powers by examining the effect of institutional constraints (such as remuneration systems) on activity levels and the mix of services. Results clearly indicate that physicians have the ability to cushion the impact of reduced fees by increasing the quantity of services provided and altering the mix, thereby maintaining their target income (270–274).

In general, therefore, physicians' discretionary powers are neither myth nor reality. They have the potential to be used if certain conditions prevail, and are related to the method of remuneration, to the supply of physicians, to the system of reimbursing patients and to other institutional variables. In particular, they are more likely to be significant when there is greater uncertainty about medical efficacy.

Two other problems connected with fee-for-service systems are "fee-creep" and "input substitution". Fee-creep refers to manipulation of the fee schedule by the physician in order to maximize income. Given the payer's imperfect information, the negotiation process is likely to lead to a biased fee structure, some procedures becoming more lucrative than others. A comparison of the prevalence of vaginal delivery versus Caesarean section, for instance, has indicated that the higher fees for Caesarean section can be a significant factor in the choice of delivery (275). Input substitution refers to the fact that, in fee-for-service payment systems, physicians do not delegate to other health care providers (nurses in particular) as readily as if they were salaried or paid by capitation.

PROSPECTIVE PAYMENT SYSTEMS

Prospective payment systems seek to offer physicians incentives to control spending and to develop a more cost-effective style of practice. Payments per head sever the link between numbers of services provided and financial reward, and hence involve minimal distortion of purely professional medical judgement (276). Research in the United States that consistently pointed to lower spending per patient for recipients of prepaid care than for comparable patients under fee-for-service health care systems (277) has been corroborated by more recent evidence from the Medical Outcomes Study (278). In addition, these systems give physicians incentives to introduce preventive measures, and may lead to a better geographical distribution of professionals.

By contrast, prospective payment may encourage providers to reduce the value of the treatment for which they receive a unit of payment, either by curtailing consultation time, by excessive prescribing or by overreferral to hospital. Also, prospective payment systems can lead to lower motivation (279) and reduced courtesy to patients. In addition, they may provide an incentive for providers to select out the sicker patients who will prove unprofitable (280).

Moving towards performance-related payment systems

The above review of the relative merits of prospective versus retrospective payment systems suggests that neither system is ideal, although the perverse effects in each case may be exacerbated by the environment in which physicians practise. Logically, a solution might be found in mixed prospective and retrospective systems of payment that combine incentives for performance and cost control.

In general, cost-containment problems in fee-for-service systems and low staff motivation in salary-based systems have produced a trend among European countries for adopting mixed payment systems, combining increased productivity with greater concern about patient satisfaction and adequate control over costs (2). The review of the various reforms of payment systems for physicians seems to reveal a common diagnosis: the need to reduce the perverse incentives embodied in the two main types of remuneration (prospective and retrospective). This common dilemma has been aptly termed the "transformation problem": "how should social conditions in health care be shaped in order to ensure that physicians' professional behaviour on the micro-level results in cost control on the macro-level?" (281).

There are, however, differences in the initial situation. Countries with open-ended systems where fee-for-service payment prevails have had to give priority in their reforms to macro-efficiency objectives. Rather than moving towards mixed prospective and retrospective payment systems at physician level in order to combine both macro-level and micro-level efficiency objectives, however, they have had to cap expenditure or set targets in order to pursue macro-level efficiency at a collective level. The reason for this lies in the initial situation: a fee-for-service system rarely allows regulators enough room for manoeuvre to enforce such mixed payments. All that can be negotiated is a limit on overall spending by physicians. Conversely, countries that already had closed systems with either salary or capitation have addressed micro-level efficiency problems by moving towards mixed payment systems.

Thus, what appears to be a move in opposite directions is, in practice, motivated by the same desire to combine both micro- and macro-level objectives, though starting from different situations. To a certain extent, the therapy can also be said to be a common one: the use of tailor-made incentives closely tied to performance. Yet in the first case, the relationship between performance and incentives is negative, i.e. volume increases are matched by downward revisions of fees. In the second case, the relationship between performance and incentives is positive.

In order to combine macro- and micro-level objectives, countries with fee-for-service systems have introduced a number of measures, including price regulation, controls on the quantity and mix of services, or restrictions on overall expenditure. France and Germany offer examples of how these regulating mechanisms can be employed to modify the behaviour of physicians. These include adjusting fee scales, e.g. by altering the relative value of some diagnostic services; introducing care protocols such as the "medical references" system in France (see Chapter 3, page 83); and changing authorizing behaviour by, for example, imposing penalties for over-utilization of certain procedures or giving physicians responsibility for drug budgets. In addition, capping budgets and setting target levels are effective in controlling over-all costs.

Since 1991, the French government has attempted to change the system from an open-ended system of reimbursing physicians' expenditure to a prospective one *(282)*. Starting with the capping of expenditure, the reform slowly moved towards spending targets.

Of the European countries that have recently adopted expenditure controls, in addition to price controls in the 1980s, Germany has the most developed approach. Physicians are paid fees for services, subject to a schedule of agreed fees and to a global budget constraint for all physicians in the region. The fee schedule comprises a tariff of "points" for 2500 items determined at federal level, together with a price per point at regional level. If the regional budget is exceeded, there is a retrospective reduction in the price per point.

In systems relying on fee-for-service payments, macro-level objectives will not be met unless negative incentives are implemented, such as capping of expenditure. In most cases, this will imply collective capping, which may sometimes be unfair and inefficient. In fact, a parallel can be drawn with the experience of global budgets for hospitals: capping ensures cost-containment, but little is known about the impact of such regulation in terms of quality and equity at the micro level.

In their search for micro-level efficiency, countries with prospective payment systems include positive, *ex ante* incentives in the form of direct financial rewards. These incentives are commonly used in addition to the existing payment systems (capitation or salary) to encourage a particular line of action. The payment of GPs in the United Kingdom offers a good example of the use of a mixed system that manages the behaviour of physicians. The introduction of upward adjustments on capitation to account for socioeconomic deprivation, and target payments for reaching certain levels of preventive coverage, appears to have been effective.

In general, however, it is difficult to predict the outcome of economic incentives. Depending on the initial situation in terms of payment systems, on physicians' preferences and on the size of the change, the introduction of financial incentives may or may not lead to the expected result. For instance, a study on the effect of changes in the fees paid to British GPs on maternity and cervical cytology services over 22 years did not find that annual changes in real fees influenced the quantity of services provided *(283)*.

Various Scandinavian countries have also tried mixed payment systems. Some counties in Sweden have combined capitation and salary mechanisms; personal doctors in Finland receive 60% salary, 20% capitation, 15% fees and 5% allowances; and in Norway family doctors are paid 50% capitation, 30% fees and 20% co-payments by patients. While a number of experiments with mixed payments have been evaluated in several countries, particularly in managed care organizations in the United States *(284–286)*, the effects of such systems are still inadequately documented.

For systems based on capitation or salary, mixed payment systems are a good solution but a difficult balance to achieve. There is no clear consensus on the *ideal* mix: it may well be that only a small share of total activity should be under fee-for-service payment. Indeed, as noted by Robinson *(284)*:

> every movement toward prospective reimbursement increases incentives for unbundling, undertreatment and risk selection. Every compensating movement back toward retrospective reimbursement revives the traditional incentives for cost-unconscious practice styles. Mixed payment mechanisms have much to recommend them ... but experience over recent years suggests that the problem is one that cannot be solved by payment mechanisms alone.

Non-price incentives, such as utilization review and selective contracting mechanisms, are additional approaches that need further investigation.

Conclusion

No single payment system can meet all the desired policy objectives. In general, studies indicate that mixed payment systems (with a large prospective component) are more successful in combining macro- and micro-level objectives. Nevertheless, a number of issues need to be taken into consideration when reforming a payment system.

Mixed payments allow more objectives to be achieved, but trade-offs remain inevitable and ought to be made explicit. The most difficult trade-off stems from the dual agency relationship, i.e. the conflict between individual and collective preferences. Depending on the emphasis placed on different objectives and incentives, physicians will be inclined to give more weight either to patients' preferences or to the interests of third-party payers. The easiest trade-off to make explicit is that between equity and freedom of choice. Patients in countries such as France have not been willing to forgo the freedom to consult specialists directly. Yet the implicit cost of this preference is the need to retain user charges, which are known to be regressive (see Chapter 3), as a way of reducing moral hazard to both the physician and the patient. There is also a potential trade-off between simplicity and tailor-made mixed payments: the increase in freedom through the use of mixed payment systems may be lost to the complexity of implementation.

Incentives display a number of characteristics that make them a mixed blessing for decision-makers *(287)*. First, incentives may be manipulated by those whom they are intended to affect, in an effort either to obtain the reward or to avoid the punishment without adopting the desired behaviour. Second, incentives do not coordinate themselves, making it difficult to standardize behaviour across sectors. Third, incentives often have unanticipated consequences, or may generate effects quite opposite to those intended. Finally, incentives may be costly to employ since some form of monitoring will be required.

To be credible, policy choices concerning the payment of physicians should recognize that all objectives cannot be met and that some objectives – and clearly some groups' preferences – will necessarily dominate others. It then becomes important to find a politically legitimate way of making such choices explicit. It is also important to recognize that choices between payment systems have implications for subsequent decisions. For instance, the adoption of fee-for-service payments will determine features of the future system: some form of expenditure capping or target will be necessary to contain expenditure, and out-of-pocket payments may become unavoidable. Also, certain choices are harder to reverse than others; it is difficult, for example, to move from fee-for-service systems to mixed payment ones. Finally, national solutions have to be identified, in the recognition that history and cultural factors are often the strongest determinants of behaviour and must be accommodated.

In countries without a gatekeeping arrangement, PHC services may be in direct competition with some specialist services (particularly maternity and paediatric services) as if they were substitutes for PHC rather than complements. Clearly, any reform of the payment system will need to address the changes that may be triggered in relationships with other health care providers. Similarly, reforms will need to take demand features into account as well. For instance, it would be difficult to introduce expenditure capping with no concomitant regulation of demand in countries, such as France, where moral hazard is believed to be strong for some groups of patients.

Finally, it should be emphasized that payment systems are only one among many determinants affecting physicians' behaviour. The standard of medical ethics, access to further education, the structure of professional prestige and standards, local peer review, selective contracting and physicians' expectations are important additional factors. Regarding the latter, if physicians are paid less than they feel they deserve in relation to similar professions, they will be more likely to respond opportunistically in order to increase income (171). Ultimately, however, the ideal payment system does not exist: "Under any system of payment it is the ethics and social commitment of the doctor which matter most of all. Where standards are low in these respects no financial structure can induce doctors to be what they are not" (171).

PAYING HOSPITALS

Acute hospitals constitute the largest single component of health expenditure in most developed countries. While economic pressures on health care resources provide an important impetus for reforming this system in many countries, additional factors contributing to pressure include advances in technology and services and the increasing expectations of patients. These have led to a number of reform strategies for the hospital system, which are reviewed in Chapter 6. This section concentrates on payment mechanisms for acute hospital services in the European Region.

Several key points concerning the payment of individual professionals also apply to hospitals. Like physicians, hospital providers can be paid either retrospectively – reimbursed for the volume of actual services provided according to a price list of services (fee-for-service payment), patient-days (per diem fees or daily charge) or cases treated (case-mix payment) – or prospectively, via global budgets provided to the hospital for a given period of time. Budgets may be calculated according to the actual costs of a provider unit, historical spending patterns, bed provision, the population covered or the volume of services to be provided (measured by volume of bed-days, or volume and mix of cases).

The predominant funding sources and payment approaches for acute inpatient hospital services for 16 European countries are summarized in Table 15. While the specifics of payment for hospital services vary between countries, Table 15 shows that they fall into two broad categories: prospective budgeting and service-based payment. There is further differentiation within each of these categories, as countries may apply system-specific adjustments in either of these broad approaches. This section explores the range of applications for prospective budgeting and service-based payment by reviewing the systems in use in the countries of the European Region.

Prospective budgeting

While prospective budgeting is not necessarily pursued the same way in each country, this approach has a number of common characteristics: payment levels for service provision are determined in advance; the payment commitment is limited to a predefined period; and the time and payment constraints for service providers are specified prospectively.

As shown in Table 15, prospective budgeting is not associated with any particular funding source. Health systems in Denmark and Norway are funded from decentralized tax-based systems, those in Ireland, Italy and Poland are funded from centralized, tax-based systems, while social insurance prevails in France, Germany and the Netherlands. One factor that distinguishes these countries is whether or not some adjustment for hospital activity is applied within the prospective budget.

TRADITIONAL APPROACHES TO PROSPECTIVE BUDGETING

Denmark and Poland are two countries listed in Table 15 that take a more traditional approach to prospective budgeting. Prospective global budgets for Danish hospitals are mainly determined on a historical basis, with adjustments for salary and price increases, service quality and planned efficiency improvements. Some commentators believe that the use of global budgets by the county councils explains the Danish hospital sector's success in controlling costs (288). Greater flexibility in the more traditional approach was considered necessary, however, when attempting to address the problem of waiting times for elective services. In 1994, the introduction of the "free choice of hospital" scheme to reduce waiting times for elective surgery made the hospitals more responsive to patients' needs. In addition, the scheme engendered a degree of competitiveness between hospitals, as additional funding could be acquired for providing the services needed to reduce hospital waiting times (288). When patients are treated outside their county of residence, the basis for payment is negotiated between the two county councils involved and is generally on a fee-for-service or per diem basis.

While hospital services in Poland continue to be financed from tax revenues, the 1994 policy document *Strategy for health (289)* supports the introduction of a mixed insurance–budget system of paying for health care. At the provincial *voivodship* level, the annual budget is divided between pay and non-pay expenditure, with resources allocated on a historical basis. While the allocation to the *voivodship* is

Table 15. Predominant approaches to funding and paying hospital operating costs for acute inpatient services in selected countries in the European Region

Country	Source of funding	Approach to paying operating costs	
		Prospective budgeting	Service-based financing
Austria	Social insurance funding		Social insurance funding based on length of stay, with lump sum subsidies provided by the Ministry of Health
Denmark	Decentralized tax-based funding	Prospective global budgeting	
Finland	Decentralized tax-based funding		Service-based reimbursement by municipalities
France	Social insurance funding	Prospective global budgeting	
Germany	Social insurance funding	Prospective "flexible" budgeting	
Hungary	Social insurance funding		Performance-related payment system based on diagnosis-related groups
Ireland	Centralized tax-based funding	Prospective global budgeting	
Italy	Centralized tax-based funding	Prospective global budgeting incorporating tariffs based on diagnosis-related groups	

Table 15 (contd)

Country	Source of funding	Approach to paying operating costs	
		Prospective budgeting	Service-based financing
Latvia	Taxation		Daily charge and service-related payment
Netherlands	Social insurance funding	Prospective "functional" budgeting partly based on activity	
Norway	Decentralized tax-based funding	Prospective global budgeting	
Poland	Taxation	Annual global budgeting	
Slovakia	National health insurance	Daily charge per bed-day	
Slovenia	Compulsory health insurance	Annual prospective funding based on contracts incorporating payment per bed-day and service-related funding	
Sweden	Decentralized tax-based funding	Prospective departmental budgeting combined with activity-based payment	
United Kingdom (England)	Centralized tax-based funding		Activity-based payment determined by purchaser/provider contracts

fixed, this authority may determine the internal distribution of funds. Changes in staffing levels and in the traditional approach are limited, but some attempts have been made to experiment with different methods of resource allocation with the intention of improving efficiency and directing resources to where they are most needed. One *voivodship*, experimenting with alternative models of resource deployment, allocated non-pay expenditure to hospitals in 1994 and 1995 on the basis of patient numbers and costs by specialty. This *voivodship* is considering a proposal that would allow the authority responsible for service provision to become the budget holder and to buy hospital services where they are available at the best price.

The experiences of Denmark and Poland, with traditional approaches to prospective budgeting, suggest that, while this method has performed adequately for resource allocation and cost-containment purposes, more flexibility may be needed in order to pursue wider objectives. In particular, efficiency is difficult to measure in a system based on historical spending. The potential for offering the necessary incentives to facilitate change, such as reducing waiting lists, has also been found to be limited. While continuing to support the traditional approach to prospective budgeting for hospital financing, some regions in Denmark and Poland recognize the need to integrate it into a more flexible payment model in order to achieve their broader health policy objectives.

ACTIVITY-ADJUSTED PROSPECTIVE BUDGETING

Traditionally, in contract-based social insurance systems, hospitals were reimbursed at a daily rate that covered all running costs, sometimes with the exception of payments to physicians. In integrated (national health service tax-based) systems, hospitals were given an annual budget to cover their running costs, often based on traditional incremental patterns. Neither system encouraged efficient provider behaviour. Open-ended reimbursement systems based on bed-days encouraged hospital providers to increase lengths of stay in order to maximize income. Similarly, historical budgets without any activity or performance measures do not have any incentives for faster patient throughput or for shorter lengths of stay: the higher the turnover, the higher the risk of overspending. During the 1980s and 1990s, several contract-based systems in western Europe, such as those in France and Germany, adopted prospective global budget systems, incorporating some measure of hospital activity such as bed-days or cases. This had a significant impact on containing costs.

France and Germany took different approaches to introducing activity-adjusted prospective budgeting. As both countries have social insurance systems, adjustments to the budget model should facilitate application in a wide variety of institutional environments. The potential for greater autonomy at institutional level that may exist within these systems may, in turn, facilitate greater innovation in approaches to resource deployment at this level.

In France, public hospitals and private non-profit hospitals affiliated to the public sector have been paid on the basis of prospective global budgets since 1984–1985. In this system, hospitals receive an annual global allocation based on the proportion of expenditure to be supported by the sickness funds. Budgets are based on historical spending levels and are intended to cover hospital operating costs. Because hospitals treat patients covered by a number of different insurers, the budget share required of each insurer is determined on the basis of the number of bed-days used in the insurer's catchment area *(188)*. The process for determining the global budget allocation involves extensive negotiations between the hospital, the supervisory authorities and the sickness funds. As these negotiations are part of an annual process, an average rate of increase *(taux moyen d'évolution)* may be applied, fixed centrally by the ministries concerned with the economy, the budget and health. About 90% of public hospital expenditure is met by the global budget allocation, the remainder coming from charges to individual patients.

A recognition of the need for greater integration and solidarity between the constituent components of the hospital sector, together with the need to upgrade the approach to paying for services, provided the main platforms for the hospital sector reform legislation passed in 1991. Following the enactment of this legislation, the budgetary process has been subjected to detailed review in the interests of improving its speed, flexibility and efficiency. In addition, provision has been made to enable the global budget to be revised during the fiscal year, to reflect volume changes assessed on the basis of accepted measures of medical activity *(290)*. As part of this reform, experiments are also being conducted in a number of hospitals to test a charge-based approach to payment according to a French version of diagnosis-related groups, known in France as *groupes homogènes de malades*. The objectives of greater efficiency and improved performance, together with the application of a standardized measure of workload for budgeting purposes, are expected to continue to be pursued in France as part of a continuing process of hospital sector reform.

In Germany, a "flexible" prospective budgeting system was introduced in 1985, on the basis that full cost coverage would be restricted to those hospitals assessed as working efficiently. Budget negotiations take place between the individual hospital, the regional association of the statutory sickness funds and the organizations of private health insurers *(291)*. The negotiations refer to the services the hospital expects to provide, and to the associated cost. The prospective daily rate and the hospital budget are agreed at the same time. Under the flexible budget system, when a hospital delivers fewer than the anticipated number of patient-days, it still receives 75% of the daily rate for the missing days in the next round of budget negotiations. Hospitals delivering more than the planned level of patient-days were expected to refund 75% of the excess daily rates.

The health sector legislation of 1993[21] enforced an income-oriented policy on growth in individual hospital budgets between 1993 and 1995. Taking the 1992 budget as the baseline, budget increases were limited to the income growth of the sickness funds. After 1996, the flexible budget mechanism applied from 1985 onwards will be reinstated *(291)*. While prospective budgets will continue to cover more hospital services, the legislation foresaw a greater role for other payment

---

[21] In Germany, cost-containment has been a major political issue since the mid-1970s. Nearly 60 cost-containment measures were introduced in eight acts in the period up to 1989 *(257)*.

components, including special daily rates for hospital departments, special fees for expensive services and case-based lump sum payments.

The 1993 legislation was the first major reform to go beyond health spending issues and review the basic structure of the health care system, although problems such as the crudeness of the daily rate as a payment unit persist. The health sector legislation is seen as a substantial move towards more fundamental reform, given the need for strengthening the budgeting process, developing links to income development, and expanding performance-related financial mechanisms (291).

Along with continuing reform of their respective health care systems, France and Germany have both chosen to continue the use of prospective budgets to pay for acute hospital services. While there are differences in the budget models used, some adjustments are made for activity. Both countries recognize the need to improve current payment approaches in order to enhance flexibility, efficiency and performance-related incentives within their hospital systems.

CASE-MIX-ADJUSTED PROSPECTIVE BUDGETING

Differences in hospital activity and severity can be taken into account by including some type of case-mix adjustment within the prospective budgeting model. As shown in Table 15, hospital systems in Ireland, Italy and Norway have taken this approach to budgeting. In reviewing their specific strategies, it is interesting to note that, despite choosing a similar case-mix measure, countries differ in the approaches adopted for implementation.

Since 1993, a global budget framework incorporating a case-mix adjustment has been used for allocating resources to regional health boards and to the large hospitals responsible for providing acute hospital services in Ireland. In this model, hospitals are classified by teaching status and the relative costs of hospital case-mix are estimated using the diagnosis-related group system (292). In this context, relative costs are assumed to indicate relative efficiency. An agreed proportion of a hospital's budget is determined on the basis of the case-mix adjustment, which may be negative or positive depending on hospital's efficiency in relation to others in the reference group. The hospital may deploy at its own discretion any extra funds gained as a result of this process.

The Irish approach contrasts with that proposed for Italy, where the 1995 reforms propose that health service payment be shifted to a tariff basis (293). For hospital services, tariffs based on diagnosis-related groups are to be set on a prospective basis within predetermined budget constraints, but some discretion is left to the regions about how this tariff system will be implemented. This could mean that the choice for regions might range from a fee-for-service type of system to one whereby tariffs would only be used to provide compensation for cross-border movement. The aim is that hospitals will be funded on the basis of the volume and quality of services actually delivered. As an additional incentive for increased efficiency, it has been proposed that local units should retain any budget surpluses, which would then be deployed according to objectives agreed with the region.

Payment for hospital services in Norway was historically based on a system of fixed grants, until a population-based global budgeting approach was introduced in 1980. Political concern about waiting lists and hospital efficiency was an important impetus for introducing reforms in the 1990s. In determining the organizational response to these problems, it became clear that a more flexible and incentive-based system was required. A pilot scheme in 1991, expanded in 1993, tested an approach to hospital service payment that combined fixed grants with a payment scheme based on diagnosis-related groups. An important outcome of this scheme has been improvements in the availability and quality of hospital cost and output data, owing to their being linked with service payment *(294)*.

Despite Norway's experiment with a case-mix approach to hospital payment, the lack of controls on hospital expenditure continues to be a problem. The absence of any general monitoring or control programme to ensure that spending limits are not breached means that deficit budgeting for hospitals can still be found in some counties. Increasingly, however, in many areas, hospital deficits result in deductions from the following year's budget. While such measures may be effective in the short run in facilitating expenditure control, a fundamental reform of payment for hospital services is likely to be required before the necessary incentives for improved efficiency become operational.

In choosing to apply a case-mix adjustment for hospital financing, the diagnosis-related group system was the measure of choice for Ireland, Italy and Norway. As each of these countries chose to reform its approach to hospital payment in the early 1990s, efficiency and productivity issues had an important influence on the types of reform introduced. The recognition that efficiency can be best assessed where resource deployment is directly related to service production was an important factor in the choice of payment model. The correct application of a case-mix measure may both facilitate efficiency measurement and offer positive incentives for service operation.

Service-based payment

The use of a generic term such as "service-based payment" should not be allowed to obscure the fact that there is considerable diversity in the approaches to hospital service payment among the countries in this general category. This diversity makes it difficult to identify common characteristics between the approaches adopted.

The basic approach involves payment based on service volume, so that the total level of investment and the period covered may be open ended. The facility for relating resources to specific services may enhance the potential for measuring and improving technical efficiency. For instance, where services are priced individually, this mechanism may be used to provide incentives for delivering particular types of service, e.g. screening, or the use of alternative sites for care. On the other hand, the open-ended nature of these systems may have negative effects on cost-containment.

There is, however, a wide diversity of approaches to service-based payment among the countries in this category. For instance, some countries may view the increased use of contracting as one way of addressing the problems caused by open-ended systems. As contracts may be based on the required service quantity or type, and/or the price and/or period covered, there is some scope for placing constraints on investment. Contract-based systems place heavy demands on information systems, however, and thus also require considerable administrative resources to develop, implement, manage and monitor. Contracting systems are therefore quite different from budgeting systems; contracts tend to be institution specific, and they represent the outcome of negotiations between the purchasers and the providers. A full discussion of contracting can be found earlier in this chapter. The specific approaches adopted by a number of countries using service-based payments are summarized in Table 15, and are briefly reviewed here.

In Austria, hospital payment is based on length of stay. In addition, the Ministry of Health provides a lump-sum subsidy to hospitals, determined according to the number of beds, special functions provided and any deficit carried forward. While in theory any shortfall in operating costs should be supported by the hospital, in reality "the hospital itself makes no losses, and there are also no sanctions" *(295)*. The increase in hospital costs in Austria is perhaps not surprising given the perverse incentives associated with financing a service on the basis of length of stay, and the absence of any incentives for cost control. Against this background the Ministry of Health has come to recognize the importance of developing new regulatory mechanisms for financing hospital services. In pursuing this objective, it is anticipated that a planned market can be developed for Austrian hospital services *(295)*. One alternative hospital financing model based on a diagnosis related group classification system is now being developed *(295)*.

In 1994, Latvia adopted a hospital payment system based on the services delivered. A mixed system is currently in use, as hospitals are paid on the basis of a daily charge and services delivered. The local sickness fund and the hospital administration agree on the range of services and on payment rates, depending on local financial resources. State-sponsored specialized treatment centres and state hospitals are partly financed by the State Sickness Fund (for a basic service package) and partly by the Department of Health (for special programmes). With the introduction of these financial reforms, the hospital administration has more freedom to determine the numbers and categories of staff and services delivered.

In Slovakia, since the establishment of the National Health Insurance Company in 1993, hospitals have been paid on the basis of a daily charge for a bed-day classified according to hospital type. The fees cover all services and expenses, and do not vary according to treatment. The application of a fixed charge may be positive or negative for the hospital, depending on the type of service provided. This system has not encouraged cost-containment initiatives. A system based on diagnosis-related groups has recently been introduced on an experimental basis in six hospitals.

While hospital services in Austria, Latvia and Slovakia are financed on the basis of bed-day charges or service-related payments, additional or alternative approaches are being considered or tested in each system. Given the problems experienced with cost-containment, attempts are being made in each case to introduce limits into the system while at the same time encouraging health institutions to exercise greater autonomy.

Owing to these problems, a number of countries are shifting to contract-based systems of hospital payment. Finland, for instance, has made considerable progress towards this aim. Before 1993, payment for hospital services in Finland was based on length of stay, while the municipalities were invoiced by the hospitals on the basis of the average cost of the bed-days used. After making provision for state funding and for patient charges, the balance of hospital expenditure was then provided unquestioningly by the municipality. The introduction of a new approach in 1993 was influenced by the need for cost-containment in an unfavourable economic climate, and the desire to increase the efficiency of the municipal services. Under this system, the state subsidy to the municipality for services, including health, is based on a formula that takes account of the age structure of the population, financial capability, morbidity, population density and land area (296). The state subsidy no longer goes directly to the hospitals; instead, the municipalities combine the subsidy with local funds to buy services from hospitals.

Hospital districts in Finland differ in the type of agreement reached with municipalities for payment of services. Some hospital districts have introduced a form of prospective payment, while many districts bill municipalities on the basis of specialty-specific prices for services provided. A number of pilot projects are under way, in which hospitals and municipalities enter into contracts specifying the price and quantity of services to be provided in an agreed period. Most hospital districts have agreed on a revenue-equalization system, whereby excessively high costs incurred in treating certain types of patient can be pooled between the municipalities in the district. Finally, a form of deficit financing has been agreed on, whereby the municipalities pay off the deficits incurred by hospitals. This practice is under review, however, and may be replaced by offsetting deficits against the following year's payment. It is likely that hospital service financing in Finland will continue to be reviewed, with the aim of improving both cost-containment and efficiency within the system.

Two other countries that have already adopted contract-based payment systems are Slovenia and the United Kingdom. One of the most far-reaching outcomes of the reforms of the British NHS has been the shift from a budgeting to a contracting system as a means of paying for hospital services.

An important objective of the British contracting system is separating the roles of purchaser and provider in hospital services. There are a number of ways in which this new type of relationship may be defined, although in each case the hospital fulfils the role of service provider within price- and quality-controlled service contracts agreed with the purchasing agent. Health authorities may act as the purchasing agents for hospital services, and enter into block cost-and-volume or cost-per-case contracts with designated service providers for defined and costed ranges of services. All hospital providers have been transformed from directly managed organizations into independent trusts (297). Trusts have a statutory duty to operate within the income obtained from contracts. In drawing up contracts, they must set prices equal to average costs and ensure that there is no cross-subsidization between services (297). Trusts compete with other providers for contracts, irrespective of health authority boundaries. A more detailed review of the impact of purchasing and contracting can be found earlier in this chapter (see pages 141–152).

In Slovenia, annual hospital payments are determined on a prospective basis. Payment is therefore based on a combination of bed-days and utilization rates for expensive services. This approach to setting payment levels was introduced in 1992, and is based on a two-step process of negotiation involving representatives of the National Insurance Institute of Slovenia (NIIS), the Ministry of Health and the health service providers.

In the first stage, the three partners to the negotiation reach an agreement within which the maximum budget for each broad class of hospital service is defined. In accordance with the agreement, the NIIS pays a flat rate to hospitals per bed-day, but with certain exceptions for more expensive services and materials. For example, admissions for high-cost services such as cardiothoracic surgery, transplants and dialysis are paid at higher flat rates. In addition, hospitals that reduce their average length of stay can receive an incentive payment for empty beds. The second stage of the negotiations takes place between NIIS management and providers. Based on the resulting agreements, the public tender for contracts with each provider is put out by the NIIS.

Conclusion

While the order of priorities may vary, the objectives most frequently cited for re-forming hospital payment methods include improving cost-containment mechanisms, enhancing service quality in a more efficient provision, and achieving community-wide access. The pursuit of these objectives is made more difficult by the dynamic nature of the hospital system, in particular, and by the financial pressures exerted by continuing technological advances and the growing expectations of patients.

The methods of paying for hospital services in any health care system appear to represent more of a pragmatic response to a continuing policy challenge than a rational planning approach consistent with a clear theoretical framework. The hospital system is a visible and substantial component of all health care systems, which means that it is politically as well as economically significant. The approach to paying for hospital services must therefore attempt to meet the objectives considered a priority by any political administration within the prevailing economic environment. While the objectives of cost-containment, efficiency and open access may be almost universal, additional objectives such as reducing hospital waiting lists may also be prioritized and will ultimately influence the mechanisms adopted.

This attempt to group national systems in several broad categories was intended to clarify understanding of the respective approaches. There are substantial differences between country systems in each broad category, which might be more appropriately considered as part of a continuum rather than a dichotomy. Nevertheless, a series of general observations can be made about the impact of prospective budgeting systems and service-based payment systems.

The most prevalent characteristic of prospective budgeting systems is that limits on expenditure are determined in advance for a defined period. Tax-based systems traditionally set prospective budgets based on historically incremental norms. During the 1980s and 1990s, however, several insurance-based systems in western Europe adopted prospective global budgeting systems that incorporated some measures of hospital activity, such as bed-days or cases. Moreover, the precise approach to managing and controlling services within these constraints varies between countries, and it increasingly incorporates such factors as case-mix controls, output measures and administrative controls. The prioritization of cost control is complemented by a concern for efficiency, with a growing number of countries employing some adjustments for activity/case mix within the budget framework. Improvements in the budget mechanism may also help to enhance quality, autonomy and management flexibility. The implementation of any budgeting system must, however, be ready to address potential problems with service quality, and also be aware of the possible dangers inherent in the politicization of the resourcing process.

It is more difficult to generalize about hospital payment systems based on service volume, because by their very nature they operate at the micro rather than the macro level. While this approach is generally characterized by the association of resource use with service use at patient level, the mechanisms used to put it into operation vary substantially *(298)*. The most obvious disadvantage of approaches in this category is their open-ended nature, which makes control of costs and utilization difficult to achieve. When this volume-oriented approach is combined with prospective pricing as well as contracting, however, payers can require hospitals to achieve specific objectives such as cost control and effective resource utilization. In turn, to achieve these objectives, hospitals need more flexibility in the organizational, staffing and financial aspects of service provision.

Finally, it is worth noting that in the country systems reviewed above, the prevailing health funding model has not generally been perceived as a barrier to reforming the approaches to paying for hospital services. Prospective budgeting systems and service-based payment arrangements prevail in both tax-based and insurance-based models. This indicates that reform of the prevailing health funding model is neither a constraint nor a requirement for reforming the approaches to paying for hospital services.

Cost-effective provision of pharmaceuticals

During the 1990s, spending on pharmaceuticals has emerged as an important factor in the increasing costs of the health sector. An increase in the overall volume of use of existing drugs and the costs associated with introducing new drugs have been two important contributory elements. Policy-makers have responded with cost-containment measures that seek to influence physicians' prescribing patterns, as well as with strategies aimed at the pharmaceutical sector as a whole. These measures typically seek to alter the incentives influencing providers, in order to make them more cost conscious. The long-term effectiveness of different measures, however, remains a fundamental question.

When examining policy options in the pharmaceutical sector, some countries have to reconcile their attempts to contain costs – which make up a high proportion of health expenditure – with their efforts to increase jobs and exports. This dilemma is reflected in the price control schemes of several countries. Moreover, the useful life of different measures to contain expenditure is shorter than the time needed to identify and introduce them.

THE STRUCTURE OF THE PHARMACEUTICALS MARKET

A characteristic three-part demand system – the doctor prescribes the product; the patient consumes it, and health insurance pays the cost – creates structural imperfection in the pharmaceuticals market *(299–302)*. The demand for medicines is not controlled by the final consumer but by the physician, while the patient's costs are defrayed by the insurance system. Furthermore, the patient's ability to transform information into knowledge is limited, since many types of treatment are not repeated. Since medicines are seen as essential in ways that most goods are not, some fear that pharmaceutical companies can set whatever price they like.

The industry is characterized by continuous product innovation. All the major companies are heavily involved in research, competing on the basis of product suitability and differentiation rather than price. The ability to develop either new medicines or new vehicles for delivering them to patients is the driving force for growth in the industry. The patent system is of prime significance, providing legal protection to innovators for between 17 and 20 years in most countries. The effective life of a patent is less, however, owing to the time lag between registering a patent and bringing a product to market.

The role of marketing in maintaining a company's position is considerable. Even the medical profession depends to a significant degree on corporate marketing materials for pharmaceutical information. Companies compete for the attention of physicians. Although physicians could obtain all the essential knowledge on new products solely by reading medical journals and participating in continuing medical education on the subject, they rarely do so *(303)*. As the majority of marketing information is transmitted in terms of brand names, the pharmaceutical companies acquire still more market power.

In response to these self-interested and/or distorting influences, national policy-makers in most European countries have established various types of public regulatory agent. These are based on the assumption that profit incentives and market competition alone cannot generate a socially optimal level of information, or produce socially desirable decisions by pharmaceutical companies. The role of pharmaceutical regulation is complicated, however, by two industrial development concerns. First, the stringency of regulations on safety, prices and profits may discourage spending on research and development, leading to declining rates of innovation *(304,305)*. Second, a government's interest in increasing national income may lead it to seek to strengthen innovative companies.

Some commentators argue that the pharmaceuticals market is characterized by a supply-side monopoly. They conclude that high profits, high prices and high spending on promotion could only exist in an industry characterized by monopoly power. Other economists have suggested, in turn, that this is a "static analysis". They assert that competitive behaviour may be independent of the current structure, and propose a more dynamic analysis of the industry based on the competitive effects of product innovation. Such innovation, however, appears to be quite compatible with substantial degrees of market power, defined as the relation between prices and marginal costs.

The supporters of "dynamic analysis" also contend that the industry's profits are exaggerated and that high promotional spending, rather than being a barrier to entry, is an important means by which companies enter new markets. Supporters of the monopoly argument counter that the patent system allows monopoly supply situations, and offers the patent holder the opportunity to maintain higher prices. Patents also discourage potential new suppliers from entering the market. Some authors, however, question the importance of patent protection for achieving monopoly power in a therapeutic market *(306,307)*. They argue that any monopoly is short-term and, given substitutes, is unlikely to be absolute.

State regulation typically involves product safety, profit or price control, controls on marketing and advertising, and restrictions on overall pharmaceutical consumption. Intervention is generally exercised by a variety of agencies, in pursuit of a multiplicity of aims. The objective of these regulations is to supplement the workings of the market, but they are often concerned with means rather than with evaluating performance in relation to ends. Devising a financing system for pharmaceutical research that will not restrain development – or result in higher prices – remains a difficult task.

PROVISION OF PHARMACEUTICALS IN WESTERN EUROPE

There are large differences in the levels of spending on pharmaceuticals between western European countries. Table 16 illustrates pharmaceutical expenditure as a percentage of GDP and of health expenditure in selected countries. Pharmaceutical expenditure per head is also shown.

The high proportion of health expenditure devoted to drugs in Greece is striking, but this is based on OECD data, which greatly underestimate total health spending. Using a different estimate *(170)*, the figure comes down from 23.5% to 16.7%. Also remarkable is the fact that, in terms of US dollars, German spending on drugs per head is more than twice the level in the United Kingdom, while the difference between France and the United Kingdom is nearly as great. The main reason is the much higher volume of purchases in both France and Germany. The Netherlands has the lowest percentage of health spending on drugs in spite of its free pricing approach, which is only modified by a reference price system.

Table 16 is misleading in that it is based on final expenditure on pharmaceuticals, which in turn depends on wholesale and retail margins and value-added tax (VAT). All of these vary considerably between countries, as shown in Table 17, and therefore the above figures do not reflect uniform definitions. In most cases, margins are for the over-the-counter market as well as for the ethical market, while in others they are only for the ethical market. Differences in the levels of VAT levied and, indeed, whether it is charged at all on pharmaceuticals, are important. Retail margins also vary considerably. One factor underlying this last variation is the average population per pharmacy, as well as whether pharmacists can stock goods other than drugs.

Table 16. Expenditure on pharmaceuticals in selected western European countries, 1993

Country	Expenditure as a percentage of:		Expenditure per head (US $)
	GDP	health expenditure	
Belgium	1.4	16.7	288
Denmark	0.8	11.3	199
France	1.6	16.8	358
Germany	1.6	18.5	426
Greece[a]	1.3	23.5 (16.7)[b]	98
Ireland	0.9	14.0	123
Italy	1.5	18.0	268
Luxembourg[c]	1.0	14.6	274
Netherlands	1.0	10.9	193
Portugal[a]	1.2	17.0	115
Spain	1.3	18.2	194
Sweden	1.0	12.7	204
United Kingdom	1.1	14.9	173

[a] 1992.

[b] Based on the country estimate.

[c] 1991.

Source: OECD (49).

If the percentage of health expenditure on drugs is calculated in ex-factory prices, and the same margins are assumed to apply to the ethical market, the United Kingdom at 13.0% is the highest spender as a proportion of health expenditure, even though its spending per head in US dollars was the lowest apart from Greece.

In the western part of Europe, cost-containment measures in the pharmaceutical sector aim to influence physicians' prescription patterns and to render both doctors and patients more cost conscious. Strategies aimed at the whole market have also been developed. Table 18 illustrates the different approaches to cost-containment introduced in the last ten years. Cost-containment measures are seldom introduced singly, however. Here they are briefly reviewed sequentially.

Cost sharing

Current pharmaceutical expenditure depends partly on the quantity supplied and partly on the price of the goods or the workforce used to supply it. Pharmaceutical expenditure is also influenced by the payments normally made by patients. Table 19 summarizes the out-of-pocket payments that patients normally have to make for pharmaceuticals.

Table 17. Breakdown in percentages of the final price for retail pharmaceuticals in selected western European countries, 1993

Country	Ex-factory price	Wholesale margin	Retail margin	VAT and other taxes
Belgium	56.6	8.5	29.2	5.7
Denmark	55.3	4.0	20.7	20.0
France	63.5	6.9	27.5	2.1
Germany	55.3	8.8	22.7	13.2
Greece[a]	49.9	5.7	24.0	20.4
Italy (1995)[b]	64.43	7.21	21.63	3.85
Netherlands[c]	58.1	11.6	24.6	5.7
Portugal	68.6	7.6	19.1	4.8
Spain	59.9	8.2	29.0	2.9
Sweden[b]	68.2	2.8	29.0	–
United Kingdom[d]	87.5	7.5	5.0	–

[a] 1994.

[b] Prescribed medicines only.

[c] 1992.

[d] Prescribed medicines within the NHS.

Sources: Interministerial Prices Committee *(308)*; Vartholomeos & Tinios *(309)*; MEFA *(310)*.

All western European countries use cost sharing to reduce demand (see Chapter 3, pages 83–100). Usually, there are exemptions for those with low incomes, and for other categories that vary between countries. The proportion of the cost paid by the patient varies by type of drug in Denmark, France, Greece, Italy and Portugal, and for certain classes of drug in Belgium. In Germany, it now varies according to pack size. The co-payment is a flat rate in the United Kingdom and for some drugs in Belgium, and is a standard proportion of the cost in Spain. There is no co-payment in the Netherlands. There are extensive exemptions in Belgium, Denmark, Germany, Italy, Spain and the United Kingdom.

Positive and negative lists

Positive and negative lists for drugs have been introduced in a number of western European countries. Positive lists are found in Belgium, Denmark, France, Greece, Italy, the Netherlands and Portugal, though in Greece the list is not effectively enforced *(171)*. There is no positive list in Spain, but one is planned. In Italy, a committee was appointed in 1993 to formulate a new positive list. After 1993, non-allopathic drugs were no longer reimbursed in the Netherlands. Some countries with positive lists may also have negative lists, but a positive list subsumes the negative one.

Table 18. Alternative cost-containment strategies in the pharmaceutical sector in EU countries

Strategies	Country examples
Supply-side strategies	
Fixed budgets for doctors	Fundholding GPs in the United Kingdom
Indicative budgets for doctors	Germany, non-fundholding GPs in the United Kingdom
Fixed budgets for pharmaceutical expenditure	Germany, Italy
Practice guidelines	France
Cost–effectiveness guidelines	United Kingdom
Prescription auditing	Several countries but not in a systematic way, except in the United Kingdom
Disease management	Experiments in France and the United Kingdom
Positive and/or negative lists	All countries
Controlling the number of products	Denmark, Netherlands, Norway
Development of a market for generics	Mainly Denmark, Germany, Netherlands, United Kingdom
Capitation or salary payment for first-contact doctor	Several countries including Ireland, Italy, Netherlands, Spain, Sweden, United Kingdom
Ceilings on promotion expenditure	United Kingdom
Paying pharmacist on a flat rate rather than percentage basis	Netherlands, United Kingdom
Demand-side strategies	
Cost sharing	All countries except the Netherlands
Health education programmes	Netherlands, United Kingdom
Developing a market for over-the-counter products	

Table 18 (contd)

Strategies	Country examples
Strategies aimed at the market as a whole	
Price controls	All countries except Denmark, Germany, United Kingdom
Profit controls	United Kingdom
Reference prices	Denmark, Germany, Netherlands, Sweden
Industry contributions when budgets are exceeded	Germany in 1993, France from 1995
Fixed or revenue budgets for the industry	France, Spain
Taxes on promotional spending	France, Spain, Sweden
Development of a market for parallel imports	Denmark, Germany, Netherlands, United Kingdom
Development of a market for generics	Mainly Denmark, Germany, Netherlands, United Kingdom

Source: Mossialos & Abel-Smith *(311).*

Table 19. Cost sharing by patients in selected western European countries, 1995

Country	Cost sharing for pharmaceuticals
Belgium	Flat rate plus zero, 25%, 50%, 60%, 80% or 100% of price
Denmark	Flat rate plus 50%, 75% or 100%
France	Zero, 35%, 65% or 100%
Germany	DM 3, DM 5 or DM 7 depending on size of pack
Greece	Zero, 10% or 25% of price
Ireland	Zero or up to £IR 90 per quarter[a]
Italy	Flat rate of Lit 3000 or Lit 3000 plus 50%
Luxembourg	Zero or 20%
Netherlands	None
Portugal	30%, 60% or 100%
Spain	Zero or 40%[b]
Sweden	Skr 160 for the first and Skr 60 for subsequent items
United Kingdom	Flat rate of £5.25

[a] Only those above the income level for General Medical Service. Families buying products over £IR 90 of value per quarter are refunded the excess amount.

[b] Patients who are chronically sick have to pay 10% up to a maximum of 400 pesetas per prescription.

Source: Mossialos & Abel-Smith *(311).*

Germany, Ireland, Luxembourg, Spain and the United Kingdom have negative lists *(171).* Ireland extended the negative list of drugs available to General Medical Service patients[22] in 1982, and is planning a positive list. Germany also removed certain minor drugs from health insurance cover in 1983 and subtracted more in 1991; it is currently developing a positive list. In 1985, the United Kingdom removed a range of drugs from the NHS – mainly those obtainable without prescription – and extended this list in 1992. In 1993, Spain removed 800 drugs from its list.

The number of products

Some countries control the number of products on the market to reduce the pressure on physicians to prescribe new ones, or to minimize the pressure on regulatory authorities when the industry asks for price increases. The numbers of active ingredients and brand-named products on the market in different countries are shown in Table 20. It is notable that Norway manages with only about 2200 brands, compared to over 23 000 in Germany and some 43 000 in the United States.

---

[22] Patients with an income below a certain level (see Chapter 4, page 122).

Table 20. The number of products on the market in selected western European countries, 1993

Country	Active ingredients	Brands
Belgium	4 150	9 000
Denmark	2 300	4 861
France	4 200	9 500
Germany	8 862	23 529[a]
Italy	4 210	8 906
Netherlands	2 200	7 924
Norway	1 100	2 216
Spain	5 400	9 500
United Kingdom	–	10 000
United States	19 000	60 000[b]

[a] Products in the *Rote Liste*; it is estimated that the number of products on the market is about 70 000.

[b] American products on the international market; the national market has some 43 000.

Source: Abel-Smith & Mossialos *(171)*.

Pharmaceutical prices and pricing methodologies

The particular character of competition in the pharmaceutical market leads many governments to intervene and fix prices. A second reason for doing this is that a substantial part of drug expenditure is paid from public funds.

Variations in the prices of the same product in different western European countries suggest that the market is fragmented *(312)*. One attempt at comparison is shown in Table 21. These data, produced by the Association of German Pharmacists, are based on only 129 products chosen in 1988 and thus exclude a number of new products. The calculation has been criticized for this, and for other reasons. For example, it includes a number of over-the-counter drugs that are not reimbursable, and excludes generic drugs. For these reasons, the results should be interpreted as only very broadly indicative. Table 21 does not reflect the major changes made in the price control systems in France and Italy since 1991, or the large price increases granted in Greece in recent years. It does, however, indicate a wide variation in prices, with France and Greece well below other countries. Germany is placed surprisingly low in view of its policy of free pricing.

Table 22 presents the OECD price index for pharmaceuticals. Between 1988 and 1993, there were virtually no price increases in France and the Netherlands, while most other western European countries experienced a steady rise. The increase in Greece is particularly marked, although prices were at a very low level in 1988.

Table 21. Pharmaceutical price levels in selected western European countries, 1988–1993 (EU average = 100)

Country	1988	1989	1990	1991	1992	1993
Belgium	88.6	91.0	92.6	100.5	107.7	116.2
Denmark	128.1	131.1	136.7	143.4	134.6	132.9
France	71.5	69.0	66.9	63.8	60.2	63.4
Germany	128.4	123.5	116.6	110.5	105.0	105.4
Greece	73.8	80.0	80.0	85.5	80.8	84.7
Ireland	130.5	129.8	132.2	129.8	129.5	133.2
Italy	79.1	83.1	89.4	96.1	102.8	95.5
Luxembourg	97.1	95.6	93.5	94.5	93.6	97.1
Netherlands	131.9	127.7	129.9	134.1	139.0[a]	148.4[a]
Portugal	67.5	61.7	57.9	57.7	60.9	67.0
Spain	71.6	70.8	76.6	83.7	89.4[a]	93.5[a]
United Kingdom	115.9	123.1	125.6	124.6	126.4	122.7

[a] Provisional figures.

Source: Bundesvereinigung Deutscher Apothekerverbände (313).

Table 22. Expenditure on pharmaceuticals in selected western European countries, 1988–1993 (1990 = 100)

Year	Belgium	France	Germany	Greece	Italy	Netherlands	Sweden	United Kingdom
1988	95.0	103.2	88.5	75.6	97.4	102.6	101.8	95.2
1989	97.8	102.5	99.9	100	98.2	100.6	99.9	97.6
1990	100	100	100	100	100	100	100	100
1991	102.6	100.5	100.8	116.7	104.9	100.4	104.9	103.0
1992	107.1	101.3	102.4	127.9	105.9	102.4	110.7	107.1
1993	–	102.0	110.5	–	110.9	102.7	–	109.4

Source: OECD (49).

What is the apparent effect of these different systems of regulating prices and/or profits on the level of drug prices in the different countries? For a number of reasons, it is not possible to make accurate comparisons. First, a high proportion of sales in one country may be for products not sold in other countries. Second, products can be similar but not identical, or identical but traded under a different name in another country. Third, package sizes, strengths, dosages and presentations vary, and ingredients may be combined. Fourth, the importance of a product in the sales of one country may be very different from that in another country. A fifth problem is determining which price should be compared: wholesale, retail (with or without discounts), hospital, or the gross or net price to the consumer. Margins for wholesalers and retailers differ between countries, as do the level of VAT and whether or not it is levied on these products. Finally, there is the problem of varying exchange rates and the imperfection of attempts to develop purchasing power parities.

The methods of regulating or influencing pricing are shown in Table 23. The underlying mechanisms are shown in the left-hand column, even though they have recently, as in France, been superseded by budgets. Presumably, if the budget system does not work effectively or if the industry is unwilling to continue it, France will revert to its old system.

Most western European countries, except Denmark, Germany, the Netherlands and (partially and indirectly) Luxembourg, control either the prices or the profits of the pharmaceutical industry. Denmark, Germany, the Netherlands and Sweden have introduced a reference price system for non-patented medicines.

It is notable that countries have been introducing multiple systems for controlling pharmaceutical expenditure over the past few years. Despite their basic systems, such as price control, profit control or reference pricing, other controls have been added. Several countries have imposed cuts on all prices, and five have budgets that have been either agreed with and enforced by the industry, with penalties for physicians, or simply laid down by the government.

There is no objective way of establishing the "real" price of a pharmaceutical product. The capital equipment costs of the company, its overheads, its research and development costs and its sales promotion costs (as several of the company's products may be promoted together) are shared among its products. The cost of production and, to some extent, the cost of packaging depend on the level of sales, as the earlier French system of price control explicitly recognized. The French system, before company revenue budgets were introduced, did not take account of production costs, but granted higher prices for products that contributed to the national economy.

Two countries that have been using price controls, Belgium and France, attempt to assess the innovativeness of the product or its advantage over existing products when setting prices. It can be difficult, however, to determine price advantage objectively. For many years, both countries had incentives for companies to produce items similar to existing products in order to obtain lower prices for the new ones.

Some countries, such as Greece, Ireland and Portugal, base their prices on those in other European countries. Italy and the Netherlands use, or are planning to establish, prices based on the average prices of other countries.

Revenue budgets for each company, introduced in France in 1994, could result in an inverse relationship between price and volume. The more a company sells, the lower the price will have to be. What is critical is how far the government takes account of the therapeutic value of what the company produces. In view of the difficulty of doing this, there may well be a tendency for companies to set targets that are based on previous sales. This may discourage the search for really innovative drugs, because if a company is drawing sufficient revenue from existing products it would not have the incentive to

Table 23. Methods of regulating or influencing prices of pharmaceuticals in selected western European countries

Country	Basic mechanism for regulating or influencing prices	Price cut	Budget
Belgium	Prices based on improvement over existing products	–	–
Denmark	Reference price system excluding patented drugs	–	–
France	Prices fixed on medical effectiveness and negotiations with companies	–	Revenue maximum per company to achieve 3.2% growth in expenditure in 1994
Germany	Reference price system excluding patented drugs	5% cut ending 1994	Indicative budgets for each physician for each region (physicians at risk for DM 280 million)
Greece	Prices fixed based on cost, transfer price and the three lowest prices in the EU	–	–
Ireland	Average price of the same product in the United Kingdom and a basket of EU countries (Denmark, France, Germany, Netherlands and United Kingdom)	3% in August 1993 and price freeze ending July 1996	–
Italy	Average prices of France, Germany, Spain and United Kingdom	2.5% or 5% cut ending 1995	Laid down by the government
Luxembourg	Prices set with reference to the price of the product's country of origin	–	–
Netherlands	Average prices of Belgium, France, Germany and United Kingdom and reference price system including some patented drugs	5% cut ending June 1996	–
Portugal	Upper ceiling corresponding to the lowest prices in France, Italy and Spain	–	–

Table 23 (contd)

Country	Basic mechanism for regulating or influencing prices	Price cut	Budget
Spain	Prices based on "cost"	3% cut ending 1997	7% growth in expenditure to be enforced by the industry in 1995
Sweden	Reference price system excluding patented drugs	–	–
United Kingdom	Profit regulation	2.5% cut ending autumn 1996	Indicative for non-fundholding GPs but firm for fundholders

Source: Mossialos & Abel-Smith *(311).*

produce new ones, apart from imitations. It has been reported in the French press that companies have been told that they will be treated more favourably if they invest in France and if they are willing to develop generic drugs. This is intended to ensure that, as a generics market develops, it will be stocked with French rather than imported products.

The United Kingdom is the only western European country that operates a profit control system. Prices are set by the pharmaceutical industry, and are indirectly controlled through the Pharmaceutical Price Regulation Scheme. This is a non-statutory agreement negotiated between the Department of Health and the Association of the British Pharmaceutical Industry (ABPI). The scheme has been in operation in various forms since 1957, and it regulates the profits that companies make from their sales to the NHS *(314)*. The scheme does not cover generic products. While the general agreement is negotiated between the Department of Health and the ABPI, individual company details are negotiated between the Department of Health and the company concerned. The scheme operates at the level of a company's total business with the NHS, rather than in relation to individual products, and it measures profitability in terms of the return on capital employed. For companies that do not have any significant capital in the United Kingdom, it is assessed on the basis of return on sales. The use of return on capital employed reflects the regulator's objective of preventing pharmaceutical companies from making excessive profits from the NHS.

Reference price systems

Reference price systems operate by grouping similar products and specifying the price that will be fully covered by insurance, subject to co-payment. The use of a reference price as a reimbursement benchmark implies that the government will pay only that particular price; any excess has to be paid by the insured person. The key issue is the criteria that are used to select the reference price. The earliest scheme appears to have been tried in New Zealand. In Europe, this system was initiated by Germany and it now applies to about half of pharmaceutical expenditure. It was introduced in the Netherlands in 1991 and in Denmark in 1993, and is also used in Norway and Sweden. Reference pricing has been proposed in Finland, Greece, Italy and Spain, but has not been implemented.

There are three stages in the introduction of a reference price system. The first covers identical preparations and the second equivalent products or combinations. The third was originally defined as covering preparations that had pharmaceutical and therapeutic similarity, but this was later modified to therapeutic similarity. A difficulty with this system is that, if one or more products are still under patent, the reference price system cannot be applied to them.

The effect of the reference price system in Germany was that spending on pharmaceuticals by the sickness funds fell by 20.6% in the first half of 1993. Monthly increases in expenditure resumed after the initial reduction. Another effect was that prescribing switched to expensive products not covered by the system, such as new antibiotics. Advertising by the pharmaceutical companies encouraged this trend.

The reference price system is to be extended, so that it is expected to cover 80% of 1989 consumption, or 60% after a positive list has been introduced. The selection criteria for this list will be effectiveness, efficiency and quality, and the list will be chosen by a new body including representatives of sickness funds and physicians, together with independent members. Manufacturers were required to reduce the prices of their non-reference-priced drugs and over-the-counter drugs by 5% during 1993 and 1994, and prices were then frozen for two years.

In July 1991 in the Netherlands, a reference price system was introduced for products considered to be interchangeable (taking into account any side effects) according to five criteria, and judged by an independent committee of experts reporting to the Association of Sickness Funds. The consumption of products clustered in this way rose by only 5% in a year, while that of other products rose by 20%. It was then decided that new products that could not be clustered would not be covered by the health insurance schemes, while older unclustered products would be brought into the reference price system. Patients have to pay any costs above the reference price, the amount now payable being about an eighth of what they paid when the scheme began.

Denmark introduced a reference price system in July 1993. It covers 20% of the drug market in terms of consumption. The groups of products selected are identical, both in chemical and pharmaceutical terms. They are grouped on the basis of type of pack, and the reference price is fixed as the average of the two cheapest products in the group. There are no plans to extend the reference price system beyond these identical products. The expected savings are just over 1% of gross drug consumption, including over-the-counter products.

Price freezes or across-the-board price cuts

Germany, Greece and Italy have often utilized unilateral price cuts. Recently, the United Kingdom imposed a three-year price freeze that ended in autumn 1996. Italy and Spain have also imposed across-the-board price reductions. Some other common methods used by EU member states to control prices are the following.

Some countries, such as Italy, establish the initial selling price of a new product, while others, such as France, establish the initial reimbursement price. The United Kingdom requires government approval for price increases. In France and Sweden, new products considered to compete with a similar existing product are automatically assigned a price 10% below the original or the last approved price for the existing product. In Greece, such products are given a price 14% below that of the existing product.

Another form of indirect price control is for a government to demand from the entire industry that it propose a plan to "pay back" or "not charge" a particular sum for a given year. In France, drug expenditure in 1995 was expected to increase by 8.5%, i.e. well above the established target. The result was that the pharmaceutical industry was asked to make a single provisional contribution of FF 2.5 billion on terms to be negotiated with the industry.

Ceilings and taxes on promotional expenses

A tax on total expenditure for pharmaceutical promotion is levied in France. The most complicated system is in the United Kingdom, where expenses above a certain level, defined by a formula for each company, are disallowed for the purposes of calculating company returns for the profit control system.

Companies have argued that taxes on overall promotion have the additional drawback of penalizing those companies that launch new products more frequently than others, and therefore need to spend above-average amounts on marketing and information. This system, however, can also discourage the introduction of new chemical entities that are no better than existing products, since companies will have to direct allowable expenses for promotion to a limited number of products.

Expenditure ceilings

These can operate on top of other measures, such as the reference price system in Germany or the profit control system in the United Kingdom.

In Germany in 1993, the government imposed an overall budget for pharmaceutical costs on each area covered by a regional physicians' association. Up to DM 280 million of any spending over these budgets had to be paid back by the physicians on a basis determined by each association, and any further excess up to DM 280 million had to be met by the pharmaceutical industry. A fixed budget was again laid down for the following year. This time, any overspending up to DM 280 million would have fallen only on the physicians.

In France, the government has reached an agreement with the pharmaceutical industry, which is intended to impose controls on the volume of sales in return for greater flexibility in fixing prices for some medicines. Under this agreement, concluded in January 1994, national targets will be set for pharmaceutical expenditure. A target of a 3.2% increase was set for 1994, well below the 7.5% increase in 1993.

Influencing physicians' prescribing

Prescribing is examined in most western European countries, and high authorizers may be warned, threatened or subjected to financial penalties. Another way of influencing prescribing behaviour is to promote the use of generics or to allow generic substitution. These policies have come under sustained attack from the pharmaceutical industry. Within the EU as a whole, generic medicines accounted for about 6.5% of the total ethical pharmaceutical market in 1992, and generated revenues estimated at US $2.5 billion (315). Over 80% of these revenues came from sales in four markets: Denmark, Germany, the Netherlands and the United Kingdom. The potential for generic substitution remains considerable, and is likely to grow. It has been calculated that the potential generic market is 77% of the drug market in France, 64% in Germany and 63% in the United Kingdom (316).

Some countries are also seeking to change authorizing behaviour by giving physicians responsibility for budgets, as in the United Kingdom where GPs have been authorized to become fundholders, or by offering physicians part of any savings, as in Ireland. Fundholding practices, which have a prescribing allowance within the firm budgets allocated to them, already have this incentive, plus the advantage of the ability to shift funds between drugs, staff and treatments.

Parallel imports

Parallel trade arises because of the large differences in prices between western European countries. The scale of parallel imports is not yet large, in spite of the large price differentials.

Investment inducements

Many of the regulatory measures introduced create opportunities to discriminate in favour of national pharmaceutical companies, contributing to national investment or employment. Governments often try to balance prices for particular products with other economic benefits that a particular company performs for the country, such as exports, employment and research and development. With this practice, the product is not judged on its merits.

Competition exists between governments in their attempts to attract foreign investment in local pharmaceutical production. This results in investment incentives in the form of state support or other incentives such as tax concessions or cheaper property.

PROVISION OF PHARMACEUTICALS IN THE CEE AND CIS COUNTRIES

The majority of problems facing the pharmaceuticals sector in the CEE and CIS countries can be traced back to the former highly centralized delivery systems, with their strong emphasis on quantity. The consequence was a poorly maintained and equipped, overspecialized, overstaffed and inadequately coordinated system that now confronts deep structural problems. When the acute shortage of drugs and medical devices is added, along with budget shortfalls (resulting in a lack of money in the hospital sector, i.e. non-payment for drugs), the lack of proper reimbursement and pricing mechanisms, and the absence of adequate legislation and regulation, the extent of the crisis in the pharmaceutical supply system becomes apparent.

In most CEE and CIS countries, governments realize the nature of their inherited problems and have adopted a series of reforms. The former concepts of centralization and emphasis on budget are being replaced by principles of decentralization, privatization, quality of care, professionalism and attention to the broader issues of disease prevention and health protection and promotion. The speed of these changes, however, depends critically on the availability of funds as well as on the ability of the respective ministries to divest themselves of certain activities, while at the same time maintaining the necessary level of control over the drug supply system.

The drug supply system in transition

The introduction of a market-oriented drug supply system is accepted in most CEE and CIS countries as a necessary part of the general reform process. The decision on whether to privatize was typically taken at an early stage in the transition period, resulting in forms of ownership in the drug supply system that would not be acceptable in western Europe. Only a few countries included exceptions for the pharmaceutical sector in their legislation, and only very few of them, such as Turkmenistan, kept the entire sector in state hands. Rapid privatization, combined with a lack of proper regulation, has often led to chaotic and unmanageable development. The result has been high prices, a surplus of imported drugs, excessive margins and enormous profits, all of which reduce accessibility and affordability.

Despite these excesses, there are cases where the introducing of a market-oriented (private) sector saved a country from severe shortages of supply. In some CIS countries, the drug supply for community pharmacies was almost completely taken over by the private sector within one or two years, owing to serious shortfalls in the state budget and the inflexibility of the state-owned sector. This development was encouraged by deteriorating levels of drug production in the Russian Federation, traditionally the main supplier of the state-owned wholesalers in the CEE and CIS countries.

The process of change in the drug supply system in the CEE and CIS countries has followed several stages (Box 17). Countries have passed through these either more or less rapidly depending on the national situation and on the influence of key persons in the sector. Table 24 illustrates the difficulties experienced by government regulatory bodies in keeping up with the rapid development of the private sector.

The functioning of public regulatory bodies needs to be improved and their capabilities strengthened. The distribution system is also having difficulties, owing to a lack of funds and its small-scale structure. This lack of funds and the limited possibilities for drug reimbursement lead to high out-of-pocket payments for patients. Out-of-pocket payments of 50% or more seriously affect the availability and affordability of drugs for large sections of the population.

In sum, although most governments have expressed their intention to guarantee the supply of drugs to their citizens, regardless of income and geographical situation (sometimes in the constitution, or in a drug policy document), the goals of accessibility, affordability and equity are often not met. This reflects both problems within the public sector and the inability of the private sector (by its nature) to take responsibility for achieving these objectives.

Position of the public sector

The current position of the public sector in the drug supply system in the economies of the CEE and CIS countries is dramatically weaker than in the past, when the health ministries controlled the complete drug delivery and compensation process. This weakened position has been caused by a deterioration in the public sector, and by its inability to manage an unknown, market-oriented sector. The functioning of the public sector itself is deteriorating, owing to the following factors.

Global decisions on privatization result in health ministries losing control over and ownership of state-owned wholesalers (sometimes including an extensive pharmacy network). This may also result in the health ministry receiving inadequate information on the volume and prices of drugs sold, and mean that drug supplies to public institutions are no longer guaranteed.

Lack of funds, owing to shrinking government budgets and priority setting at higher levels, leads to:

Box 17. Stages in drug supply transition

Stage 1.   *Implicit introduction of private ownership*
Private ownership is introduced in the drug supply system as part of general measures to encourage private initiatives within the framework of economic reforms, without subsequent adaptation of relevant legislation.

Stage 2.   *Emergence of a number of private pharmacies*
Private pharmacies emerge in addition to the existing state-owned system. These new pharmacies show many ownership forms (not necessarily limited to pharmacists), but mostly do not comply with accepted standards.

Stage 3.   *Decentralization of the state-owned sector*
Privatization can take place only after decentralization of old structures and when each pharmacy has its own financial account. Some countries decentralized before the fall of the former regimes, whereas other countries are just beginning.

Stage 4.   *Privatization of the state-owned sector*
This privatization[a] takes place gradually, depending on the available funds and the will to privatize. In many cases it is financed by profits from current activities. Some countries maintain an interest in the sector to guarantee supply, and keep some pharmacies or a wholesaler under state control.

Stage 5.   *Uncontrolled market expansion*
Increased availability of imported drugs, rising prices, margins and profits, uncontrollable sale of drugs, and examples of unacceptable and irresponsible behaviour trigger the need for regulation. This is supported by emerging social problems (inequity).

Stage 6.   *Setting up of regulating authorities*
Supporting, controlling and regulating authorities are introduced (with functions previously performed by ministries or state-owned wholesalers). The initial focus on privatization is replaced by investing in legislation, regulation and control structures. This process needs key professionals and funds.

Stage 7.   *Sector regulation*
The sector is gradually regulated in terms of licensing, setting minimum standards, limits to forms of ownership, limiting the establishment of new pharmacies and guaranteed coverage in rural and remote areas, etc.

---

[a] Privatization of pharmacies predominantly by employee ownership schemes or by voucher programmes.

Table 24. Pharmaceutical sector development in selected CEE and CIS countries, March 1995

Item	Country				
	Albania	Armenia	Georgia	Tajikistan	The Former Yugoslav Republic of Macedonia
National drug legislation	Yes	Draft under discussion	Draft under discussion	No	Draft under discussion
Essential drug list	Yes, but not used	Yes	Yes	No	No
Drug registration	Limited functioning	Yes	Limited functioning	–	Limited functioning
Quality control laboratory	No	Recently established	No	–	No
Drug regulatory agency	Being established	Established	No, independent units	–	No
Inspection	Not functioning	Yes, to be improved	Not functioning	–	Yes, to be improved
Good pharmacy practice (317) guidelines	No	No	No	–	No
Distribution system	Limited functioning	Limited functioning	Poorly functioning	Chaotic	Limited functioning
Privatization	Started	Started	Started	Discussed	Started
Licensing of pharmacies	Yes	Started	Started	–	Yes

Source: Walt (318).

- underfunding of the health care system;
- insufficient funds for hospital drugs;
- underpayment of officials, resulting in a large turnover of personnel;
- personnel moving from state-owned companies to the private sector in search of higher pay;
- insufficient funds to maintain proper control and inspection; and
- large out-of-pocket payments and co-payments for drugs.

The workforce and the control and inspection equipment are inadequate. Finally, tensions have built up between central-level institutes and decentralized bodies over supervision of the drug supply system.

This deterioration of public authority seriously affects the position of the state as a reliable employer and as a health care provider.

The public sector's inability to manage the new market-oriented sector can be ascribed to a number of reasons:

- the inability to withstand commercial pressures to privatize rapidly and introduce a "free market" in pharmaceuticals;
- the lack of legislation to regulate a market-oriented supply system;
- the lack of understanding of how a market-oriented system works;
- insufficient knowledge about how such systems are regulated elsewhere in the world; and
- the lack of adequate forums for discussion with representatives of the pharmaceutical industry, which isolates the public sector, even though many in the pharmaceutical sector have a professional attitude and are willing to help find acceptable solutions.

In the initial phase of the transition process, the actions of the health ministry are often left behind by the speed of events in the market-place, where the focus is on privatization and restructuring.

Overall, the state's position in the transition process in the CEE and CIS countries is quite weak. Much depends on the power of certain key people. Later, when the focus returns to drug financing, reimbursement, essential drug lists or formularies, the influence of a health ministry gradually increases. Authority is restored, however, only when the necessary instruments are in place and the sphere of influence of the health ministries and drug control agencies improves.

The position of the private sector

The private sector's position in the transitional period has been quite strong, although there has been some resistance to privatization and regulations are often quite tight.

In the drug supply system, private wholesale activities are prospering and it is sometimes surprising to see how quickly markets develop. In general, the private pharmaceutical wholesale sector has established a substantial market share in a short time. At first, there are typically many small wholesalers and traders (and many intermediaries). After one to two years, however, this intermediate trade and the number of wholesalers decrease.

At pharmacy level, a wide variety of types of ownership has emerged, ranging from kiosks to large professionally run pharmacies. Pharmacies can be owned by pharmacists, cooperatives of employees, pharmaceutical wholesalers, prescribing physicians or business people from other sectors. This range reflects the fact that it can be difficult to restrict ownership because of constitutional rights and insufficient legislation.

The private pharmaceutical sector in the CEE and CIS countries cannot in general be compared with that in western Europe. This is due to the sector focusing on: high-profit, imported drugs; a narrow range of products with few low-priced drugs; quantity instead of quality; and profit instead of a reasonable income. The low level of organization, the lack of common standards or quality levels (such as those set out in the WHO guidelines on good pharmacy practice *(317)*, and low levels of responsibility for the public service function of the pharmacist are contributing factors.

In general, once specific regulations are introduced in the pharmaceutical sector, the performance of the private sector improves: the worst cases disappear, and pharmacies with a more professional attitude are upgraded.

Key problem areas

Policy concerns raised by western European and North American consultants have focused on state policies and responsibilities, reflecting the perceived weakness of the public sector in managing the reform process adequately (see points 1–4 below). Officials from CEE and CIS countries bring up different, more technical topics, reflecting the lack of proper instruments and the complexity of the reform process in the pharmaceutical sector (points 5–9 below).

1. In its priority setting, the state is frequently more occupied with privatization than with health care financing and cost-containment. This generates inequity, impedes access and lowers affordability (high co-payments).

2. Markets are growing very fast, fuelled by rising imports. At the same time, overprescribing and polypharmacy produce a great deal of irrational drug consumption.

3. Markets develop faster than public sector capacities and actions, and the legislation process takes a long time.

4. There is a lack of a comprehensive strategy or national drug policy. Some countries have adopted a coherent strategy for the pharmaceutical sector and a framework for politicians, government officials and professionals for the future. The lack of a policy, however, leads to ad hoc decision-making, and slows down the reform process.

5. Some countries have a constitutional obligation to provide drugs without charge to large groups of the population. With an increasing volume of higher-priced imports, the levels of public drug expenditure in the CEE and CIS countries are growing far above those in western Europe. Budgetary constraints are becoming tighter and there is an urgent need for satisfactory solutions.

6. Reimbursement systems may ease the burden on both the government and the patient. Needs assessment is essential but is often not properly done, while cost-containment is often given a low priority.

7. Privatization opens the way for a wide variety of forms of ownership, but quality and professional standards are often substandard. Large investments, as well as a transfer of knowledge, are needed in order to establish a viable pharmaceutical manufacturing industry. This takes time, and requires good partners and adequate funding.

8. Patent protection, inspection and quality control are high-priority issues for pharmaceutical professionals, but are frequently hard to achieve in tandem with rapid market development.

9. Donations to charity cause numerous problems. They distort the distribution system and introduce unnecessary drugs, drugs with short expiry dates, new brands and unregistered drugs into a country.

Each of these key problem areas has an impact on the main public health policy target, which is to make essential and appropriate drugs widely accessible. Access has been positively influenced by privatization and market growth. Overall policy objectives have been negatively influenced by inefficient distribution chains, high price levels, low quality, incomplete information, budget problems and the lack of reimbursement systems or health insurance.

Developments in the CEE and CIS countries show that, while for large parts of the population the availability of drugs has increased, affordability has decreased for many groups. Unless proper funding and fair reimbursement mechanisms are in place, the social inequity within rapidly privatized drug supply systems will continue to harm vulnerable groups of the population.

Allocating capital for investing in health

One key aspect of technological change and overall growth in the health sector has been the accumulation of capital in hospitals, clinics and other facilities. The shape of today's health system and the types of service it delivers are simultaneously supported and constrained by the existing capital infrastructure. Similarly, today's investments will determine much of the structure of future service delivery options.

In both the formerly socialist CEE and CIS countries, where the primary objective of reform is to restructure the previous hierarchical system, and in western Europe, where the main objectives are deregulation, cost-containment and controlling technology, one key element on the reform agenda is dissatisfaction with present allocation of capital and use of technology. Developing and strengthening alternatives to hospital care, such as PHC and day centres, and making better use of and coordinating the existing resources within the hospital sector, are common goals. Nevertheless, there are also important differences between countries when it comes to institutional characteristics, reform policies and particular organizational issues.

CONCEPTUAL FRAMEWORK

Economists distinguish between capital, investment and depreciation. Capital refers to the existing *stock* of productive assets. Investment, in contrast, is a *flow* and involves additions to capital. Depreciation is also a flow, and refers to subtractions from capital as the value of the productive assets decreases over time. The distinction between these concepts is important, because it identifies investment as a critical dynamic activity that is adjusting the capital structure of the sector. This adjustment of capital stock usually occurs only slowly over time. Investment exceeding 5–10% of the existing capital stock would be unusual. Thus, it has taken many years to accumulate the present capital infrastructure of hospitals and other facilities in Europe.

The level of technology in health care can be defined on the basis of the ability to understand, influence and prevent diseases *(319)*. This framework provides a useful starting point for discussing past patterns of investment and present allocation of capital in the health sector. At the basic level, among the so-called "non-technologies", health services are characterized by taking care of sick people and nursing them. Knowledge of the pathological process is usually slight; in any event, there is not much there can be done to halt the progress of the illness in question. An example of care in this area would be that for patients with incurable diseases, such as AIDS, and also for those with minor diseases for which there is no effective medical treatment, such as the common cold. The next level is "half-way technology". This offers the possibility of counteracting the unfavourable effects of disease or of postponing death but, owing to insufficient knowledge about the disease mechanism, it cannot provide a complete cure. Examples are those commonly known as "high-tech" care, such as organ transplants and treatment for cancer or diabetes. At the final level, among the "high technologies", a genuine understanding of the disease mechanism does exist so that it is possible to cure the illness in question completely, or even prevent it. Vaccines for many epidemic and other diseases, and antibiotics are good examples.

This framework is limited to links between the knowledge of disease mechanisms and technologies and excludes, for example, trauma care. Furthermore, the definition of "technology" is rather narrow, and specifically based on the understanding of diseases. Despite these limitations, the framework provides a useful starting point for discussing the dynamic links between technology, costs and capital in the health sector.

A DYNAMIC PROCESS

At any given point in time, health services comprise a mix of different forms of technology, based on the current knowledge and understanding of disease and trauma. Using the three levels described above, some services are based on non-technologies, others are half-way technologies, while others are based on high technologies. The mix of different forms of technology is directly linked to capital spending.

In most cases, however, technological breakthroughs develop from non-technologies to half-way technologies. It is plausible that the cost function associated with a disease, as knowledge grows from non-technology to high technology, is in most cases an inverted U *(320)*. This means that spending is highest on the half-way technologies. Of course, new techniques that entail lower costs per patient may also result in a greater volume of services performed, owing to more widespread use of the technology, and thus may generate an increase in total spending.

In an ideal relationship between investments, health technologies, capital and health sector reforms, one should first make certain that investments are allocated to the right form of capital, i.e. that they are carefully balanced between different forms of care. This allocation should be guided by given levels of technology and knowledge. If a technological breakthrough allows a certain disease to be treated more cost-effectively in outpatient settings, or even prevented through the use of vaccines or other measures, the inpatient facilities where patients formerly received treatment should be rapidly scaled down, closed or used for other purposes, and investments made in outpatient facilities or preventive measures.

Second, investments made in the health sector should promote the move towards high technology. Costly but inefficient half-way technologies should be avoided as far as possible. This will also send important signals to private equipment manufacturers on how they should allocate their research and development budgets. Third, reinvestments in capital should be carefully balanced with operational spending, to ensure that an appropriate stock of capital is maintained over time. In the absence of such a balance, two types of problem are likely to emerge. If too high a percentage of available resources is invested in new capital stock, too little will be left for operational spending. In the worst case, there will be no money left to start up the new activity in question. On the other hand, if too few available resources are invested, capital stock will deteriorate, with negative effects on service quality and possibly on operational spending as well.

Existing indications of capital allocation make intercountry comparisons difficult. There are differences in definition and in forms of care across countries; it is difficult to measure quality, and there are differences in technology levels. For example, bed numbers are a common proxy for hospital capital. Yet in one country the number may aggregate long-term and acute beds, while in another these classifications may be separate. A bed in a small, understaffed and underequipped rural hospital is not comparable to a bed in a large, well equipped facility with skilled staff. Furthermore, it is hard to make direct comparisons between data concerning, for instance, length of stay in central, eastern and western Europe, since health service provision is based on different levels of technology.

The effectiveness of hospital services in many CEE and CIS countries is adversely influenced by the poor quality of capital stock. Many of the small district hospitals in the CIS have no more than 4–5 m² per bed. Some of the smallest hospitals also have low occupancy rates and lack radiology services, adequate heating and running water.

According to OECD statistics, occupancy rates average 60–85% among countries in western Europe. The same variances typically exist within countries, if rates at different types of institution and in urban versus rural settings are compared. In most western European countries, the average length of stay is well below ten days for acute hospitals, substantially less than in the CEE and CIS countries. As already noted, the difference partly reflects the fact that health services in the two parts of the Region are based on different levels of technology. In western Europe, for example, the widespread use of laparoscopic surgery has substantially decreased the average length of stay. Another explanation for these differences is that hospitals in the CEE and CIS countries have more of a social function, similar to that provided in western Europe by other facilities such as nursing homes and home care services. Moreover, hospitals in western Europe are on average more efficient in their provision of services.

Differences in the accumulation of capital in the hospital sector in different countries can partly be explained by different geographical and infrastructural conditions. These factors may explain why Norway, which has greater transport problems than Sweden, also has more hospitals in relation to its population. Different organizational incentives may also play a part. For example, the comparatively long lengths of stay in German hospitals are sometimes attributed to the fact that they have traditionally been paid per diem, and that before 1992 German hospitals were not allowed to provide outpatient care. When the British NHS was established in 1948, it took over some 3000 hospitals organized according to two different systems: public hospitals and private non-profit institutions. Even today, the structure of hospital care in the United Kingdom may partly be accounted for by referring to conditions that existed before 1948.

The capital allocation process for hospitals in western Europe varies according to structures of hospital ownership and styles of public regulation. In nearly every country, however, there is a detailed regulatory framework through which national or regional governments determine the location and service characteristics of major hospital investments.

The locus of control over funds for new investments is a central planning issue. In tax-financed health systems in western Europe, it has traditionally been a national (Finland, the United Kingdom) or regional (Sweden) public authority that accumulates funds and makes investment decisions.

Although the United Kingdom reforms that turned hospitals into "self-governing trusts" were originally expected to give these self-managing institutions control over their capital investments (321), political concern about the total public sector borrowing requirement has led to renewed control over new hospital borrowing by the Treasury. Trusts do receive capital depreciation payments as part of their operating budgets, and these can be put towards the purchase of capital equipment and less expensive renovations.

In health systems financed by social insurance, hospitals usually receive capital depreciation payments on their operating budgets. In the Netherlands, private hospitals retain the ability to borrow funds for new projects, while in Germany new capital is allocated by the 16 *Länder* according to public objectives. There is substantial tension in the Netherlands between the Ministry of Welfare, Health and Cultural Affairs, which administers strict national controls on new services, equipment and capital investments, and the predominantly private hospitals, each of which controls its own depreciation and borrowed funds.

SOME CURRENT ISSUES

Throughout Europe, the dynamic link between investments and future operational spending is a major concern. The forces determining the accumulation of capital stock differ in the private and public sectors. In countries where the sector has been centrally directed and predominantly publicly managed, investment in new capital has been driven by central planning, typically through a budgeting process determined by population and service capacity norms. Public budgeting does not, however, always reflect the real cost of investment. Public investment may also flow into hospitals and equipment that, for example, duplicate facilities for different populations or occupational groups in the same urban area. In the CEE and CIS countries, investment decisions made through central planning were too far removed from local environments to reflect local community needs. Reforms that separate financing from care provision will change the locus of investment control, and could create new problems in coordinating investment policy with the existing structure of capital stock.

In the private sector, financial incentives determine the size and type of investment. In principle, investment flows into technologies and infrastructure that provide the greatest profits. Ideally, this response to market forces results in an efficient use of resources. There are, however, important reasons why this principle is not always achieved in capital investment in health. Market failures may restrict the efficient functioning of the market, and encourage a misallocation of capital that favours large hospitals and the indiscriminate accumulation of new technology. Information deficits make it difficult for health service payers to make appropriate assessments and investment choices. Equity is also affected if the allocation of capital is left to market forces, particularly in low-income or rural areas, or for certain medical conditions.

The form of the provider payment system establishes incentives for both public and private investment decisions in a more indirect way (320). Fee-for-service payment, especially in combination with passive third-party payers and patient choice, encourages supplier-induced demand, the costly expansion of specialist services and indiscriminate investment in new technology. On the other hand, line-item budgeting in the public sector, especially when it is applied with service norms, has also led in the past to overinvestment in hospital beds and equipment. In a number of countries, continuing health sector reforms are changing the payment system capital through case-based fixed fees, capitation systems and global budgets to encourage greater efficiency in the use of capital.

Since continuing reforms in the health sector are likely to result in more self-regulating providers, changing the ownership and management of capital will be an essential task for reforms in the CEE and CIS countries. The objective is to increase the incentives to provide efficient services. Short of privatization, greater managerial autonomy may be achieved through decentralization to regional or local government control, or through contracts for managing publicly owned facilities. In some systems in western Europe, hospitals are publicly owned but autonomously financed through global budgets or contracts. These providers face less detailed regulations, but more demands are placed on them to use resources efficiently. This also encourages more careful planning of the links between investment, capital, depreciation and operational spending, starting at local level.

In the CEE and CIS countries, as in western Europe, the scaling down and merging of hospitals into fewer units began in the 1990s. Bed numbers have been reduced since 1990. In many cases, however, closing hospitals and reducing beds have been on a small scale because of the political and practical difficulties involved in transferring resources from one use to another. Closing specialist units and integrating them into general facilities is also an important reform. In Estonia, for example, selected obstetric hospitals are being merged with nearby general hospitals, thus improving services and gaining access to the superior diagnostic, surgical and laboratory capacity of the general hospital. In Kyrgyzstan, the introduction of short-term chemotherapy and outpatient treatment for tuberculosis will make it possible to reduce the number of hospital beds, and eventually to close or change the use of specialized facilities currently assigned to the treatment of tuberculosis.

Governments and other purchasers have experienced problems in their efforts to control investment in new technologies. New investments are typically driven by the present system and incentives, with the result that additional resources are allocated to areas and types of care that already have a large stock of capital. To break this pattern of past investment, the cost–effectiveness of services must become an important principle of health sector reform. Many analyses have demonstrated the cost–effectiveness of PHC, prevention and public health services in comparison with hospital services. The cost–effectiveness of additional preventive programmes is not always better than that of treatment, however. This is especially true in well developed countries that already devote substantial resources to preventive measures. Thus the question of cost–effectiveness does not inevitably lead away from investing in hospitals, but it can support investment in hospital quality and availability as part of the need for a balanced distribution of resources.

CONCLUSION

Over the last few decades, the bulk of investment in the European health sector has been in half-way technologies in hospitals. In western Europe, with higher incomes and more resources allocated to the health sector, the accumulation of beds has been accompanied by rapid technological change, resulting in more intensive forms of care and increasing costs. In the CEE and CIS countries, the growth in hospital beds has been accompanied by slower technological change and slower cost increases, but has also meant less innovative and appropriate care, underfunding, inadequate maintenance of facilities and lower-quality services.

In contrast to the rapid development of new health technologies, adjusting the capital stock takes time. Once built, hospitals or other health care facilities are politically difficult to close. Thus, the pattern of capital infrastructure in the health sector is subject to substantial inertia.

In a stable environment, the problem of inertia would assume minor importance. The health care sector is, however, associated with rapid developments in new possibilities for treatment and diagnosis, and this in turn is linked to the optimum allocation of capital. Thus, health sector reforms should seek to introduce incentives for purchasers and providers that result in optimum decisions regarding cost-effective investments in new technology. Reforms should also stimulate the critical examination of existing patterns of capital allocation.

6 Delivering Services Efficiently

In the late 1980s and early 1990s, health care reforms in Europe have paid increasing attention to the organization and behaviour of service providers at the micro (institutional) level. These changes have concentrated mainly on improving managerial efficiency and health outcomes. There has also been a growing concern to develop quality of care programmes and, where possible, substitute more appropriate for less appropriate forms of care, which requires restructuring both the internal and external organization of hospitals as well as enhancing the capacities of PHC. Related changes have also been introduced in the area of human resources.

Improving outcomes and quality of care

As noted in Chapter 1, the development of health policy has traditionally focused on the financing of health care and on the organizational structures within which that care is provided, while quality issues have largely been left to the individual health care professional. Now it is increasingly recognized that health care reform should also address the quality of care provided. The former deference to professional (particularly medical) judgement about how best to deliver health care interventions is giving way in the face of growing recognition of widespread variations in quality, volume and practice. Early studies demonstrating large variations in the rates of many non-urgent surgical procedures and results, both within and between countries *(322)*, has led to other work showing how indications for particular treatments differ widely *(323)*. This variation reflects a number of factors, including differences in the prevalence of disease, culturally determined preferences for particular forms of treatment, the patterns of structural and financial incentives, and clinical uncertainty about the most appropriate treatment in any given circumstance *(324)*.

THE OUTCOMES MOVEMENT

More recently, this clinical uncertainty has given rise to what has become known as the "outcomes movement". The movement has drawn not only on growing awareness that there are large gaps in knowledge of which treatments are effective and for whom but also on the fact that, even when research-based evidence is available, it is frequently neither well known nor acted on. For example, the evidence that streptokinase is effective in reducing mortality from heart attacks (had the available studies been appropriately combined) was present several years before the treatment became widely used *(325)*. The movement has also drawn on the knowledge that many clinical interventions do not achieve their intended objectives, such as the treatment of children with glue ear that failed to improve their hearing *(326)*. Furthermore, many people in countries with comprehensive health systems, particularly those with chronic conditions such as cataract and prostate disease, are not receiving treatment that could benefit them *(327)*. Finally, the outcomes movement recognizes the importance of understanding how to change professional behaviour, in order that more effective and efficient treatments can be provided.

In its most developed form, this movement encompasses systematic reviews of available evidence on selected topics, the dissemination of evidence on what is known to be effective and in which circumstances, the development of a research agenda to fill the gaps, and support for creating an appropriate infrastructure, including a cohort of coordinators of quality of care in practice and of validated research methods to measure outcomes in relation to the process and structure of care. This approach is different from the traditional responsive model of medical research, which is typically dominated by basic medical scientists.

Certain points require emphasis. The term "systematic review" has a specific meaning, as it is now recognized that traditional literature reviews are often misleading *(328)*. Studies that produce negative findings tend either not to be published or to be published in less accessible journals. The methods used in individual studies must be taken into account. For example, in a trial comparing an intervention with a placebo, if the researchers are aware of which treatment each individual has received, they can overestimate the effectiveness of the treatment being studied. The populations on which studies are undertaken may be unrepresentative of those for whom physicians have to make treatment decisions. For example, many trials of treatments for heart disease have excluded women and elderly people.

Examples of systematic reviews have changed perceptions of which treatments work, for whom and in which circumstances. For example, the comprehensive review of interventions in pregnancy and childbirth undertaken by the National Perinatal Epidemiology Unit in the United Kingdom demonstrated that a large number of commonly used forms of care are likely to be ineffective or even harmful (Box 18) *(329)*. Other examples include WHO's initiatives and reviews on diabetes, oral health and obstetric care *(330–332)*.

The outcomes movement differs from the traditional model in its use of a variety of disciplines, including clinicians, statisticians, sociologists and economists. It also

---

Box 18. Forms of obstetric care clearly demonstrated to be ineffective or harmful

Contraction stress cardiotocography to improve perinatal outcome

Ethanol or progestogens to stop preterm labour

Routine enema and/or pubic shaving during labour and delivery

Rectal examination to assess progress of labour

Requiring a supine (flat on back) position during labour

Routine restriction of mother–infant contact

Routine nursery care for babies in hospital

Routine supplements of water or formula for breastfed babies

Source: Enkin *(329).*

employs a range of methods, including: randomized trials, in which participants are typically allocated at random to either the treatment being studied or to a placebo; observational studies, in which use is made of natural variations in intervention rates; and qualitative research, which can generate hypotheses and explore the meaning attached to the variables collected in quantitative studies. It also distinguishes between efficacy, which is how an intervention works in ideal circumstances, and effectiveness and cost–effectiveness, which are how it works in routine clinical practice *(333–335)*. This movement represents the next generation of quality-oriented research. As such, it brings a range of existing activities together in an integrated form, including health technology assessment and quality assurance *(336)*.

HEALTH TECHNOLOGY ASSESSMENT

There are various examples throughout Europe of different components of health technology assessment. Some western European countries have organizations specializing in health technology assessment, although their detailed structures vary widely *(170)*. Others, in addition to assessing technologies, also promote their appropriate use *(335,337,338)*.

Governments typically play a major direct or indirect role in the development of health technology assessment. This reflects a desire to ensure that advice is independent of commercial influence, in the light of concern about some research undertaken by the pharmaceutical and medical equipment industries *(339)*. In some cases, agencies have been established within or closely linked to government, such as the French Agence nationale pour la développement de l'évaluation médicale or the German Abteilung für Angewandte Systemanalyse. In other countries, agencies are also linked to government but have been established at regional level, such as the Catalan Oficina Técnica d'Avaluación de Tecnología Médica. In more decentralized models, research is undertaken by universities, other research centres and by the providers *(331,335,337,338)* within a national framework commissioning research. Finally, in some countries, agencies have been set up by those responsible for paying for health care, such as Assistance publique de Paris or the Dutch Ziekenfondsraad. Other countries have introduced collaborative mechanisms between third-party payers and health professionals. These include Mutuelle chrétienne in Belgium, Kupat Holim in Israel, and sickness funds in Germany, Poland and the Russian Federation (St Petersburg and Samara).

These systems seek to evaluate emerging and existing technologies, collect and synthesize available evidence about their cost–effectiveness, undertake appropriate evaluative research, and disseminate their results *(340)*. The extent to which these organizations are linked to the process of implementation varies considerably, and is often related to the existence of policies for controlling the diffusion of technology. Despite the considerable volume of activity in technology assessment, the rapid growth of health care technology and the frequently changing indications and context within which it is used have meant that much of clinical practice is still inadequately evaluated.

It is impossible to give a simple answer to the question of which arrangement is best. Information on the extent to which the diffusion of certain technologies has been controlled does show large differences (see Table 25), though these reflect a variety of factors, including some related to health system financing rather than to technology assessment activities *per se*. Comparisons also often fail to distinguish between appropriate and excessive levels of particular technologies.

In several countries, technology assessment has influenced the overall mix and level of high-technology equipment. It is argued that the results of technology assessment seem to have little influence on decision-making by health care providers, either in the utilization of health care technology or in the quality of care provided. An alternative approach for technology assessment that addresses these concerns is to involve providers in systematic data collection and interpretation by comparison of practices. This is discussed below.

Rather than seeking to prescribe the optimum structure for a technology assessment system, it may be more useful to consider the tasks that should be undertaken. These include a systematic identification of priorities based on national circumstances and a review of existing information; commissioning reviews of existing evidence and carrying out basic research; a means of ensuring that the results are collated in accessible form; and mechanisms for disseminating and implementing them. Implementation can take many forms, including regulation, financial incentives and education. The most appropriate approach will depend on the circumstances and on the pattern of ownership of health facilities.

Table 25. Numbers of computerized tomography scanners per million population in selected countries in 1993

Country	Scanners per million population
Australia	20.0
Germany	16.8
Sweden	13.8
Netherlands	11.7
Canada	9.2
United Kingdom	5.8

Source: Battista (341).

One example of the new approach that seeks to span the spectrum from research to practice is the Research and Development Strategy in the British NHS. National priorities are established by a control committee, but supplemented by a network of supporting committees in each region and by other central bodies, such as the NHS Centre for Reviews and Dissemination (342). This process is also linked to commissioning, as health authorities are required to ensure that the services they purchase are supported by evidence of effectiveness.

QUALITY ASSURANCE

The collection, synthesis and dissemination of evidence is the basis of improving the quality of clinical care. It is equally necessary to establish mechanisms to ensure that the available evidence is used. These constitute what are usually described as quality assurance activities, although other terms such as quality development and audit are also used.

At the outset, it is important to define what is meant by quality. Quality has been interpreted in different ways. Maxwell (343), for instance, has suggested six aspects of quality of care: access to services, equity, relevance to community need, social acceptability, effectiveness, and efficiency and economy. The components of high-quality health care can be described as: a high degree of professional excellence in relation to present knowledge and available technologies, efficiency in the use of resources, minimal risk to the patient, satisfaction of the patient and the final health outcome *(344)*. Others have taken a more restricted view, but the key point is that quality is multidimensional. Four critical dimensions can be identified: effective and appropriate care, efficiency in the use of resources, patient satisfaction and health outcomes. These dimensions are clearly linked. For instance, appropriate and effective care will result in higher patient satisfaction and improved health outcomes. Similarly, if care is efficient it implies that it must be effective.

Quality assurance has three important dimensions: its continuous nature, the different ways of measuring quality, and the differentiation between internal and external approaches *(345)*.

The first dimension acknowledges that strategies for improving quality cannot be based on single events. The audit cycle is often referred to as the classical model (Fig. 20). It involves selecting a topic, establishing a criterion that can be used to measure quality (based on operational research evidence), setting a standard (the level realistically achievable), measuring the level actually achieved and comparing it with the standard; implementing change, and adjusting the standard, either by increasing it to encourage further improvement or by relaxing it in recognition that the original value was unrealistic. Finally, the cycle is repeated. In practice, activities

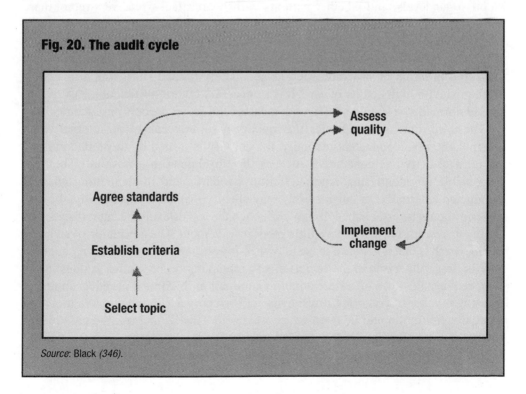

Fig. 20. The audit cycle

Assess quality

Agree standards

Implement change

Establish criteria

Select topic

Source: Black *(346)*.

described as quality assurance often fail to complete the cycle, thus failing to achieve the optimum level of quality

The second dimension indicates that quality can be measured in terms of structure, process and outcome *(347)*. Structure refers to the treatment facilities, including factors such as the quality of staff, the availability of appropriate technology and the standards of accommodation. Process relates to what is done to the patient, such as the interval between diagnosis and treatment or the use of appropriate medications or interventions. Outcome is the extent to which the intended result of treatment is achieved. In an ideal world, all assessments of quality would be based on outcome measures, such as whether patients survive treatments or whether they are restored to full health. Process measures inevitably suffer from the relative lack of knowledge about the precise nature of the link between an intervention and its outcome. There are difficulties in basing quality assurance activities on outcomes alone, such as when small numbers of a particular type of patient make it impossible to know if a poor outcome is due to the treatment or to the underlying disease process *(348)*.

Although the methods available to assess outcome are continuously improving and, in particular, the range of health status measures is increasing, it is often more feasible and informative to measure process *(349)*. This is when such measures are based on research-related evidence that correlates with a good outcome, even if this cannot easily be measured in routine practice. Commonly used examples of process measures are: assessing whether patients with diabetes are achieving good control of blood sugar levels, and whether patients with heart attacks receive streptokinase within an hour of reaching hospital. In the former case, for example, work coordinated by WHO has shown widespread diversity in blood levels of Hb A_{1c}, a measure of diabetic control, both between and within countries *(350)*. Finally, quality can be measured in terms of structure, such as adequately trained staff, which is a basic prerequisite for high quality of care. It is a necessary but not sufficient measure, and should normally be supplemented with measures of either process or outcome.

The third dimension indicates that quality assurance can be an internal or an external activity. Conducted internally, the activity is owned by those undertaking the clinical activities concerned, such as the physicians in a hospital. They are responsible for identifying criteria, setting standards and implementing change. Conducted externally, an outside body may specify that some means of quality assurance should be established; it may influence the topics examined and discuss the aggregate results, but it will have little other involvement. The advantage of an internal approach is that it fosters a sense of ownership among those undertaking it, and it may be less vulnerable to the opportunistic manipulation of results. It does, however, require a culture of reflection and examination in clinical practice. In an increasing number of countries, physicians are gradually accepting the idea that their clinical activities should be open to comparison. This is far from the case everywhere, however, and much will depend on whether quality assurance activities are adopted in a supportive format. In European countries, professional bodies have played a major role in promoting a more open culture *(351,352)*.

There is a growing body of experience with quality development policies in the Region. Some western European countries, such as Belgium and Denmark, have adopted nationwide policies, and many more are in the process of doing so. Several of the CEE countries, such as the Czech Republic, Poland and Slovenia, have been establishing quality development policies, especially for obstetrics and perinatal care. It is important that these policies are followed up with a clear strategy for implementation, including the necessary training and computing support. In France, the Netherlands and the United Kingdom, participation in quality assurance activities is a legal or contractual obligation for some physicians working in the public sector. The scope of such activities during the 1980s has now widened to including the establishment of national associations and, in a few cases such as Hungary, government funding for bodies to implement policies.

The external approach typically focuses on structural measures. This is largely because these are so much easier to measure than process or outcome, although existing accreditation programmes recognize the limited nature of this assessment and are attempting to develop supplementary measures of process and outcome. Hospital accreditation is a typical example. Originally developed in the United States, it has now extended to several western European countries such as France, the Netherlands and the United Kingdom (353). In different formats, accreditation has also been adopted in a number of CEE and CIS countries, including Estonia and Georgia. Accreditation is important for countries seeking to establish mixed provision of private and public health services, since it offers a means of reassurance that facilities meet agreed minimum quality levels. Once these basic standards have been achieved, however, it does little to encourage further improvements in the quality of care.

THE IMPLICATIONS FOR SERVICE PROVISION

A better understanding of the factors underlying differences in quality often has implications for service organization. In many cases, it will become apparent that a different configuration of services will lead to improvements in the effectiveness, efficiency or accessibility of care. For example, in some countries, recognition of the deficiencies of traditional models of providing outpatient care have led to the development of so-called "one-stop clinics", in which patients with common symptoms are comprehensively investigated in a single day (354).

In some cases, however, there will be trade-offs. One example is the issue of regionalization. There is now growing evidence that hospitals and physicians undertaking large volumes of particular procedures obtain better results than those who undertake only a few (355), although there is still substantial debate about the precise nature of the relationship between volume and outcome and the extent to which other factors have been taken into account (356). Also, the results may vary with the local circumstances. While concentrating services in a few large hospitals may improve outcome, however, it may do so at the expense of access if patients are deterred from seeking treatment because they live too far away. In practice, several countries, such as the Netherlands, Sweden and the United Kingdom, have adopted a policy of centralization for certain services. These are often supplemented by provisions that reduce the problem of increased travel, such as satellite clinics. Consequently, a focus on policies for quality of care may lead to quite significant changes in the structure of service provision.

Implementing quality assurance can, in some circumstances, also influence the provision of health care by releasing resources. An example repeated in many countries is the issue of hospital-acquired infections. In one review in the United States, it was estimated that quality assurance programmes have been associated with a 32% decrease in infections (357). This leads to shorter stays in hospital and fewer readmissions. Similar findings have been reported in Europe (358).

CLINICAL GUIDELINES

The development of clinical guidelines represents a way in which technology assessment and quality assurance have been linked. They have been defined as "recommendations issued for the purpose of influencing decisions about health interventions" (359). On the basis of a systematic review of evidence, supplemented where necessary by expert opinion, guidelines are drawn up for managing particular conditions. There is now an extensive body of literature on the most appropriate means of developing guidelines, as well as on how they should be used (360). Ideally, they should be firmly based on evidence, and they should involve practitioners in their development. The extent to which they are followed may be used as a measure of process in quality assurance.

Guidelines are being developed by government agencies, physicians' organizations, insurance companies and others. Guidelines can be voluntary or mandatory, flexible or rigid, and linked to rewards or sanctions, such as financial penalties. As noted above, they should be based on good information on both quality of care (efficacy) and patient preferences, but information on both of these issues is often lacking.

Several studies have shown that the dissemination of guidelines is, in itself, insufficient to change behaviour (361,362). The main reason is that decisions made by physicians and patients are shaped by a range of factors, such as different attitudes to and perceptions of risk and different values placed on particular outcomes (363). Important factors include the use of feedback, opinion leaders, education and the local development of evidence-based guidelines (364).

Concerns have also been expressed about the costs of developing and disseminating guidelines. These concerns should not be interpreted as suggesting that guidelines are of no value. They can be effective in the right circumstances, as part of an integrated programme to improve quality, as has been shown, for example, in the Netherlands (Klazinga, N., unpublished data, 1993) and in pan-European work on the quality of care in diabetes.

CONTINUOUS QUALITY OF CARE DEVELOPMENT

WHO has been involved in a specific initiative in the European Region: continuous quality of care development (QCD) programmes. These take a comprehensive,

integrated and dynamic approach to quality development, acting at various levels of
the health care system and involving different health care actors. QCD is based on
the following principles: explicit definition of quality goals, the identification, dissemination and use of best outcomes ("best practice"), continuous professional self-
assessment and self-regulation, and patient and community involvement. It com-
pares outcome results between similar settings, identifies and disseminates best practice, and encourages implementation. The model involves seven steps:

1. identification of the problem
2. establishment of priorities, indicators, criteria and standards
3. collection of data
4. assessment of quality
5. feedback to providers
6. implementation of change
7. re-evaluation and quality monitoring.

This ongoing process, based on "benchmarking" and "feedback", is not new in
industry, and is now becoming a trend in health care. Initiatives include breast
cancer, oral health and vascular surgery programmes in Denmark, and obstetric and
perinatal care in Belgium, the Czech Republic and Slovenia (332,335,365).

The development of national policies on quality of care seeks to address two key
issues in health care reform: improved effectiveness of interventions, and increased
clinical accountability and responsiveness to patients.

QCD places responsibility for implementation on the different actors and levels
of health care. Quality development can be seen as a mechanism to ensure that
providers are involved in policy formulation and decision-making. This approach
makes the assumption that health professionals are in the best position to evaluate
and monitor the quality of care they provide, and that they should therefore be given
the responsibility to carry out quality initiatives. The need for QCD has particular
significance for health professionals and medical organizations. In a collaborative
project between the European Forum of Medical Associations and the WHO Regional Office for Europe, the principle of QCD was seen as an ethical obligation for
the medical profession (366).

While the role of health professionals is essential to this initiative, its success will
depend on a coordinated approach involving patients, managers, third-party payers
and government health officials. Implementation of the model requires a broad
framework of enabling measures, including: financial and professional incentives;
information systems, such as the development of national databases on outcome
indicators, clearing houses or clinical databases; the introduction of quality markers;
the setting up of dissemination and feedback mechanisms for providers; the introduction of telematics; and legislation. Regarding the last measure, some commentators have contended that legislation and regulation should be limited to those areas
that are ill suited to professional self-regulation, such as regulation of formal complaints procedures, technology assessment or patients' rights (367,368).

Measuring outcomes as an integral element of the routine work of health care providers is central to QCD initiatives. This requires the development of information systems based on carefully selected quality indicators. Some proponents of QCD believe that these information systems should be developed primarily by professional organizations themselves, with support from governments or other third-party payers.

In addition, QCD requires a coordinated approach involving managers and providers at local level, as well as international, national and regional authorities. Countries such as Belgium, Denmark and Slovenia have developed national policies on continuous QCD in collaboration with the Regional Office *(344,369,370)*.

At the international level, experience of what constitutes a successful approach is growing *(331,334,335)*. Significant progress has been made in identifying common quality indicators in fields such as perinatal and obstetric care, mental health, diabetes, hospital-acquired infections, use of antibiotics and oral health. Pilot European databases on common outcome indicators have been designed for perinatal and obstetric care *(371)*, diabetes management *(372)*, oral health care *(373)*, hospital-acquired infections *(374)* and mental health *(375)*. Based on this approach, further progress has been made in areas such as diabetes and oral health management *(330)*.

RECENT EXPERIENCE IN EUROPE

The various components of evidence-based health care, from research through dissemination to implementation, are now in place in several countries. In many others, however, there is still very little activity, with health policy discussions still tending to focus on issues of financing and organization. The difficulties facing countries seeking to integrate evidence-based health care with health sector reform should not be underestimated. One set of problems relates to the ability to undertake research. Few countries have an adequate research infrastructure and, in some, the lack of information systems (whether in hospitals, in PHC or in other fields such as geographical information systems) also presents obstacles. Necessary outcome measures, such as for health status, may not always be available in the appropriate language, or cultural factors may limit their relevance. Even in the largest countries, the sample sizes necessary to evaluate certain treatments may involve international collaboration, and this presents a further challenge.

There is considerable scope for international collaboration. This is already well established through mechanisms such as the Cochrane Collaboration, an international network of individuals preparing and maintaining systematic reviews of available evidence (in particular ensuring that studies reported in languages other than English are not overlooked), agreeing standardized methods and disseminating information *(218)*.

The growing complexity of modern health care has major implications for many aspects of health service provision, particularly optimum settings for health care and the configuration of services. Furthermore, evidence of both ineffective care and underprovision means that failure to address these issues will lead to wasted resources, missed opportunities and, ultimately, avoidable morbidity and mortality.

Linking policy and practice decisions to continuing assessment is still a relatively new concept. Health care systems need to measure their performance directly, ensuring the collection of better data on health outcomes by the professions. In the long run, health care can only make a greater contribution to health outcomes if more is known about the value of interventions, and if this information is used more systematically in decision-making. The development of a research infrastructure and mechanisms for implementing its results can no longer be seen as a luxury.

Decentralized provider management

The decentralization of management to provider institutions, coupled with the development of more effective management by strengthening expertise, introducing improved information systems and increasing financial autonomy, form part of a notable reform trend across the Region. They reflect a general movement towards decentralization, which in some countries includes the introduction of provider markets and the separation of the purchaser and provider functions. Increasing managerial autonomy and reducing bureaucratic control are intended to encourage more innovative practices and increase responsiveness to purchasers' and patients' demands.

In several publicly operated health systems in western Europe, the traditional hierarchy of health authorities – at regional, area or local level – and hospital providers is being replaced by more decentralized management arrangements. In some cases, they take the form of quasi-autonomous nongovernmental organizations (quangos) or self-governing hospitals. These have been introduced in the United Kingdom, and similar arrangements are under consideration in several other countries. In social insurance systems, managerial autonomy in hospitals has been strengthened by the recent introduction of more market-oriented incentives in the relationship between the insurer/purchaser and the provider. In several of the CEE and CIS countries, responsibility for hospitals has been decentralized to local public authorities and, in some cases, these have the power to contract directly with insurers. Self-governing schemes, however, are still at an early stage of development in both the western and eastern parts of the Region. Key issues include public accountability, the representativeness of management boards, and legal liability.

In some health systems, hospital decentralization and more effective hospital management include the involvement of clinical staff in management. For decentralized structures and contractual arrangements to operate efficiently, hospital management and clinical providers need to cooperate. This cooperation has been encouraged in the United Kingdom and some Scandinavian countries through the development of new management structures such as clinical directorates, and by devolving budgetary responsibility to groups of clinicians at department or specialty level.

IMPROVING MANAGEMENT

One major trend has involved adopting management techniques from other sectors in order to improve hospital performance. These include benchmarking, business process re-engineering, patient-focused care, quality improvement techniques and internal contracting models. Evaluation of the impact of these techniques, however, is largely lacking.

A second trend has been to develop management capacity, including the improvement of general management expertise, supported by more sophisticated information systems to facilitate better decision-making in clinical, financial and other managerial areas. Several countries in western Europe have made significant investments in information systems. Denmark, Greece, Spain, Sweden and the United Kingdom have introduced systems that provide a higher degree of local autonomy including, in some cases, rewards for managers and the freedom to reinvest savings. Nevertheless, approaches that concentrate on managerial efficiency targets present several dilemmas. They divert attention from improved efficiency in health care delivery, and tend to preoccupy managers with marginal rather than strategic changes in delivery systems.

Shifting boundaries: hospitals, PHC and community care

Patterns of health care organization and delivery across care settings (hospital, primary, community and home) are increasingly being reconfigured to reflect changing circumstances on both the demand and supply sides of services. Pressures to review current practices reflect a variety of factors, including a concern to contain overall system costs, new demands for resources resulting from epidemiological changes related to demographic structures, and the increased expectations of patients and providers. New technologies in fields such as genetics, imaging, miniaturization, pharmaceuticals and information have had a substantial impact on the appropriate mix of preventive, diagnostic and treatment practices. There is close scrutiny of how resources are used, and growing scepticism over earlier assumptions about the appropriate roles of different care settings. In particular, the future role of hospitals is increasingly being questioned, given the possibilities of providing diagnostic and treatment procedures elsewhere.

Health systems have adapted to these pressures through a process of substitution.[23] This term can be defined as the continual regrouping of resources across and within care settings, to exploit the best and least costly solutions in the face of changing needs and demands. In other words, health sector staff, skills, equipment, information and facilities can be reorganized in order to achieve better clinical, financial and patient-related outcomes.

Substitution is not a new phenomenon. In health services, there are continuous development and adaptation of clinical practice and organizational patterns. One earlier example of substitution was BCG vaccination, which helped to eliminate the tuberculosis sanatorium with profound consequences in terms of resources. The new option – in this case a technological innovation – changed the actors, the method, the timing, the location and even the reason for care. A later example, which may also

---

[23] This expression was first used in the 1988 Dekker report in the Netherlands *(261)* in which substitution was recognized as a key policy instrument for health care reform.

have profound consequences, is the move towards using H_2-receptor antagonists instead of surgery for peptic ulcer; further substitution is now taking place through the testing for and eradication of *Helicobacter pylori*.

A SUBSTITUTION TYPOLOGY

Numerous shifts in treatments, procedures and organizational patterns can be included under the category of substitution. A useful typology differentiates them according to three kinds of substitution: moving the *location* at which care is given, introducing *new technologies*, and changing the *mix of staff and skills*. There may be other substitution types according to different combinations of these three *(376)*. Fig. 21 sets out a framework of care delivery, indicating the main health care settings and the types of substitution between them.

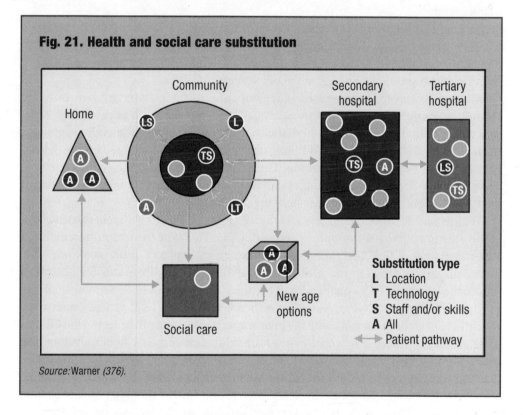

Fig. 21. Health and social care substitution

Source: Warner *(376)*.

In moving to home care from secondary hospital care all (A) substitution types apply, e.g. hospital at home schemes, hospital outreach programmes, enhancement of long-term care, blood transfusions and renal dialysis.

Again, in moving to home care from primary or community care, all (A) substitution types apply, e.g. self-care programmes and diagnostic patches (a newly emerging technology using monoclonal antibodies).

Moving to primary or community care from secondary hospital care may involve substitution in:

- location (L) only, such as that for physiotherapy or chiropody;
- location and technology (LT), such as those for electrocardiography and desk-top laboratory activities;
- location and staff and/or skills (LS), such as nurse practitioners, community pharmacy advice on prescription drugs newly designated for over-the-counter sale, shared care protocols and community-based mental illness services; and
- all *substitution types* (A), such as ultrasound applications and genetic testing and counselling.

Many elements of substitution that begin as locational shifts often have more profound implications. These arise from additional requirements for increased skills as clinicians experiment with new technologies, particularly in primary and community care.

As noted above, there is evidence that more successful outcomes can be obtained when clinicians undertake procedures many times each year. Thus location and skill mix (LS) in combination become important in moving from a secondary to a tertiary (specialist) hospital, e.g. specialist cancer surgery *(377)*.

Many activities that earlier took place only at tertiary level have been shifted to secondary hospitals in a straightforward locational shift (L), such as cardiology services. Other activities, such as renal dialysis, have shifted across the entire spectrum. In this case, PHC has had, in addition, to acquire new knowledge (LS) as home-based dialysis became more common. These shifts can be expected to increase both as technology becomes more mobile and as secondary hospitals take over more of the functions previously the preserve of the tertiary sector.

Within each location, pressures to achieve greater efficiency dictate substitutions in the location of both technologies and staff (TS). This type of substitution includes cases in which: a new technological process either replaces a previous one (e.g. micro-surgery or drugs in place of traditional surgery) or substitutes for personnel (e.g. in the laboratory); less qualified staff take over the functions of those more qualified (e.g. practice nurses for GPs); and self-care becomes possible (e.g. patients purchasing over-the-counter drugs or tests with the pharmacist's help, rather than seeing the GP).

The interface between social care and health care remains underdeveloped in many European countries. Some governments are seeking to redefine health service functions in order to transfer them to the social services, thus separating the "cure" and "care" processes. In some cases, the motivation behind this type of substitution lies in the fact that, while health services are free of charge, social services are subject to some form of cost sharing, thus becoming a case of substitution of private for public finance. In other areas, social and health care services are pooling resources, particularly in the provision of services for elderly people.

The formulation of new options blurs the boundaries between the various aspects of the care system. The new options emerging are very diverse, including general care for the elderly involving health and social support, open access by GPs to diagnostic services and self-standing treatment centres for day surgery of a specialist nature, such as cataract or varicose vein surgery.

THE POTENTIAL FOR SUBSTITUTION

A number of major shifts or substitutions identified here have been under way in different parts of Europe for some years, often with major implications for the PHC sector. Some early examples of *location substitution* include: the Santé service Bayonne et région in France, started in 1961 as a home nursing scheme for cancer sufferers, and expanded to include care of elderly and/or physically handicapped people; the "home-based home care post-discharge" scheme in Motala, Sweden, which began in 1967 as "a hospital bed in the patient's own home" for elderly people; and the community-based "Hospital at home" scheme in Peterborough in the United Kingdom, launched in 1978, to facilitate early discharge or to prevent admission.

In terms of *technology substitution*, one Dutch study *(378)* identified a number of key technologies that could potentially be transferred to the home. They include infusion therapies, adjustable beds, home monitoring of risky pregnancies, enteral and parenteral nutrition, traction for congenital dysplasia of the hip, and photo-therapy for neonatal jaundice.

The potential advantages of substitution policies include increased patient satisfaction, improved clinical outcomes, greater efficiency and more appropriate management of certain diseases. There are substantial differences between the various substitution schemes, however, and in many cases there is little evidence about their impact on health service objectives. Furthermore, the advantages of substitution may be reduced or lost if policy-makers adopt new schemes in an uncoordinated manner or without clear strategic objectives. Too often, substitution involves simply changing the location, without an appropriate shift in skills and technology or without a reallocation of resources.

Successful substitution relies on a comprehensive analysis of current service delivery patterns in each country, good information on the merits of individual substitution policies, and a detailed understanding of the changes required in resources and mix of skills. Table 26 summarizes both obstacles to and opportunities for encouraging the substitution process in health care reforms, whereby greater emphasis would be placed on the development of PHC.

Financial approaches employed by insurance or purchasing agencies often lack incentives for PHC to substitute for secondary care. Funding is allocated according to inputs rather than outcomes, while in many cases the flow of money through different health care organizations discourages cooperation and coordination. It fails to recognize the holistic and complex nature of patients' problems, which may remain unresolved or be looked after in a duplicative and inefficient way.

Restructuring hospitals

Inpatient care typically consumes 45–75% of resources dedicated to health care. As discussed above, there is an increasing perception that there are more cost-effective alternatives to the care currently provided in hospitals, and that consequently there is scope for a further reduction in hospital services. A number of other pressures are also triggering changes. The trend towards subspecialization, the need for expensive

Table 26. Substitution: obstacles to and opportunities for health reform

Obstacles	Opportunities
Financial incentive for PHC to substitute for secondary care is insufficient.	Finance according to patient needs. Finance tasks, not institutions.
Funding is related to input of people and resources.	Fund according to outputs and outcomes required. Emphasize measures of health and social gain, for both quality and quantity of life.
Funding does not recognize the holistic and complex nature of people's problems.	Fund coordinated or managed care: move from vertical to horizontal financing across multiple providers working together, from primary and secondary care, the voluntary sector and social care.
A major shift of funding to PHC would be absorbed but not used to the best advantage.	Develop evidence-based PHC management. Actively implement internal workforce substitution. Undertake systematic evaluation of ability to shift technologies and personnel from hospital to PHC and home care. Blur boundaries between PHC and secondary care. Give special attention to using nursing skills.

technologies, the perceived existence of economies of scope and scale, and cost pressures have all have been interpreted as being likely to lead to fewer, larger hospitals providing acute or high-technology care, with increased support from PHC or from subacute hospitals that may be more similar to nursing homes.

Policy-makers face questions about the long-term role of the hospital, its future configuration and how changes in hospital systems can be implemented. This section examines trends in hospital provision, and some of the policies that have been or can be adopted to bring about change. Hospital reimbursement and financing policy is a key part of any attempt to reform the hospital sector, and considered in Chapter 5. Hospital policy needs to be guided by two other elements of policy analysis: the insights from organizational theory that suggest that hospitals are complex, adaptive systems that respond in unexpected ways to changes in the external environment; and a strategic vision of the role of the hospital sector in health care, how it is expected to perform, its overall size and the nature of its relationship with primary, social, long-term and other forms of care.

TRENDS IN HOSPITAL CARE

Direct comparison of hospital data between countries is difficult, since there are substantial differences in the availability, completeness and denominators of national statistics, as well as in the role and the mode of hospital provision. Factors influencing these differences include reimbursement systems, the relationship between PHC and secondary care, the provision of PHC and its role as a gatekeeper, and the role and availability of social care. Comparisons between the western and eastern parts of the Region are even more difficult, owing to institutional and other differences. These include the roles of some hospitals and hospital beds, the state of development of the social care sector, and public expectations regarding the role of hospitals.

The total number of hospital beds has fallen significantly in recent years in almost all western European countries, mainly at the expense of acute inpatient beds (see Fig. 22). The reasons for these changes are not well documented, but they probably reflect a combination of cost-containment policies, changes in technology or methods of treatment, and changes in the roles of PHC and social care. Also, in most countries, there has been an increase in admission rates, together with a reduction in average length of stay. The latter trend has accompanied changes in the management of patients, improvements in clinical techniques such as minimally invasive surgery, and incentives to reduce lengths of stay and ensure that patients who no longer need acute care are discharged to other settings.

In general, the CEE and CIS countries have more beds than western Europe, mainly as a result of the large number of comparatively small hospitals. These numbers are associated with notably higher admission levels than those in western Europe. Although there may be a genuinely higher level of morbidity in these countries, the differential in bed use and provision is more likely to be the result of a heavier reliance on hospitals, public preferences, lower levels of private transport, and the reduced role of the social sector. Also, a substantial part of the difference in admissions can probably be accounted for by supplier-induced demand and, in some cases, the proximity of patients to hospitals.

As shown in Fig. 22 and Table 27, there are major variations between CEE and CIS countries in the number of beds per 1000 population. The range between the highest and lowest figures has remained largely unchanged since 1980. There has been some reduction in the number of hospital beds, although the fall has not been universal and has been less pronounced than in western Europe. In a few countries, there has been a small increase. In many cases, the bulk of the changes have taken place since 1990 (see Table 27), reflecting changes in policy towards bed provision and changes in health sector funding. There is still considerable scope for closing hospital beds and entire hospitals in the CEE and CIS countries.

As shown in Table 28, CIS countries such as Armenia, Azerbaijan and Georgia have experienced an apparent collapse of admissions, which is likely to be attributable to health budget cuts. The trend in length of stay is a downward one,

Fig. 22. Numbers of hospital beds per 1000 population in the WHO European Region, 1980 and 1994

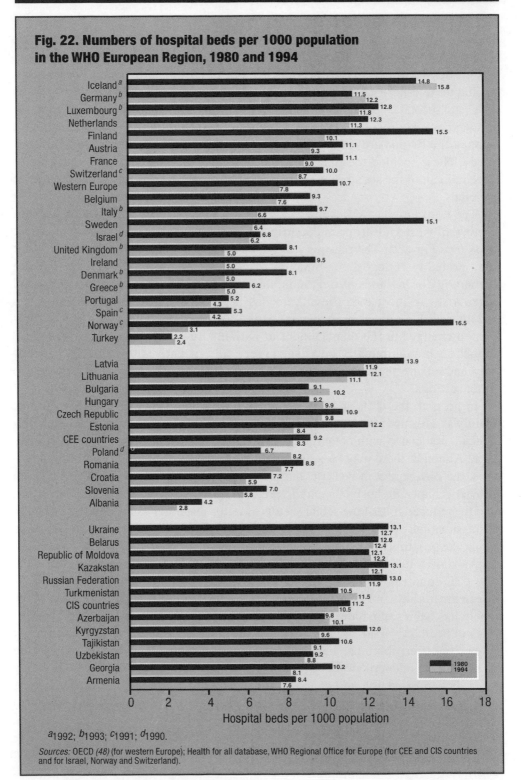

Hospital beds per 1000 population

[a]1992; [b]1993; [c]1991; [d]1990.

Sources: OECD *(48)* (for western Europe); Health for all database, WHO Regional Office for Europe (for CEE and CIS countries and for Israel, Norway and Switzerland).

Table 27. Numbers of hospital beds per 1000 population in CEE and CIS countries, 1980–1994

Country	Hospital beds				Change 1985–1994	Change 1990–1994
	1980	1985	1990	1994		
CEE countries						
Albania	4.18	4.01	4.03	2.77	−31%	−31%
Bulgaria	–	9.11	9.79	10.24	12%	5%
Croatia	7.23	7.45	7.38	5.91	−21%	−20%
Czech Republic	10.85	11.01	10.92	9.81	−11%	−10%
Estonia	12.19	12.27	11.60	8.35	−32%	−28%
Hungary	–	9.61	9.84	9.92	3%	1%
Latvia	13.89	14.31	14.04	11.93	−17%	−15%
Lithuania	12.07	12.78	12.44	11.09	−13%	−11%
Poland	6.67	6.59	8.22	–	–	–
Romania	8.78	8.94	8.92	7.70	−14%	−14%
Slovakia	–	–	7.46	–	–	–
Slovenia	6.95	6.33	6.04	5.78	−9%	−4%
CIS countries						
Armenia	8.40	8.70	9.09	7.58	−13%	−17%
Azerbaijan	9.75	9.90	10.10	10.06	2%	0%
Belarus	12.55	13.07	13.23	12.42	−5%	−6%
Georgia	10.17	9.97	9.80	8.09	−19%	−17%
Kazakstan	13.09	13.59	13.67	12.14	−11%	−11%
Kyrgyzstan	12.01	12.03	11.98	9.59	−20%	−20%
Republic of Moldova	12.05	12.22	13.15	12.22	0%	−7%
Russian Federation	–	12.98	13.06	11.94	−8%	−9%
Tajikistan	–	10.64	10.69	9.11	−14%	−15%
Turkmenistan	10.46	9.74	11.49	11.47	18%	0%
Ukraine	–	13.14	13.56	12.75	−3%	−6%
Uzbekistan	9.18	11.83	12.48	8.81	−26%	−29%

Source: Health for all database, WHO Regional Office for Europe.

but at a slower pace than the reduction in bed numbers. This suggests that occupancy may have increased, but that there are still significant opportunities for improving efficiency.

Policy strategies

While there are various approaches to restructuring hospital services, most policies aim to achieve one or more of the following objectives:

Table 28. Changes in key hospital indicators in CEE and CIS countries over the period 1990–1994

Country	Hospitals per unit of population	Hospital beds per unit of population	Admissions per unit of population	Length of stay
CEE countries				
Albania	−70%	−31%	−	−33%
Bulgaria	20%	5%	−7%	−1%
Croatia	−37%	−20%	−17%	−10%
Czech Republic	10%	−10%	14%	−16%
Estonia	−6%	−28%	−3%	−18%
Hungary	−	1%	0%	−10%
Latvia	−5%	−15%	−6%	−5%
Lithuania	0%	−11%	8%	−11%
Poland	−	−	−	−
Romania	1%	−14%	5%	−10%
Slovakia	−	−	−	−
Slovenia	10%	−4%	0%	−7%
CIS countries				
Armenia	−10%	−17%	−42%	5%
Azerbaijan	−2%	0%	−40%	−1%
Belarus	−2%	−6%	−1%	0%
Georgia	−17%	−17%	−60%	3%
Kazakstan	−9%	−11%	−23%	5%
Kyrgyzstan	−	−20%	−26%	3%
Republic of Moldova	0%	−7%	−8%	5%
Russian Federation	−5%	−9%	−5%	1%
Tajikistan	6%	−15%	−	−
Turkmenistan	−12%	0%	−16%	−3%
Ukraine	0%	−6%	0%	3%
Uzbekistan	−9%	−29%	−21%	−3%

Source: Health for all database, WHO Regional Office for Europe,.

- a general improvement in the efficiency of service delivery, which if success-ful, will reduce the need for beds and allow changes in the size, configuration and cost of hospital systems;
- appropriate use of hospital services, which is expected to lead to a reduced number of admissions and demand for beds; and
- change in the shape of the network of hospital services to achieve a more efficient and effective configuration.

IMPROVING THE EFFICIENCY AND APPROPRIATENESS OF HOSPITAL CARE

Approaches to improving the efficiency and appropriateness of hospital services can be grouped into four main categories: payment systems, quality-of-care strategies, management techniques and clinical performance strategies. The first three have already been explored in previous sections. This section will therefore focus on clinical performance strategies, including shifting to day case treatment, improving the appropriateness of admissions, expediting the discharge of patients and applying utilization review techniques. Many of these strategies involve either substitution in the hospital service by introducing new technologies or by changing the mix of staff and skills, or substitution of location for PHC and community care services, often accompanied by the substitution of technologies and/or staff and skills.

Day case and minimal access procedures

Day case procedures have been adopted as a major source of improved efficiency in several countries *(171)*. Similar improvements are expected from minimally invasive surgery, and from the growth in diagnostic and interventional imaging techniques *(379)*. It is often assumed that this work represents a pure substitute for inpatient care. It is probable, however, that at least some of this growth is additional work that is made possible by extra capacity and the availability of new techniques, in particular endoscopy and magnetic resonance imaging. Furthermore, if the capacity released by these new approaches is not closed, there may be opportunities for admitting more patients as a result of supplier-induced demand. In these cases, new techniques are likely to increase both the hospital admission rate and the overall cost. Procedures that formerly required a stay in hospital and are now increasingly conducted as day cases include inguinal hernia repair, breast biopsy, varicose vein stripping, cystoscopy, arthroscopy, myringectomy, cholecystectomy, laparoscopy and termination of pregnancy. Early experience suggests that the growth of minimal access techniques requires a shift in the production function of hospitals from beds to operating theatres and from inpatient care to community aftercare.

Improving the appropriateness of admission and care

A key part of a strategy for changing the role of hospitals will be a set of approaches designed to reduce the number of admissions. Clearly, successful primary prevention of disease offers the prospect of reducing disease-specific admission rates. There are, however, three types of strategy for reducing the likelihood of admission of those already ill: primary care substitution, raising admission thresholds and preventing admission by providing appropriate alternatives.

The diffusion of technology into PHC (largely in the form of pharmaceuticals) has made possible the safe and effective management of a growing range of conditions. For some conditions, PHC can act as partial substitute for secondary care services, thus reducing admissions. Issues related to substitution across settings are explored in more detail in the next section.

It is also possible directly to prevent admission to hospital by raising the threshold of severity that must be met before a patient will be admitted. Technology has an important role to play in this area. The development and expansion of day or out-patient surgery are an example of a fall in surgical admissions due to technological advances. Cruder supply-side changes may also result in shifts in the admission threshold: when faced with a reduced bed stock due to bed closures,.clinicians have little choice but to raise their admission thresholds. Clinical, management and policy interventions can be designed to target those thresholds. Short-stay observation units may safely separate out "borderline" patients who will not actually require admission (e.g. by ruling out acute myocardial infarction) *(380)*. The observation unit approach does not always reduce admission rates (e.g. in asthma) *(381)*, however, and when demand is high it may become little more than a pool of extra beds. Professional education and training on specific issues can be shown to reduce admission rates in certain circumstances: for example, a training pro-gramme for senior house officers in an English hospital led to a significant drop in child asthma admissions *(382)*. In Italy, a combination of diagnostic and ther-apeutic protocols, clinician training, observation beds and financial incentives for medical staff succeeded in reducing admissions in a large general hospital *(383)*.

A third set of strategies consists of developing alternative interventions that will reduce the need for admission. The provision of non-hospital specialist services can be facilitated by technological innovation or by deliberate policy changes in operat-ing methods. Some approaches that have been shown to achieve a reduction in ad-mission rates include the introduction of community clinics and domiciliary visits by teams of specialist physicians and nurses *(384)*. In Israel, weekly home visits by a physician to elderly patients with severe congestive heart failure appeared to cut annual admission rates by more than half *(385)*. In Canada, enrolling elderly people in a programme to provide health and social care at home or in nursing homes appeared to result in reduced admission rates to acute hospitals *(386)*. It may even be possible to use planned admissions to hospital-based respite care to avert admit-ting certain elderly patients with chronic conditions to acute care *(387)*. Annual comprehensive home health checks by specialist geriatric nurses in both California *(388)* and South Wales *(389)* did not, however, result in any reduction in admission rates in those over 75 years of age.

Several of the approaches outlined above offer the prospect of preventing acute admissions, but they may also involve relatively resource-intensive interventions. The evidence that might compare the costs of community-based care with those of admission is still substantially lacking. Intensive home care may or may not be more cost-effective than admission but, even if cheaper, it may offer less real scope for resource savings than has hitherto been assumed.

Expediting discharge from hospital

There are two main approaches to improving discharge rates and thereby achieving reductions in length of stay: improvements in clinical management, and measures to expedite discharge once the patient has recovered. These may be indirectly influ-enced by measures such as the development of diagnosis-related groups or other case-mix systems (the Czech Republic, Germany and Hungary), statistically based targets (Slovakia) and/or targets incorporated into plans for the provision of services (United Kingdom). Target-based systems often offer considerable scope for manipulation and may encourage suboptimal practice if inappropriate mean lengths of stay are set.

More success appears to be achieved by providing less detailed direction, while offering incentives for physicians to develop audit and managerially based approaches to reducing length of stay. The integrated care or anticipated recovery pathways developed in the United States are examples; some parts of the United Kingdom are also experimenting with these. The expected pattern of care for a patient is documented, variations monitored, and improvements developed as a result. The advantage of these systems is that they provide more clinically and locally meaningful information.

The most effective measure for reducing the demand for beds appears to be improving the hospital system's ability to discharge patients who are no longer benefiting from the services of a fully equipped general hospital. As shown below, many studies have found that a large number of hospital bed-days are used by these patients. There are number of approaches to this problem.

First, home nursing and, more recently, hospital-at-home schemes have been introduced in Denmark, Ireland, Spain (the Basque Country) and the United Kingdom. The suitability of housing for this purpose is an issue for many people in the CEE countries and in parts of western Europe.

In Belgium, hospitals have been able to redesignate beds from acute care to nursing home use. Similar measures are being considered in Hungary. Many countries are converting small hospitals into nursing homes. As part of the resource allocation process in the United Kingdom, regression analysis found that nursing home provision had a significant effect on admission rates and bed-days used. The growth in the nursing home sector in Ireland and the Netherlands has probably played a significant role in reducing hospital admissions.

Measures have been introduced in Ireland and the United Kingdom to improve coordination between the health and social care sectors through joint planning. Denmark and Sweden impose financial penalties for delays in placing patients who need social care. In western Europe, responsibility for the two sectors is usually separated, but experience suggests that joint management, as in Ireland and Northern Ireland, or a single purchaser, as in Hungary, does not guarantee improved coordination.

Finally, the development of nursing home provision can be promoted by changing provider payment systems.

A particular problem with these policies is that they generally involve shifting costs to individual users or their families. This can occur either directly, in the form of co-payments, which are often needed for nursing home care, or indirectly, by requiring family members to provide some of the care. The growth in the number of women in the workforce, an increase in the proportion of people living alone, and changing public expectations will make such policies more difficult to introduce, particularly if a "contract" to provide various types of state support for the elderly or chronically sick has been established by years of payment into some form of state insurance scheme.

Utilization reviews

Utilization reviews are an increasingly popular technique for examining the appropriateness of admissions and the use of inpatient beds. These reviews seek to assess whether admission was necessary, and whether care could have been provided in another setting.

The initial techniques were developed in the United States in the 1960s, and were first applied to control spending in the Medicare and Medicaid programmes *(390)*. In 1972, the federal government imposed a requirement for concurrent admission and length-of-stay review by a Professional Standards Review Organization (PSRO) *(391)*. In the 1980s, the techniques were developed further by insurers aiming to improve efficiency *(392)* by reducing length of stay, thus allowing an increase in workload and income without increased bed capacity *(391)*.

Evaluations of the PSRO programmes have not produced consistent findings. Some studies reported a 10–15% reduction of hospital inpatient admission rates, while others did not detect any significant effects. The projections of cost savings also differed considerably. Although utilization reviews may initially lead to reductions in length of stay and in admission rates, these effects seem to be greatest during the period following the review and decrease over time *(392)*.

Differences in the application of utilization reviews in other countries can be explained by the differences in health care provision and the ways in which it is financed. In the United States, for instance, economic incentives such as fee-for-service systems and clinical and legal incentives (defensive medicine) have encouraged physicians to make intensive use of hospital services *(390)*. This has led to the introduction of pre-admission authorization, and patients who fail to obtain this are often subject to financial penalties, although hospitals and physicians are rarely sanctioned.

Table 29 lists some examples of published utilization review studies, and indicates the dimensions of inappropriate bed use. These results also demonstrate the need for a more standardized and validated approach. Although some of the tools have been validated in the United States, their applicability to other health systems has not been established, and they should be used with caution *(393,394)*. The uncritical use of utilization reviews could introduce barriers to appropriate care.

Linking initiatives

It has generally been found that unexpected consequences and opportunities for manipulation often result from attempts to apply a single set of incentives to hospital systems. Many of the measures described above are complementary, and the challenge for policy-makers is to build these into an integrated system that can increase the appropriateness of hospital use and the efficiency of the system, but that also remains flexible enough to allow innovation.

Table 29. Inappropriateness of bed use: selected studies

Study	Location	Results
Baré et al. *(395)*	Barcelona, Spain	9.1% of admissions 29.2% of bed-days
Victor & Khakoo *(396)*	Central London, United Kingdom	0.7% of admissions
Victor et al. *(397)*	Central London, United Kingdom	14.6% of admissions
Namdaran et al. *(398)*	Edinburgh, United Kingdom	19% of beds for all specialties 33.1% of beds for geriatric orthopaedic rehabilitation 29.6% of beds for geriatric rehabilitation and assessment
McClaran et al. *(399)*	Montreal, Canada	19% of beds
Apolone et al. *(400)*	Greater Milan, Italy	41% of bed-days for all specialties 12% of bed-days for surgery 20% of bed-days for cardiology 60% of bed-days for psychiatry, geriatrics and neurology
Hynes et al. *(401)*	Dublin, Ireland	46% of beds for all specialties
Anderson et al. *(402)*	Oxford, United Kingdom	62% of bed-days
Coid & Crome *(403)*	Outer London, United Kingdom	10% of bed-days for all specialties 22% of bed-days in medicine 2% of bed-days in surgery 9% of bed-days in orthopaedics
Popplewell et al. *(404)*	Australia	3.7% of admissions 9.2% of length of stay
Seymour & Pringle *(405)*	Dundee, United Kingdom	4.2% of bed-days of all patients 10.2% of bed-days in patients aged 65 and over
Murphy *(406)*	Central London, United Kingdom	16% of bed-days
Rubin & Davies *(407)*	Liverpool, United Kingdom	4.5% of beds

Source: Baré et al. *(395)*.

Although reducing length of stay and increasing day case work allows additional work to be performed and/or beds to be closed, the impact of these changes on costs is complex. To achieve shorter stays, additional resources such as therapists, nurses or staff with other specialist skills may need to be deployed. Furthermore, unless the fall in length of stay results from technologies that reduce patients' dependence (e.g. minimally invasive surgery), those who remain in hospital will increasingly need skilled nursing care.

Unless bed closures keep pace with the fall in length of stay or measures to control admission are introduced, it is probable that admission thresholds will fall and that admission rates will rise. For instance, a threshold change appears to explain part of the major increase in emergency admissions experienced recently in a number of British hospitals. In this case, hospitals are discharging patients who have a low-cost per diem and replacing them with high-cost patients who require a range of treatment and investigations. As a result, the total costs of the hospital system could increase.

Measures for improving hospital efficiency and reducing length of stay also need to take into account the impact on other parts of the system. If patients have high levels of dependency when they are discharged, they are likely to make demands on PHC services or may even, on occasions, need readmission. This may reduce the willingness, or the ability, of the PHC system to prevent other admissions. The problem is likely to be more acute where there are institutional barriers between different types of care delivery, such as in a number of CEE countries, where outpatients are generally followed up after discharge by physicians who were not responsible for the period of hospital care.

An integrated approach may help to achieve savings from lower lengths of stay and reduced admissions. A strategy is needed, however, for identifying cost savings or reallocation. Savings may be significantly reduced by high technology and by the larger numbers of highly skilled and hence more costly staff at the bedside, in clinical support and in management, that are needed to achieve improved performance. The fixed costs of health provision are high, and a significant percentage of these are associated with infrastructure. For this reason, marginal reductions in bed numbers may be of little assistance in making savings.

CHANGING THE SIZE AND CONFIGURATION OF THE HOSPITAL SYSTEM

A number of issues need to be taken into account in changing the configuration of the hospital system. These include the appropriate distribution of specialist services, the shortage of evidence to guide hospital planning, the appropriate benchmark (beds or hospitals) and the management of change.

The distribution of specialist services

The distribution of services for specialties such as cardiac surgery, neurosurgery, plastic surgery and cancer gives cause for concern. The current situation, where treatment and diagnostic facilities are often duplicated, owes much to history and perpetuates significant disadvantages in terms of fragmented research effort, lost economies of scale and potentially poorer clinical outcomes.

Many countries have systems for controlling the purchase of expensive medical equipment. In some cases, these controls extend to private providers. Systems have also been set up to control the development of specialist services, but these may not have the capacity for dealing with the existing problems of suboptimal distribution.

It does not appear that markets are an efficient mechanism for addressing the overprovision or duplication of specialist services. Indeed, the non-price competition for hospital care found in most markets will tend to encourage the development of such units. In more planned systems, there are other incentives that make the restructuring of specialist services difficult. Here, there are three key issues.

Specialist services often have a high profile and enjoy a high level of public support, creating political barriers to change.

The rationalization of such services often requires substantial investment in the hospitals chosen as the site for centralization, and the writing off of capital assets in other hospitals. This means that hospitals need access to bridging finance, or the ability to predict income over a long period, in order to be able to spread implementation costs. The lack of this type of "banking" function is a particular problem in some countries in the European Region.

Specialist services in general hospitals make a substantial contribution to covering overhead costs. If a unit is closed, purchasers and/or owners may have difficulty replacing these funds from existing revenues. This means either that the entire hospital's viability could be threatened, or that the total cost to purchasers could rise.

A shortage of evidence

There are gaps in the evidence needed to guide hospital planning. There is, for example, considerable uncertainty about the existence of economies of scale. If there are major advantages to greater size, the centralization of hospital services (subject to considerations of accessibility) would be a sensible policy direction. There have, however, been few conclusive studies on the effects of scale on efficiency. Studies in this area suffer from difficulties in obtaining comparable information about inputs and in assessing the value of outputs, as well as in identifying the correct level for analysis, i.e. the whole hospital or individual departments. The analysis available is so complex that it is hard to translate into locally applicable policy (408).

Further uncertainty surrounds the relationship between the quality of outcomes and the volume of work undertaken (377,409). There is some positive evidence in this area (355,410–417), although the relationship is less strong than might have been expected and in some cases is nonexistent (418). The problem for policy-makers or health care purchasers is that, while there is clearly an intuitive link, in the absence of data on risk-adjusted outcomes it may be difficult to require change in the case of an individual hospital. Determining whether the relationship concerns an individual physician or the organization's competence presents further difficulties (419–421). Finally, some users might be willing to trade increased waiting or travel times for a lower risk of a poor outcome.

Although the literature about clinical effectiveness is increasingly well developed, there is little research-based evidence about the components of effective hospital management. There is no agreed definition of what constitutes an effective hospital. There are also reasons to doubt whether the examples of excellence drawn from general management theory are applicable on any but the most superficial level. Hospital managers and purchasers of hospital care have insufficient understanding about the mechanisms for changing hospital services.

A final area of uncertainty concerns the impact of new technology on the way that care is provided. Improvements in technology may act as a spur to centralization owing to the need for high-cost equipment, or they may allow the wider dissemination of a whole range of techniques now only found in central hospitals *(422)*. Although there is an extensive literature on technology assessment, little consideration has been given to how technology will be used and, in particular, what the broader impact of some of the expected developments might be. This applies to new medical technologies (for example, molecular medicine and minimally invasive techniques) but also to the development of informatics, including remote diagnosis, improved information for self-care and telemedicine.

The small but growing literature on the future of hospitals predicts that there will be fewer, larger, high-technology hospitals serving very large populations, possibly supported by community hospitals, outpatient centres, PHC and home care. This may involve the regionalization of major trauma treatment. There has not, however, been a debate about the availability of other models, and it may be that a highly pluralistic system of hospital organization is needed in order to reflect different cultures, clinical models and geography. The costs and benefits of alternative methods of providing acute care have not been fully explored, and there is a danger that bold statements about hospitals at home, day hospitals, subacute beds and other alternatives may be made and acted on in the absence of convincing evidence about their true capabilities.

Beds or hospitals: which is the correct yardstick?

Most substitution policies aim to reduce the use of individual beds. Beds, or even wards, however, may not be the correct units to analyse in formulating policy. Hospitals might be a more logical choice. The following key issues should be considered.

At least 30% of the costs of hospitals are associated with buildings and other fixed facilities. A significant percentage of overhead costs is tied up in "indivisible" assets, and in staff whose numbers are, at best, only indirectly related to bed numbers.

Some beds recorded in statistics may exist only on paper, or may be largely unoccupied. In a number of CEE and CIS countries, a considerable number of beds could be eliminated with little impact on the system's capacity, since they may be technically available but are not in fact either staffed or used.

Repeated small cuts can damage staff morale, particularly in efficient hospitals that may be less able to make further savings.

To have the greatest impact on the costs of the hospital system, however, whole hospitals need to be closed rather than small adjustments made to the total bed stock.

Managing change

The history of managing change in hospital systems is not encouraging. The political and financial costs of closing hospitals are an important reason for this. In a number of systems, these are exacerbated by the lack of a banking function or by the inability to hold reserves, which means that it is difficult to fund a large single expenditure such as capital investment or compensation for staff redundancy. The perceived importance of hospitals in the public mind is a further problem, as it makes even small changes contentious.

In a number of countries, it is not clear who leads the process of changing hospital systems. The creation of insurance funds in a number of CEE countries, and the complex relationships between these bodies, health ministries, owners, finance ministries and parliaments, allows several institutions to assume that they are leading the process. Organizations that control mechanisms for effecting change may not have a clear policy framework to help them to define what that change should be.

The history of the forces driving change in hospital systems is poorly understood and, although there have been a number of interesting policy developments and natural experiments, these have often not been either evaluated or documented. They include issues such as: obtaining support for change from key stakeholders; developing mechanisms for communicating with the public, and explaining the reasons for change; and approaches to managing change. These are discussed in more depth in Chapter 7, in the context of implementing health care reform.

STRENGTHENING HOSPITAL POLICY-MAKING

The development of hospital policy and policy-making in Europe would benefit from a stronger theoretical framework. A combination of market and planning mechanisms, operating on both the demand and supply sides of the system, may be needed. It is rarely enough to rely on only one policy instrument, such as reimbursement systems. Table 30 outlines a framework of approaches to changing the hospital systems.

Although there is a shortage of evidence, a number of policy elements appear to be required in order to ensure a coherent and realistic strategy for hospitals. These include:

- clear and unambiguous responsibility for the overall management of change at government level, but also in hospitals themselves;
- a clear set of financial and managerial targets for the hospital sector, including incentives for managers and clinicians to improve hospital efficiency and make other managerial changes;
- opportunities for managers to learn good practice from each other, and systems for disseminating successful initiatives to improve efficiency;
- a clear budget for the hospital sector, with appropriate financial targets (these will probably need to be combined with other performance-based targets);
- if targets are set, ensuring that policies allow for innovation and encourage the search for efficiency;

Table 30. Policy approaches to changing the hospital system

Supply side	Demand side
Indirect mechanisms	**Indirect mechanisms**
Cost sharing	Payment systems
	Provider markets
	Evidence-based purchasing
Demand management	**Changing service delivery**
Appropriateness and utilization review	Developing management capacity
Disease management	Performance management techniques
Substitution policies: primary, community,	Cost reduction/efficiency programmes
home and social care strategies	Treatment protocols
Prevention strategies, including self-care	Quality improvement techniques
and PHC interventions	
	Planning approaches
	Hospital closure
	Reorganization programmes

- establishing a set of sensible case-mix-adjusted targets for improvements in length of stay, day case work, admission rates, etc., and ensuring that an integrated approach is taken to the way these targets are set and their achievement managed;
- a performance management system with penalties and appropriate rewards, in a political context in which institutions that fail will not necessarily be rescued;
- a strategy for managing and improving integration between hospitals, PHC and social care;
- a plan for releasing real expenditure and costs when bed closures are being considered (in many cases, closing whole sites or hospitals may be more effective than closing beds);
- an approach for dealing with distortions in provision, and for managing the distribution of specialist services;
- techniques for managing the implementation process, including strategies for communications and for recruiting support, particularly from medical staff;
- ensuring that funding for implementation is adequate, including provision for some form of bridging finance; and
- a contingency plan for dealing with the unintended consequences of policy change.

A renewed role for PHC

The four strategic elements of PHC, as defined in the Declaration of Alma-Ata, may be summarized as follows *(423)*.

- the need to reorient health services so that PHC is at the core of the health care system, while secondary and tertiary care act as supporting, referral levels;
- a concept of health policy that includes lifestyle and the environmental determinants of health, i.e. an intersectoral approach to health policy;
- community and individual involvement, both in terms of participation in the decision-making process and of greater individual responsibility for one's own health; and
- appropriate technology and cost–effectiveness, including the efficient allocation of resources and their redistribution away from hospitals and towards PHC.

The broad acceptance of the principles of PHC has brought about a new health culture, which includes but transcends narrowly biomedical determinism. Many countries in the European Region have taken decisions to develop their PHC services, and have adopted policies to promote health through intervention in the environment and in the lifestyles of their population. The new public health movement, whose principles were stated in the Ottawa Charter for Health Promotion *(143)*, added new impetus to this effort (see the section on the evolving role for public health in Chapter 2, pages 65–78).

Relating community involvement to individual responsibility has also achieved some success, as health promotion and education have raised awareness of the health-related risks of modern lifestyles and environments. On the other hand, community participation in the decision-making process has so far been minimal.

New low-cost technologies have been developed that can support a PHC-led health strategy. Desktop computers as well as biochemical and other diagnostic laboratory equipment are being used extensively in a growing number of countries.

THE ORGANIZATION OF PHC SERVICES ACROSS EUROPE

Debate continues over the most appropriate way to structure the delivery of PHC services. Among European countries, there are arrangements based on solo general practice, on group practice and on multidisciplinary health centres. There are different approaches to placing patients on lists, and different views on whether patients need to be referred to specialists.

In terms of dividing patients into discrete populations to receive PHC services, the pattern is mixed. Theoretically, a family or personal list system increases the likelihood of a personal relationship developing between doctor and patient, and ensures continuity of care. Alternatively, some countries define catchment areas, whereby patients are assigned to GPs and/or health centres according to their place of residence. Advocates of patient choice, however, tend to view the geographical approach in a negative light.

Patient lists

GEOGRAPHICALLY DEFINED POPULATION

PHC physicians serve geographically defined populations in Bulgaria, Croatia, Estonia, Finland, Greece (in rural areas, where general practice exists), Hungary,

Iceland, Israel, Lithuania, Norway, Poland, Portugal, Romania, Slovakia, Slovenia, Spain, Sweden and Turkey (in theory). In several countries, such as Bulgaria, Israel, Portugal and Spain, they also have patient lists.

The introduction of patient lists is a common policy objective; Finland, Hungary, Norway, Romania, Slovakia, Slovenia and Turkey are all introducing such lists. This aim is closely connected with changing remuneration from salary to capitation, and with reinforcing the gatekeeping role of PHC physicians. The political character of this change in remuneration strategy is evident in Sweden, where the "old" salary system may be returning after a period of emphasis on capitation and patient lists. The opposite is true in Finland and Norway, where the "personal doctor programme" (PHC physicians with patient lists) is well under way.

PERSONAL OR FAMILY LISTS

In Denmark, Ireland, Italy, the Netherlands and the United Kingdom, each GP has a list of specific individuals. GPs are paid by capitation, and are self-employed, independent contractors. Some geographical limitations typically apply. The main difference in countries, such as Portugal and Spain is that GPs are salaried. Acting as a gatekeeper is possible in both systems: GPs in Portugal, Romania and Spain are gatekeepers to secondary care *(424,425)* as they are in Denmark, Ireland, Italy, the Netherlands and the United Kingdom.

In Denmark, Group 2 patients (3% of the population) have no obligation to be on a specific GP's list. This is the case in Ireland for categories 2 and 3 (the 60% of the population that is better off). In the Netherlands, publicly insured people (61% of the population) are obliged to be on a GP's list, while privately insured people do not have an obligation to register (although, in practice, most are on the list of their choice). In Italy, children under the age of 14 are registered with a PHC paediatrician.

There are no patient lists for defined areas in Austria, Belgium, the Czech Republic, France, Germany, Luxembourg and Switzerland. In Belgium, there is a movement in favour of patient lists (and capitation) and GPs can opt for this method. In Austria, some provinces have a semi-capitation payment. The Czech Republic has changed to a "no defined population" system, whereby patients have direct access to all physicians. Where there is no patient list for a defined geographical area, patients can consult as many doctors as they wish (either GPs or specialists), though in practice most patients stay with one GP. A "no defined population" approach usually implies a fee-for-service form of payment *(425)*. See Chapter 5, pages 158–159, for a detailed discussion of fee-for-service payment systems.

Referral restrictions

The gatekeeper is a defined point of entry to secondary care. When PHC physicians act as gatekeepers, they function as agents of their patients: doctors decide when and to whom to transfer responsibility for care of a specific problem. In a few countries, the doctor has absolute discretion on this matter. In others, it is the patient who decides when and to whom to be referred even before visiting the doctor.

GATEKEEPING

GPs are gatekeepers in Croatia, Denmark, Finland, Ireland, Italy, the Netherlands, Norway, Portugal, Romania, Slovenia, Spain and the United Kingdom. Medical care from casualty (accident and emergency) departments does not, however, require prior referral by the GP.

In Croatia, Romania and Slovenia, children and workers have their own "general specialists" and women have direct access to gynaecologists and obstetricians, thereby weakening the GP's gatekeeping role. In Denmark, Group 2 patients have unrestricted access to specialists.

In Italy, there is direct access to ophthalmological, dental, gynaecological and obstetrics services (plus paediatric care, because of the paediatric patient list). This is also the case in Spain, except that there is no direct access to gynaecological services. In Italy, Portugal and Spain, in urban areas and for the economically better-off, it is common to contact the GP after having seen a private specialist, in order to gain access to diagnostic and therapeutic procedures such as official prescriptions and sickness certificates. This is known as "inverse referral". Many people in Portugal and Spain use the emergency services as a way of gaining access to specialist care in public hospitals.

In the Netherlands, people with dental problems can apply directly to a PHC dentist. When specialist care is provided in an emergency, without referral, the authorization is obtained retrospectively ("posterior referral"). Continuing care by the specialist after one year needs further authorization ("extended referral"). Both extended and posterior referral are commonly authorized indirectly, without consultation. Indirect referrals are also common in Italy and Spain. In the Netherlands, midwives undertake around 40% of normal deliveries, and their fees are covered by a public health insurance scheme. Patients insured privately are reimbursed at a higher level, so they can afford to pay the fee of a GP or obstetrician (426).

In Ireland, patients belonging to categories 2 and 3 have direct access to specialists. In the United Kingdom, patients with sexually transmitted diseases have direct access to specialists; people with dental problems can also consult a dentist directly, although NHS dentists now have patient lists. In Norway, specialists can officially be consulted only through referral (although 10% of all patients receive treatment without being referred). Choice of specialist is only available in private practice (426). In Spain, too, GPs cannot choose specialists in the public system. Patients are referred to a designated specialist (outpatient or hospital) in the geographical catchment area.

DIRECT ACCESS TO SPECIALISTS

Patients have direct access to specialists in Andorra, Austria, Belgium, Bulgaria, the Czech Republic, Estonia, France, Germany, Greece, Hungary, Iceland, Israel, Latvia, Lithuania, Luxembourg, Poland, Slovakia, Sweden, Switzerland and Turkey.

In Belgium, France, Luxembourg and Switzerland, patients are free to choose their GPs and specialists, and can also choose between private and public institutions and between outpatient and hospital settings. In Germany, patients need a referral from an office-based physician (GP or specialist) for hospital care. In all these countries, the tasks of primary and secondary care are not well defined, and this results in overlapping activities and strong competition between physicians.

In Hungary, since the 1992 reforms, GPs serve as gatekeepers and can choose the specialists to whom they wish to refer their patients, though the system is still in its early stages. To some extent, this will eventually be the situation in Poland, where the system has not yet been implemented. In the Czech Republic, since the reforms, patients have direct access to all physicians, including specialists. Health care in Bulgaria, Estonia, Latvia, Lithuania and Slovakia relies heavily on specialists, specialist care being provided by both hospitals and polyclinics on an outpatient basis. In rural areas throughout Europe, PHC physicians can be gatekeepers because specialists and hospitals are scarcer and people consult their local doctor first.

PHC AND HEALTH CARE REFORM

PHC has had a rather fitful relationship with the continuing process of health care reform in Europe. On the one hand, reform documents typically refer to the importance of PHC, and efforts to increase effectiveness often involve strengthening the role of PHC in service delivery. On the other hand, however, many reforms have focused predominantly on cost-containment, limiting the flow of revenue to providers or, where relevant, to insurers. In these exercises PHC, like public health, has sometimes been perceived as only a marginal player.

The largest role for PHC may be in health reforms in the growing number of countries that seek to give it control over part or all of other delivery sector budgets. The best known example has been the United Kingdom's five-year-long development of GP fundholding, in which a growing number of GP practices were given responsibility for hospital elective surgery and outpatient visits, and subsequently for outpatient pharmaceuticals and community care. Indeed, the United Kingdom has begun a further extension of GPs' responsibilities into what is termed "total fundholding", whereby general practices control budgets for all patient spending in the health and community care sectors.

Similar efforts to give PHC control over resources in the hospital sector can be seen in Finland, in several counties in Sweden (most notably Dalarna), in several regions of the Russian Federation (notably Kemarova) and in a new experiment in a social-insurance-financed health system in the city of Berlin in Germany. These initiatives give different PHC actors responsibility for their budgets; in Finland and Sweden, for example, they are boards of locally appointed or elected public representatives, respectively. They also carry different degrees of budget responsibility (from 20% of hospital expenditure for regular GP fundholding in the United Kingdom, to 100% in Finland and Sweden). Despite the variety, all these mechanisms serve to enhance the position of PHC.

These efforts to give more responsibility to PHC are still controversial. In the United Kingdom, although some evaluations have been positive (426), critics are concerned that fundholding is leading to adverse selection of patients and to greater social inequities in service delivery. In Finland, a debate is beginning about whether municipal PHC boards are competent to purchase hospital health services efficiently and effectively. Nevertheless, it is in this area, as budgetholder, that PHC may well be most actively involved in European health care reforms.

In the CEE and CIS countries, PHC has been an important focus of reform. Most countries have replaced or are seeking to replace their Soviet-style polyclinics with some type of PHC physician. Although these efforts were initially hampered by the lack of trained GPs, or even of appropriate training programmes, the process of establishing a new model of PHC delivery is well under way in central and eastern Europe and, increasingly, elsewhere.

The integrative role of PHC

To meet the challenges that lie ahead successfully, PHC needs to build on its strengths and provide a service that fragmented, vertical services cannot offer. This should be done by developing PHC's role as a provider of integrated services to and with the patient and the community. This integrative role has three complementary dimensions: functional, organizational and educational.

Functional integration implies that the episodic management of disease should be superseded by an integrated approach to the health needs and problems of individuals, the family and the community. Community-oriented PHC has shown that it can achieve considerable improvements in health in an effective and efficient manner *(427–429)*.

Organizational integration focuses on how health centres function, both internally and in relation to other services. The concept of the multidisciplinary health team should be reinforced so that different PHC professionals work together and are not simply sharing the same roof. Integration with different agencies providing services to the patient implies that PHC should clearly define the limits of its mandate and work closely with clinical specialist services, social and welfare services and public health services to improve the quality of patient care.

Educational integration can generate the knowledge, skills and attitudes currently lacking in many training programmes for health professionals. Key initiatives here include undergraduate training in PHC, specialist training, and continuing education for GPs and family practitioners and other members of the PHC team.

The implications of substitution

SHIFTING SPECIALISTS INTO PHC

As noted above, a significant pathway of substitution involves specialists shifting their activities into PHC and/or community care settings. This is already happening in some European countries – in some places at significant levels. In systems where money follows the patient, hospitals might well be able to convince their populations that "ease of access" is a good reason for specialist outreach.

Marinker *(430)* outlines the distinction between GP and specialist with great clarity:

> The diagnostic task of the specialist is to reduce uncertainty, to explore possibility and to marginalize error. This contrasts sharply with the diagnostic task of the general practitioner. This is to accept uncertainty, to explore probability and to marginalize danger.

To put it more strongly, if specialists are allowed to dominate PHC, thus reducing continuity of care and the GP's responsibility for the most common health problems, patients generally will suffer. Starfield, in her review of PHC in 11 developed countries *(431)*, concluded that "restriction of specialists to hospitals and their payment by salary is generally associated with better system performance for the population as a whole".

Nevertheless, there may well be a case for outreach activities, and PHC will certainly need extra support if it is to meet the new demands placed on it. Changing relationships between nursing and general practice are likely to play a part in future developments.

THE PHC NURSE/PHYSICIAN INTERFACE

Box 19 contains a statement about a "nursing constant". This logic could be applied to general practice as well. In certain respects, the activities of both groups, with their emphasis on pastoral care, differ in degree more than by type. Nursing is certainly challenging medicine in the PHC area, and this relationship may represent a rich vein for substitution.

In practice, the skills of nurses in Europe are not always well matched to the task. Substitution may thus be a double-edged sword, threatening PHC physicians on the one hand but also acting as a threat to nurses, who can in turn be replaced by aides and other health workers. The role of nursing and reform is addressed below in the section on developing human resources.

TEAMWORK

By suggesting a greater integration of activity at the community level, teamwork raises the difficult issue of coordinated or "seamless" care. The scenario suggests the coexistence of health and social care; in practice, the two often merge together.

Substitution can occur within and across professions in one sector, and across sectors as well. This will call for professionals to relax their boundaries – not something

---

Box 19. The PHC nursing/general practice constant

The work of the PHC nurse and GP is based on skills and values and includes:

- a thorough knowledge of the patient's social context
- a coordinating function
- a teaching function for carers, patients and professionals
- developing and maintaining programmes of care
- technical expertise, exercised personally or through others
- concern for the sick, but also for those currently well
- a special responsibility for the frail and vulnerable.

Source: Department of Health *(432)*.

they find easy to do, apart from delegation, because of ethical issues. Rigid work hierarchies would become inappropriate, and line management challenged. A matrix of skills across the spectrum will most likely bring the best results, but this demands new organizational forms – teams – if it is to work as intended.

The term team should not be understood narrowly. In practice, "working together" can take many forms: a formal team; a loose collaboration; a group subcontracting to another team; a gatekeeper, calling on others; or a partnership with carers.

Beyond these options there is the further dimension of core and extended teams. These require greater coordination, and pose major leadership problems. Multidisciplinary review might help to ensure a more balanced provision of care. Better communication will also be important. Expanding clinical teams in PHC alone will demand accelerated development of information systems.

COMMUNICATION AND INFORMATION TRANSFER
The sharing of care between PHC and hospital sectors is likely to increase. Information systems that are accessible to all team members will be required; access policies will need to be determined in the light of confidentiality; and the system must be able to incorporate care protocols and guidelines, and to present clinical information in a problem-oriented way. Given the increase in health service activities that take place in PHC settings, information systems will need to meet epidemiological and management requirements at population level, as well as to support providers of direct clinical care to individual patients. Substitutions of all types, occurring in an increasingly flexible way, will place major demands on information system development.

Developing human resources
The largest proportion of recurrent expenditure in health care systems is typically staff costs, making human resources a critical factor to be addressed in any reform of health care delivery. Successful health care reform involves careful consideration of key human resource implications, such as planning staffing levels and skill mixes, educational training and accreditation, incentive policies and industrial relations.

The health sectors in the CIS and southern European countries are overstaffed with physicians (see Fig. 23). In 1994, the numbers of physicians per 1000 population in Georgia, Ukraine and Azerbaijan were 4.4, 4.3 and 3.9, respectively, with the CIS average at 3.5 per 1000. In western Europe, the highest numbers of physicians per 1000 population are in Italy (4.7), Spain (4.0) and Greece (3.9). The higher employment ratios for physicians in these countries can be explained by the lack of medical resource planning, and by the late introduction of limits on the number of medical school places. This has also led to higher levels of unemployment among physicians. Whether the higher numbers of physicians in some countries are the result of tradition, the lack of control over medical school places or a tendency to substitute staff for capital-intensive approaches, this overcapacity needs to be addressed. Market forces and unemployment among the medical professions do not

Fig. 23. Numbers of physicians and nurses per 1000 population in the WHO European Region, 1994

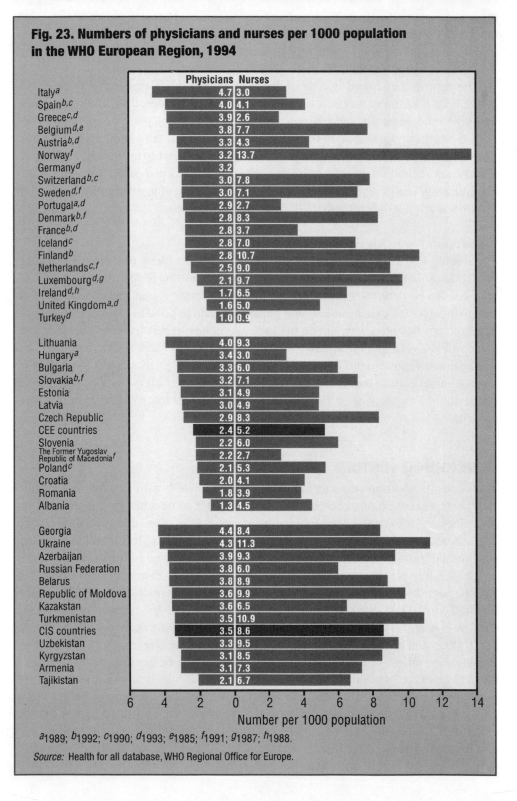

	Physicians	Nurses
Italy[a]	4.7	3.0
Spain[b,c]	4.0	4.1
Greece[c,d]	3.9	2.6
Belgium[d,e]	3.8	7.7
Austria[b,d]	3.3	4.3
Norway[f]	3.2	13.7
Germany[d]	3.2	
Switzerland[b,c]	3.0	7.8
Sweden[d,f]	3.0	7.1
Portugal[a,d]	2.9	2.7
Denmark[b,f]	2.8	8.3
France[b,d]	2.8	3.7
Iceland[c]	2.8	7.0
Finland[b]	2.8	10.7
Netherlands[c,f]	2.5	9.0
Luxembourg[d,g]	2.1	9.7
Ireland[d,h]	1.7	6.5
United Kingdom[a,d]	1.6	5.0
Turkey[d]	1.0	0.9
Lithuania	4.0	9.3
Hungary[a]	3.4	3.0
Bulgaria	3.3	6.0
Slovakia[b,f]	3.2	7.1
Estonia	3.1	4.9
Latvia	3.0	4.9
Czech Republic	2.9	8.3
CEE countries	2.4	5.2
Slovenia	2.2	6.0
The Former Yugoslav Republic of Macedonia[f]	2.2	2.7
Poland[c]	2.1	5.3
Croatia	2.0	4.1
Romania	1.8	3.9
Albania	1.3	4.5
Georgia	4.4	8.4
Ukraine	4.3	11.3
Azerbaijan	3.9	9.3
Russian Federation	3.8	6.0
Belarus	3.8	8.9
Republic of Moldova	3.6	9.9
Kazakstan	3.6	6.5
Turkmenistan	3.5	10.9
CIS countries	3.5	8.6
Uzbekistan	3.3	9.5
Kyrgyzstan	3.1	8.5
Armenia	3.1	7.3
Tajikistan	2.1	6.7

Number per 1000 population

[a]1989; [b]1992; [c]1990; [d]1993; [e]1985; [f]1991; [g]1987; [h]1988.

Source: Health for all database, WHO Regional Office for Europe.

appear to be reducing the supply of physicians at a sufficient rate, and some countries are still reporting increases in the number qualifying. There is a need, therefore, to review recruitment to medical schools, particularly those in the private sector.

A related issue is the need to review traditional definitions of medical roles and the division of responsibilities between the various professionals, as well as to avoid the use of overqualified and expensive personnel by devolving certain less clinically demanding tasks to more appropriate staff. The distribution of staff is also critical, with a number of countries in the Region experiencing difficulties in staffing rural areas. In several Member States, the availability of PHC physicians and other PHC staff is also a problem. Specialists continue to predominate, in terms of numbers, status and earning potential.

Reform programmes in European countries need to place more emphasis on establishing appropriate assessment and training policies for the numbers of staff and mix of skills required in reformed systems. Some reform failures have partly resulted from the lack of trained staff with appropriate skills. The areas requiring particular attention include public health, general and family practice, nursing and management training.

PHC physicians are a key professional group. In many European countries, the role, status and training of these physicians have been neglected in favour of specialist medicine. PHC reforms have emphasized the cost-effective role of the PHC physician as gatekeeper and first point of contact with the system, providing continuous, individual care with a community orientation.

Training family physicians and GPs has become increasingly important. In some countries, family or general practice is now considered a specialty in its own right. Most western European countries have vocational training programmes for general practice. Estonia has rapidly developed a specialization and training programme with an up-to-date curriculum. In some CEE and CIS countries, however, slow progress in this area has undermined the introduction of appropriate PHC-based reform.

THE CONTRIBUTION OF NURSING[24]

As the single most numerous group of health care professionals in the Region, nurses play a significant role in the health system. Around five million people work in the nursing services of the Member States, half of them in the CEE and CIS countries. In many countries and many settings, nurses are the first, last and most consistent point of contact that patients have with the health care system. The contributions of this professional group are increasingly recognized, and there is widespread agreement about the need to strengthen and develop its functions. Nursing[25] is seen as a cost-effective resource for delivering health care services, particularly in the fields of public health and PHC. Thus, nursing development is part of the more general trend to increase the cost–effectiveness of health care delivery.

---

[24] This section draws upon the WHO Regional Office for Europe publication *Nursing in Europe: a resource for better health* (Salvage, J. & Heijnen, S., ed; WHO Regional Publications, European Series, No. 74 (in press)).

[25] "Nursing" is used here as a general term. Terminology and definitions vary from country to country. The terms "nurses" and "nursing" should be understood to mean all health workers doing nursing work, including nurses, midwives and feldshers (for a definition of the latter, see page 244).

In the CEE and CIS countries, nursing development stagnated for many years in disease-oriented health care systems heavily based on medical specialization. Despite broad intercountry diversity in the degree of progress that has been made (or not made) in overcoming such barriers, a reappraisal of the whole of nursing is taking place throughout the European Region.

The nursing workforce

An analysis of the nursing workforce is complicated by the variety of staff grouped under the broad heading of "nursing personnel" and the frequent lack of differentiation between grades, qualifications and competences in human resource planning and deployment. For instance, in many CEE and CIS countries, auxiliary and/or unqualified staff perform nursing duties, comprise 50–90% of all nursing personnel and are included in the statistics on "nurses".

The number of nurses per 1000 population varies widely in the European Region. In western Europe, rates range from 0.9 in Turkey to 13.7 in Norway (see Fig. 23). In general, these rates follow a north–south divide, with relatively higher rates in northern countries than in southern Europe. The low number of nurses, combined with a high rate of doctors in some southern countries, has led to a very low nurse:doctor ratio in Greece, Portugal, Spain and Turkey. The ratio of nurses to the population appears more closely related to income indicators such as GDP rather than to health care need. Shortages of nurses, particularly in rural areas, are reported in Greece, Israel, Italy, Malta, Portugal and Turkey. Difficulties in recruiting qualified staff are common throughout this group, owing mainly to low pay, poor working conditions and a lack of career opportunities. Only 5–10% of the workforce is male, except in Italy, Malta and Spain, where men comprise about a quarter of the total nursing workforce.

Problems with matching supply and demand for nursing staff are reported throughout the Region. Shortages of well educated nursing staff and difficulties in recruiting suitably qualified nurses are common in the CEE and CIS countries. Recruitment of new staff is difficult in rural areas, the main reasons being low status, poor salaries and bad working conditions, which lead to migration and/or reduction of the nursing workforce. Many people seek better jobs in the private sector. In some situations in the CIS, auxiliaries are employed in qualified posts. Workloads can be very high: 1 nurse and 3 support staff may care for as many as 80 patients. High turnover rates are reported in several countries, including Azerbaijan, Belarus, Georgia, the Republic of Moldova, the Russian Federation and Tajikistan.

Recruitment and turnover ratios vary significantly in western Europe and are highly correlated with status and working conditions, as well as with demographic factors, government policies and national and local labour market conditions. The picture can also change relatively quickly, making generalization or the mapping of trends difficult. Some countries report shortages of nurses and nursing students as well as high turnover rates, while elsewhere spending cuts have reduced the number of posts and mopped up surplus staff. Recruitment for specialist posts may still be a problem.

The opening of Europe's borders, with some voluntary migration out of the CEE and CIS countries as well as the movement of displaced people (particularly from the former Yugoslavia), is creating new phenomena. Nurses in the CEE and CIS countries tend to move to richer CEE or western European countries (especially Germany) seeking better wages and working conditions. Some western European hospitals actively recruit foreign nurses, even though locally qualified staff may be unemployed.

PHC nursing in Europe

The belief that the role of nurses in maintaining health is as important as their role in caring for the sick can be traced back to the 1950s. The view is that nurses should not only care for individuals, but also for families and communities. The idea of the public health nurse, who performs a generalist role within a PHC framework, has also steadily gained acceptance. Nursing in Europe has been influenced by a range of philosophies and is characterized by several different approaches; hence the role of the nurse differs significantly across the Region.

In some CEE countries such as the Czech Republic, Hungary and Slovakia, nurses are beginning to be recognized as independent health care professionals, but in other countries they are still subordinate to physicians. In Albania, Bulgaria, Poland and Romania, nurses are regarded as medical assistants and their role is determined by medical doctors. In Poland, the nurse's role is determined by the physician in charge of the unit, who may give written permission for nurses to undertake certain tasks. In Romania, professional nursing training was abolished in 1978 and the role of nursing subsequently declined into that of medical assistant, i.e. the most common term in Romanian to describe the "nurse".

In the CIS, nurses work in a variety of settings including hospitals, polyclinics, maternity homes, children's homes and kindergartens. They work under the instruction of physicians, providing a service to other professionals rather than to patients, which is an obstacle to developing the nursing function. There is evidence, however, that professional roles and functions are being re-examined, and that the role of nurses is increasingly perceived as vital for providing cost-effective care. Training, continuing education and increasing responsibilities may also prove effective tools for improving the status of nurses.

In the CEE and CIS countries, the number of health professionals working in PHC is generally very low. There is an enormous shortage of community nurses and physicians, especially in rural areas, owing largely to the fact that the role of nursing is not recognized or developed in PHC. There are a lack of available education, low status and poor working conditions, with long working hours and low salaries. Most nurses that do work in the community are more likely to fulfil the role of physicians' assistants, carrying out medical treatments or procedures. There are a few innovative examples of nursing care, such as in Hungary, where district nurses provide home nursing in some areas, and mother and child care nurses undertake community midwifery tasks, including health education and family planning. In some rural areas, where medical care is not available, nurses and feldshers provide all PHC.

Feldshers are health workers who operate between the traditional roles of the nurse and the physician. They have considerable independence and perform preventive, diagnostic and therapeutic tasks. In rural areas, feldshers traditionally provide all PHC and manage staff, performing a role similar to that of the nurse practitioner in the United States. In urban areas they may be employed by the emergency services (including ambulance services) and/or in a role oriented towards prevention and public health, while in some rural areas they often provide midwifery services.

In western Europe, nursing is generally considered as an independent health care discipline that complements the other health care professionals in multidisciplinary teams. In some countries such as Greece, Malta and Turkey, however, the nurse's role is still that of providing services to the medical profession. Developing or maintaining community nursing, including home visiting, is defined as a priority in many of the countries. Activities such as home visiting, however, while well established in countries such as Denmark, Finland, Iceland, the Netherlands and the United Kingdom, are relatively underdeveloped in others such as France, Ireland and the Mediterranean countries. Community nursing may involve several different roles: district nursing, health visiting (combined under the title of public health nurse in Ireland), family planning, school nursing, occupational health, community psychiatric and mental handicap nursing, paediatric nursing and health education.

Some examples from countries show the wide range of philosophies and approaches. Community nursing is well developed throughout the Nordic countries. In Sweden, for instance, nurses are trained in five main areas that take a holistic approach to patient care: nursing care, health promotion and disease prevention, planning of care, health education and development of nursing skills. In Iceland, there is an extensive home nursing service, with community nurses caring for the elderly population in a flexible way, combining care in patients' own homes and in nursing homes. Nursing in Spain has developed from the purely curative function of assisting physicians, into a more autonomous role that involves health promotion and disease prevention. In the United Kingdom, rapid progress in recent years has brought greater autonomy and accountability for the nursing profession. Two relatively new PHC roles for nurses have developed: the practice nurse and the nurse practitioner. Practice nurses are generally employed by GPs to work as members of the PHC team and to provide nursing care in the doctor's clinic. Nurse practitioners may work in a hospital or the community, they can be employed by a GP or a health authority, and they have the authority to make some decisions about patient care, diagnosing medical conditions and treating and referring patients within the scope of their training.

Recent developments in nursing

Nursing practice in Europe is changing, and there are indications that the profession is altering its ways of working in response to new demographic patterns, new concerns about cost-containment and new goals and needs for health care. Great efforts are being made, especially in the CEE and CIS countries, to explore new concepts and to implement new approaches. Despite the wide differences in professional roles and functions among European countries, some common trends in reform are emerging.

First, there are efforts to measure the outcomes of nursing interventions (particularly in the United Kingdom and northern Europe) where nurses, like all other health care providers, are increasingly coming under pressure to produce value for money. A number of studies have shown that in certain areas and conditions, particularly within PHC, nursing care may be more cost-effective than care by family practitioners. A study of general practice in the United Kingdom found that practice nurses were able to provide safe and effective care of hypertension, and had more success in preventive interventions *(433)*. In the United States, a study of nurse practitioners has shown that they can provide first-contact PHC as safely and effectively, and with as much satisfaction for patients, as a family physician *(434)*. In a review of a wide range of studies, Feldman *(435)* showed that nurse practitioners, working in PHC and outpatient care settings, can provide good-quality care at lower cost.

In the United Kingdom, a review of existing research from the Audit Commission *(436)* and the Centre for Health Economics at York University *(437)* has demonstrated that there is a direct correlation between the employment of qualified nurses and better patient outcomes. The SETRHA study *(438)* demonstrated that work by nurse practitioners is diverse, is associated with a high degree of patient satisfaction, and focuses on wellbeing as well as illness. Nurse practitioners were also found to practise safely and effectively, and to generate savings in some areas. It was concluded that PHC revealed the greatest potential for developing the nursing role. Other studies *(434,439,440)* have demonstrated that appropriately trained nurses can give care of comparable quality to that provided by physicians. They are particularly effective at providing services that depend on communication with patients, and at preventive activities. Furthermore, nurses are capable of providing quality care at lower cost *(434)*.

Second, nursing is shifting its focus away from mainly task-centred practice towards care that focuses on the health needs of the whole person, and away from hospital-based services towards PHC nursing for both the sick and the well, with an emphasis on disease prevention and health promotion. Such changes should be underpinned by appropriate regulatory frameworks.

Third, changes in nursing practice inevitably mean that nursing education needs to be reviewed. There is renewed interest in nursing education in many European countries, with reforms focusing on curriculum review and reorientation to PHC; on new programme development, especially in higher education; on continuing education schemes; and on forging closer links between education and services.

Finally, there are signs that attitudes towards the position of nursing in society and its role in health care delivery are slowly changing. The perception of nursing as a low-status occupation requiring minimal training, and the associated undervaluing of humanistic psychosocial care, are beginning to moderate, though the process is slow and uneven. The issues of low pay, poor working conditions and low status need to be addressed through the introduction of career structures and appropriate financial incentives.

7 The Process of Implementing Reform

Health care reform has been harder to implement than expected *(61,441–443)*. Moreover, it has often had unintended consequences *(444,445)*. Several countries have experienced difficulties that have had little to do with the actual content, but instead reflect inadequate planning for the implementation process. Yet the reform debate has paid little attention so far to the problems of implementation, and to strategies for managing change.

This chapter begins by applying a conceptual framework for health policy analysis to examine experience to date on implementing health systems reform, in order to provide a better understanding of the role of specific contextual elements, processes and actors in reform programmes. Next, some general lessons are highlighted from the review of country experience.[26] Finally, a series of strategies to facilitate change are suggested.

A framework for the analysis of implementation

A framework for health policy analysis can help policy-makers to understand the factors that facilitate or impede change (see Fig. 24). This framework presents implementation as an integral part of the policy process. While notice is taken of policy content (the appropriate design of a social insurance system, for example), attention focuses on the context in which policy is introduced, the process by which it is formulated, implemented and evaluated, and the actors who influence policy content, context and process and who are affected by it *(446)*. Effective policy-making requires that each aspect is addressed separately as well as collectively.

CONSIDERING THE CONTEXT

The development of health care reform in a specific country is influenced by a wide range of contextual factors. As discussed in Chapter 1, societal values and economic recession have played a significant role in triggering reform in several European countries. Here, four contextual areas that are particularly influential in the implementation process are reviewed: the macroeconomic situation, the political environment, societal values and external influences.

The macroeconomic situation

For many countries, the central constraint in implementing reform is the relative strength and resilience of the national economy. This is true for the western

---

[26] The Regional Office held a workshop in Copenhagen in November 1995 to review salient experiences in reform implementation and to explore the factors both inhibiting and facilitating implementation of health systems reform. The workshop was attended by a number of policy-makers involved in health care reform across Europe, who from their own experience highlighted specific concerns about implementation and proposed strategies to deal with these obstacles. This chapter incorporates the main points resulting from that debate.

Fig. 24. Framework for health policy analysis

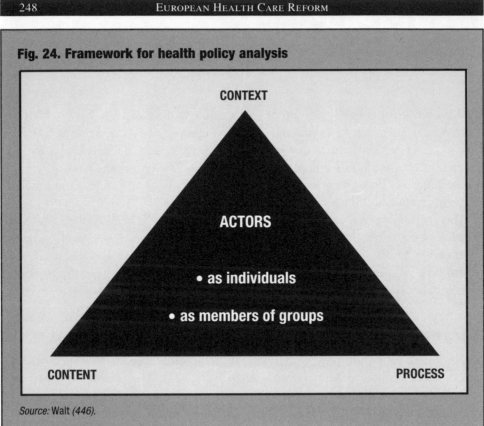

Source: Walt (446).

European as well as the CEE and CIS countries. Many current health reforms are being introduced in a period of economic retrenchment, which contrasts sharply with the preceding four or five decades of expansion. Most CEE and CIS countries have experienced severe economic recession, leading to a significant decline in the financial resources available for health services.

This has placed greater pressures on public expenditure (the search for cost-containment and efficiency) and, in some countries, has resulted in attempts to shift financial burdens from central state bodies to individuals, autonomous institutions, or regional and local authorities. In periods of economic contraction there is less room for manoeuvre, and the planning procedures associated with expansion do not work well. Planners are not motivated in the same way (447), leading to lower professional morale and creativity. In several countries, the scale and magnitude of changes proposed by reform programmes are difficult to implement against a backdrop of economic retrenchment and decreasing health budgets.

The political environment

As the new institutional school has argued (448), the structure of a country's political institutions can have a major impact on its ability to achieve health sector reform. The relative strength of private interests (individual, collective and corporate) vis-à-vis the public sector, and the history that lies behind these relationships, all influence the capacity of a government in office to introduce change successfully. This holds true whether a country is federal or unitary in structure, whether its regional or local government is strong or weak in relation to that of the state, or whether or not it has a written constitution that limits the role of the state. As a direct consequence, the appropriate locus for undertaking health reform will vary from country to country. In some instances, responsibility may be national, as in the United Kingdom. In others, it may be shared between the national and regional authorities (Denmark and Sweden) or between the national and municipal authorities (Finland). Elsewhere, the power to introduce health reform may lie at the interface of self-governing statutory institutions and regional and national government, as in Germany. In each instance, different weight is placed on the relative importance of the process as opposed to the outcome of political debate, and each country approaches health sector reform within its own particular framework.

The relationship between these different institutional characteristics and the implementation of health reform is complex. For example, while the United Kingdom has demonstrated the ability to force through major structural reform, Sweden has shown itself to be more capable of testing a variety of different reform ideas simultaneously through demonstration and pilot projects. In countries where the political system favours multiple-party coalitions (e.g. the Netherlands) or a "checking" role by a second national legislative body (e.g. the Bundestag in Germany), health reform (like all public policy) must be negotiated by multi-party or sometimes all-party coalitions, in turn typically leading to more measured or incremental reform. How one evaluates these different arrangements, of course, depends on one's view of the importance of radical as against incremental measures of reform in the health sector. The political changes sweeping the CEE and CIS countries have created several institutional obstacles to implementing health system reform. One key obstacle has been the emergence of governments hamstrung both by weak multi-party coalitions and/or complicated relationships between a president, the parliament and regional governments. These new and sometimes unstable institutions tend to approach health care reform with strongly ambivalent feelings, seeking to achieve western European service standards but without worsening the difficult health and employment situation. The mix of new institutions, various degrees of intra-institutional competition, and an ambivalent approach to reform often combine to produce erratic and sometimes inconsistent policy-making. Another constraint has been that, as in many western European countries, health ministries have generally been accorded a comparatively low position in the political hierarchy, and consequently health policy has ranked low on the reform agenda.

In some countries, administrative staff at all levels of the policy process have been purged, and their replacements have been unprepared and/or unqualified for the tasks before them. When new institutions have been set up, with new administrative and political authority, they have often lacked personnel with relevant skills and experience, thus exacerbating uncertainty. Where administrative staff have not been removed, efficiency has declined as former rigid hierarchies and party discipline are replaced with a different and to some extent alien decision-making culture *(449)*.

The absence of an independent administrative (civil) service often means that, as the parties in power change, the administrative machinery replicates the inbred inefficiency of the former system *(450)*.

Societal values

Value systems are seldom explicitly taken into account when policy implementation is considered. Yet, in relation to health care reform, there is evidence of considerable conflict in values between policy-makers, professionals and the public, as well as within each of those groups – for example, over the use of market mechanisms in health care. Where values clash with reform objectives, there may be considerable resistance to executing policies. Hence, understanding value systems is paramount if governments are to develop reform policies that are both acceptable and workable.

Value systems are embedded in political structures. In the liberal democracies of western Europe that established "welfare states", the introduction of health sector reform (often in concert with other social policy reforms) has been relatively unpopular with the public and with influential professional groups *(451,452)*. In these countries, where large public social programmes have been central features of the political landscape, the health system achieves high coverage of the population and is popularly perceived to be working relatively satisfactorily. There may be some dissatisfaction with quality, but there is little support for reductions in care – still less if these are achieved by the imposition of market mechanisms. There is a fundamental difference between a government seeking to extend benefits to large numbers of people and one seeking to take those benefits away *(451)*. Moreover, where the objectives of reform are tax containment and cost sharing, couched in ideological, pro-market terms, governments have had to face direct opposition from groups strongly attached to public health policies or to collectivist, non-market values.

On the other hand, where a government's *raison d'être* for reform is based on improving access to, or the quality of, health care, basic social values may be shared and widespread. Even where the motivation for reform is perceived to be positive, however, there are still pitfalls between policy formulation and implementation caused by the need for trade-offs between public and private control, restrictions on freedom of choice due to budgetary constraints, and availability versus affordability *(453)*. Implementation may be highly affected by the extent to which governments can persuade the public that their reform programmes are driven by positive intentions rather than purely by economic constraints.

In political systems that have undergone a change of regime, such as those in the CEE and CIS countries, reform may be welcomed by the new middle class and by some health professionals because it is perceived as an opportunity to challenge overcentralized, bureaucratized, initiative-stifling health systems. While reforms may be seized on as an opportunity, however, they may be difficult to implement because they are opposed by significant groups that see themselves being placed at a disadvantage – the elderly, for example. Furthermore, reforms may be undermined by tensions between the old and new guard, among both professional groups and citizens.

External influences

Exogenous factors have played an important role in the development of health system reform. One key influence is the transference of reform models and ideas across national boundaries. For instance, the creation of the national health services in the late 1970s and early 1980s in Greece, Italy, Portugal and Spain was influenced by the British NHS model *(454)*. The most recent reform of the NHS, based on the notion of competitive contracting imported from the United States, has in turn exercised considerable influence on the content of health care reform in several countries, not only in the European Region but also in Latin America, Africa and Asia.

Importing reform models from other countries has not only a clear influence on the formulation of new reform programmes but also significant implications for implementation. New reform strategies are often embraced by policy-makers on ideological grounds, with little understanding of the technical resources required to put them in place. This hampers implementation, particularly when the receiving countries have less developed health systems. For instance, the Russian Federation has imported some ideas for reform without adequately considering their applicability in the specific local context *(241)*. Transferring ideas without skills will add to the problems of implementation, as discussed below in the context of the technical capacity to manage reform.

In some cases, reform policies have suffered from low credibility when they were perceived to have been imposed from outside, and as a result have encountered greater implementation difficulties. Reforms led by multilateral and national development agencies and linked to financial aid concessions can experience these problems. In some Latin American countries, for instance, reforms have been seen as externally imposed *(455)*.

MAKING SENSE OF PROCESS

How the implementation process itself – i.e. the stages or steps required to introduce change – is conducted constitutes a key element in achieving change. The success of this process may be directly affected by the system of government, and by the distribution of power and authority between central and local levels.

Distribution of power and authority

Almost all governments transfer some authority or devolve some power for public planning, management and decision-making from national to subnational levels, or from higher to lower levels of government *(456)*. In practice, however, as discussed in Chapter 2, the system of decentralization varies substantially between countries. At one end of the spectrum, the centre exercises tight control over the lower levels of the administrative system through legislative and financing mechanisms. At the other end, lower-level authorities may have considerable discretion in interpreting central policy and may exercise some control over expenditure, especially where they have the right to raise revenue. Policy implementation is clearly affected by the prevailing system and by the extent to which the centre can expect lower-level authorities to follow its guidelines. Implementation will depend on how much political authority is vested in the system of government, and which mechanisms the centre can use to influence subnational authorities. Such mechanisms may include regulations, legislation (whether discretionary or mandatory), financial inducements and sanctions.

The status of the centre, its authority and its legitimacy are key factors in implementation. In several CEE and CIS countries, the decentralization of authority to health insurance agencies and/or the regional or local level has left health ministries with accountability for implementation but with little authority and/or mechanisms to drive reform. In the Russian Federation, for example, a considerable degree of health care reform has been conducted by regional authorities, with only weak guidance from the centre *(241)*. Similar difficulties in Kazakstan have led to a drive for recentralization of health policy control in the hands of the national government *(76)*.

In many countries, health ministries are weak in comparison with social security or health insurance agencies. The latter allocate funds to health programmes, often paying little regard to the priorities established by the ministries. In the same way, in countries whose systems are funded from general taxation, finance ministries tend to play a major role in resource distribution. This role of finance ministries is also important in several health systems funded by social insurance, as in the Netherlands.

Operationalization of reform policies

While the distribution of authority between central and local institutions influences implementation, there are other factors involved, mainly related to how the process is conducted. If it is unclear how to make policy objectives operational, implementation may falter.

Many governments develop lofty policy objectives in devising health care reforms, but find it more difficult to spell out how these objectives are to be achieved. This may reflect the tendency of most political systems to give greater rewards to "shrewd deployment of symbols and generalized arguments" than to detailed forecasting and analysis *(457)*. Many analyses of health care reform point to the gap between policy intent as against strategies for making policy work. For example, Bulgaria has introduced a new national health insurance system that will be monitored by the Ministry of Health, but there has been little discussion about how the state will consult and collaborate with the institutions in the new scheme *(458)*. Yet health reform is "process oriented", being aimed at restructuring relationships between public and private sectors, managers and policy-makers, providers and consumers. Any restructuring depends on understanding how change should be implemented, and who is likely to favour or resist reform.

The introduction of reform in the health sector has specific characteristics that make bridging the gap between policy intent and action particularly difficult. Technically, health care reform is complex. It needs a sound infrastructure with good information systems and management skills, together with the substantial additional resources needed to put new organizational arrangements into place. Also "to reform", by definition, implies a challenge to the status quo. To be successful, reform needs collaboration or some form of consensus between a multitude of different actors in both the public and private sectors. Moreover, as pointed out above, reform programmes tend to have multiple objectives, some of which may conflict with political and societal values. In Table 31, a model of the factors that facilitate implementation has been used to summarize the difficulties that may confront the introduction of health sector reforms *(459)*.

The pace of implementation

There are substantial differences in the way that countries have approached the process of reform implementation. One important aspect of this process is the pace at which countries introduce change. The ability to introduce rapid change is closely related to political factors such as the type of government, or the role of social actors supporting or opposing change.

In 1991, the British government introduced a comprehensive and radical set of reforms in the NHS, which were implemented in a very short time. By the mid-1990s, most of the planned changes were in place, in what has been termed a "big-bang"

Table 31. Factors affecting the implementation process

Facilitating factors	Current health care reforms
Clearly stated policy goals One main objective avoids confusion or conflict.	**Reform goals often in conflict** Multiple objectives, some of which conflict with political and societal values.
Simple technical features Knowledge and technology exist. No new resources are needed.	**Highly complex features** Experience is lacking. Training is needed. Expensive information and costing systems need to be developed.
Marginal change from status quo Easier to get incremental change agreed.	**Reforms require major change from status quo** Major change may be strongly opposed.
Implementation by one actor Collaborating across sectors complicates process.	**Reforms often pluralist** Public and private sector collaboration is difficult.
Rapid implementation Short duration limits build-up of resistance and distortions of policy.	**Reforms complex and execution slow** New systems (procedures and institutions) have to be devised and established.

Source: Cleaves *(459)*.

approach to health care reform *(460)*. The strategy involved the centralized, top-down development of a grand reform plan, which was enacted without pilot projects and in spite of strong opposition from the British Medical Association and a substantial proportion of the population. Indeed, such was the government's belief in the appropriateness of the reforms that it "proceeded without demonstration projects and with a minimum of consultation" *(461)*. The United Kingdom's case underlines the power of a strong majority in a unitary national government to implement reform: "If Britain did not have a political system designed to give the government of the day an automatic majority in the legislature, then clearly the 1991 reforms of the NHS could never have been introduced" *(460)*.

The restructuring of the health system in New Zealand, a country with a British-style constitution, followed a similar pattern. The New Zealand reforms were contentious, and faced considerable opposition, but were none the less swiftly implemented *(462)*. The reforms parallel those of the British NHS but are acknowledged to have gone further, with an even faster pace of change *(462)*. Some commentators contend that the introduction of health system reforms in both New Zealand and the United Kingdom owed more to ideology than to policies based on sound empirical evidence *(463,464)* and conclude that their swift implementation was explained by the nature of their political systems.

In some CEE countries, particularly the Czech Republic, the pace of reform has also been relatively fast. These health systems have undergone a radical transformation, with the introduction of new financing arrangements based on social insurance, changes in the remuneration methods for health care personnel and a decentralized organizational and administrative structure.

In contrast to this centralized approach to health system reform, changes in Finland, Germany, the Netherlands and Sweden have been more measured. In keeping with its shared public–private and national–regional structure of institutions, Germany adopted a gradualist strategy of incremental change based on the progressive introduction of legislation aimed at containing costs. Reform implementation in Germany has been strongly defined by the traditional values and principles of the statutory health insurance system, and by the organizational features and financing mechanisms related to these principles. The pace of implementation has varied, depending on the type of legal regulation being introduced. While regulations that became effective immediately (such as the budgetary constraints in the 1992 reform law) had a substantial impact, those due to be implemented through the contractual process between sickness funds and provider groups have sometimes met with substantial resistance.

In the Netherlands, the 1988 Dekker report *(261)* set out an ambitious plan for restructuring the health care system, which, in effect, "advised the government to drop its comprehensive health care planning approach and to rely on market forces for effective cost containment of health care expenditure" *(67)*. Shifting coalitions in the national government, however, coupled with political, institutional and public opposition, meant that only partial implementation had occurred by 1994. As de Roo *(67)* wryly observed, "we are witnessing an ongoing process of pragmatic socio-political adaptation of a political value to new social conditions". Thus in the Netherlands, as in Germany, the institutional structure together with basic social and political values has generated a more cautious, incremental approach to reform.

Health care reform in Finland and Sweden has been predominantly incremental, although each country has introduced national system-level changes that have fundamentally altered previous institutional arrangements. In both countries, the shared health sector roles of municipal (Finland) or national and regional (Sweden) governments, as well as a pragmatic emphasis on cross-party political coalitions to ensure continuity, have made it possible to introduce coherent, nationally formulated reforms that can be implemented effectively by broadly independent county or municipal governments.

In Sweden, for example, national legislation in 1992 shifted ownership and responsibility for all residential care for elderly people – including nursing homes – from the 26 county councils to the 284 municipalities. The shift encouraged a closer link between residential care for the elderly and social services run by the municipalities (including home care services) and is considered by most observers to have been a success *(465)*. There have also been occasions, however, when national and local policies have been in conflict, particularly on cost-containment issues. For several years in the early 1990s, Parliament unilaterally imposed a "tax freeze" on the counties, preventing them from raising new revenues for the health sector. Conversely, individual counties often developed their own strategies for increasing the efficiency and effectiveness of the publicly operated delivery system.

The pattern has been broadly similar in Finland. Close national–local collaboration produced the Hiltunen reform of 1993, which shifted the focus of control and changed the method of calculating national subsidies for the locally run health care systems. This reform, which was four years in the planning and needed more than 50 changes to national legislation, was implemented on schedule. Cost-control issues, which were more directly a municipal concern, have produced a variety of different initiatives for influencing provider incentives.

Overall, despite the numerous structural and cultural differences between Finland and Sweden and between these two Nordic countries and Germany and the Netherlands, there are certain similarities in the process of implementing health sector reform. Most specifically, the shared character of decision-making power in the health sector has resulted in a more deliberative approach than that seen in more centralized countries such as New Zealand and the United Kingdom.

The reforms introduced in Italy (1978), Greece (1983) and Spain (1986) also followed an incremental process of change *(454)*. Key aspects of the reform plans, such as shifting the main source of funding (from social insurance to general taxation) or developing new models of PHC, have only partially been implemented. Some of the theories advanced to explain this limited implementation include the system of patronage involving political parties and interest groups, the shortage of management skills to implement change, and the lack of a politically independent civil service to carry out reforms. In Italy and Spain, another explanation may be the continuing process of decentralization, which has given regional governments considerable discretion in setting priorities *(454)*.

A final aspect of implementation is the dynamics between intended and unintended policy outcomes. Particularly in relation to market-oriented measures, the announcement of reform proposals can trigger anticipatory movements as key players in the health system seek to position themselves for the future situation. Groenewegen *(466)*, describing the change processes in the Dutch health care system, suggests that the very debate initiated by Dekker led to change. The ideas about introducing market concepts expressed in the Dekker report *(261)* provoked specific responses from influential actors in the health care field even before the government set out its policies. Thus just the expectation of reform may lead to unanticipated and unplanned change.

THE IMPORTANCE OF THE ACTORS

In addition to context and process, actors or stakeholders are a key determinant of policy change. Four sets of actors play an influential role in reform implementation: citizens, professionals, policy élites and interest groups.

Citizens

The relative power of citizens to exert influence on health service developments, either individually or as members of interest groups, varies widely between European countries and depends on the degree of public participation in each health system. As noted in Chapter 2, participatory mechanisms are more developed in Ireland, the Netherlands, the United Kingdom and the Scandinavian countries, and less developed in southern and eastern European countries. In the Netherlands, for instance, the involvement of consumer groups is relatively formalized, with the Dutch Federation of Patients and Consumers participating in a variety of decision-making processes *(170)*.

In general, however, the views of patients on health system reforms are often lacking. Although many reform proposals formally seek to enhance the involvement of citizens, their views and those of patients have largely been ignored in much of the recent development and implementation of reform. Nevertheless, broad public support for reform can be an effective catalyst for change, just as the lack of it can be a major barrier.

Professionals

Social scientists have often described the health-related professions as playing an unduly influential role in the development and implementation of health policy. This so-called "professional dominance" reflects key characteristics both of medical professionals and of the health sector. One critical factor is the central role played by physicians in the medical enterprise, owing to their control over clinically related knowledge. The high social status of medical professionals in many European societies is a related issue. As a result, the health-related professions are able to exercise sufficient influence to ensure that professional rather than public interests prevail, that service delivery is often organized to accommodate professional interests, and that professional prestige and status facilitate their dominance of the decision-making process *(467,468)*. The medical profession, in particular, often exercises its influence through interest or pressure groups. Owing partially to the diverse functions of different medical organizations, this influence varies considerably between European countries. Some organizations, such as the French Ordre des médecins or the British Medical Association act as trade unions. Others, such as the British and the Irish royal colleges or the Bundesausschuß in Germany are more concerned with professional standards; some, such as the Colegios de Médicos in Spain, perform both functions. In the CEE and CIS countries, the number of medical organizations seeking to play a more influential role in developing national health policy has increased.

The medical profession has played a significant role in the development of reforms in a number of European countries. In CEE countries such as the Czech Republic and Latvia, the medical profession became both the driving force and agent for reform. In the Czech Republic, physicians took advantage of the changing political context to introduce their own preferred policy, whereby providers would be reimbursed on a fee-for-service basis from health insurance funds (Potucek, M., unpublished data, 1994). This particular policy change had a significant impact on the national health insurance fund, which went bankrupt less than six months after it was set up *(174)*. Also in the Czech Republic, the medical profession resorted to strikes to oppose particular reform measures, achieving a significant degree of success.

Policy élites

Policy élites – senior politicians, bureaucrats and managers who formulate and implement policy – are all important stakeholders in the health sector. Key questions often revolve around the relative powers and interests of each group. Bureaucrats, in particular, play a strategic role in implementing reforms, and their response to policies can affect the outcome. Policies with benefits that are apparent only in the long term may be perceived negatively by those implementing the reforms – the officials and managers who have to introduce new systems, break old habits and relinquish accustomed forms of security, control, responsibility or even corruption *(469)*. Bureaucrats who understand the costs long before the public sees any benefits may find ways of delaying or amending policy. To avoid such behaviour, politicians typically find it useful to mobilize support from outside the bureaucracy. In the United Kingdom, politicians were central to introducing change to the welfare state, while Department of Health officials were not crucial political actors *(451)*.

While politicians can be a force for change, they can also obstruct it. For example, despite a frequently expressed desire by politicians in Finland and Sweden to decentralize management to provider units, these same politicians have shown a marked reluctance to reduce their direct involvement in health service provision *(470)*. Therefore, in a sense, progress towards one health care reform goal has been hindered by members of the very same group that sought it.

The tendency of politicians to advocate change for everybody but themselves may be a factor in hindering the development of social policies, including health sector reform, in much of central Europe. One observer argued that "central and eastern Europe is certainly neither prepared nor willing to move directly from state paternalism to social citizenship" (Potucek, M., unpublished data, 1994). This political intransigence can pose particular problems for the implementation of health care reforms. For instance, other actors may become more influential, and the role of interest groups such as the medical profession or the insurance companies may assume greater importance.

In considering the role of policy élites, it is important to take into account the level at which they work. Bureaucrats at the centre may be relatively distanced from managers' day-to-day concerns or from the "street-level bureaucrats" at local authority level. When formulating policy, central-level officials may not necessarily consider the feasibility of its implementation and, even if they do, may not be aware of potential problems.

Finally, different groups in the policy élites disagree about some issues. For instance, in some countries, the previously influential role exerted by the health professions is being undermined – and in places usurped – by the growing ascendancy of bureaucrats and managers. Studying the effects of the changes in the British NHS on the health professions reveals increasing managerial control over professional activities. Nevertheless, health professionals still exercise considerable control over their work and over the supply of their labour (467).

Interest groups

The increased role played by interest groups is evident in a number of European countries. Not only are patients and professionals often represented by a variety of organized groups that exert significant influence on reform, but a second set of interest groups representing commercial interests, such as the pharmaceutical and medical technology industries or health insurance groups, has also had a significant impact.

In Europe, the growth in the number of such groups has led some to talk of an "overcrowded policy environment" (471) and, where they are particularly powerful, decision-making may become very difficult. The failure of the Clinton proposals for reforming the health care system in the United States demonstrates the influence exerted by stakeholders on the policy process. It also underlines the fact that stakeholders are not always (if ever) altruistic in their demands, but generally seek to protect their own interests (472).

Historically, the health care systems of the CCE and CIS countries were characterized by strong central control (174). With the demise of these centralized political systems, the new governments have been seeking for a new structural paradigm for their health care systems. One consequence of this has been the replacement of the administrative élite with untrained and/or inexperienced personnel, as well as the opening up of the health care system to the influence of a whole range of new stakeholders. "New" in this sense means that health professionals, managers and administrators, local politicians and citizens all believe that they should have a greater role to play in restructuring the health care system. Indeed, some commentators argue that changing the power structure through a pluralistic health care system is essential in order to meet new needs and demands and improve overall efficiency *(473)*.

Learning from experience

As the previous section suggests, there appear to be several attributes that make some governments more successful than others in implementing reform. This section focuses on these attributes, and on the circumstances behind them. Two important points need to be made, however, about the interpretation of "success". First, success in this context is taken to mean the ability to implement desired policies, regardless of their ultimate impact. There is no value judgement as to whether policies are good or bad, but only of whether they have been put into action. Since evaluation is central to reform, implementation strategies should also be judged on the extent to which they include evaluation and feedback mechanisms as an integral part of the process. Second, although reforms have not been fully executed in most countries, this should not necessarily be seen as a negative factor. Even a small change in the health system may be quite radical. In the Netherlands, for example, although the pace of formal implementation has been slow, considerable change has taken place informally as a consequence of the very discussion of reform.

The analysis of experience with implementation suggests seven factors that have played a central role in bringing about change: timing; financial sustainability; political will and leadership; strategic alliances; public support; process management; and technical infrastructure and capacity.

TIMING

Clearly, the existing political, social and economic environment within which reform is to be introduced will determine the probability of its success. The previous section noted the importance of contextual circumstances such as economic recession or political instability in effecting change. Choosing the most appropriate time to reform, such as when there are appropriate or specific circumstances that favour change, is a key factor in determining success.

In times of political change – which may range from war, as in Croatia, to a change of political regime, as in most CEE and CIS countries – opportunities for radical adjustment may be possible and can lead to quite dramatic reforms. A new government may have the necessary political legitimacy to execute policies that was denied to its predecessors. Periods of wide political and social transformation offer "historical windows" for introducing change. For instance, the national health service reforms in Greece, Portugal and Spain were introduced at the end of long periods of authoritarian rule, and after new constitutions had been approved that established health as a social right *(454)*. The changes under way in the CEE and CIS countries, following the fall of the previous communist regimes, offer ample evidence to support this point.

Nevertheless, a rapid pace of change may be difficult to sustain in the long term. In the Russian Federation and several other CIS countries, the early momentum for change became bogged down by the unstable economic climate. Even where the environment facilitates change and where the need for change is accepted, as in Finland or in the United Kingdom, policy-makers may have only five years at the most in which to act – the "honeymoon" period of reform. The growing popular backlash against radical change currently appearing in the CEE and CIS countries lends support to this view.

Time and timing are crucial in deciding both when to reform and how to execute changes. Policy-makers should survey the political, social and economic environments and identify those circumstances that will facilitate the introduction and implementation of reform.

FINANCIAL SUSTAINABILITY

The availability of financial resources is critical in implementing reform, as economic recession has often been a major constraint. In the CEE and CIS countries, the introduction of new funding schemes and new models of provider organization has been slowed down by health care budget cuts (up to 40% in some central Asian republics).

Even when reform measures are aimed at containing costs and/or at generating savings, their results are not likely to be felt in the short term. Additional costs, e.g. for information systems and management training, are involved in putting into place new organizational arrangements such as hospital contracting. Marginal changes in the established organization of services, such as priority shifts between areas, may need extra resources.

Policy-makers need to consider the financial implications of their proposed reforms. They may have to be prepared to invest additional resources in specific areas in order to achieve particular objectives. Introducing new approaches or making changes in the established configuration of services, even when aimed at generating savings, requires financial commitment in most cases.

POLITICAL WILL AND LEADERSHIP

Political will is a significant factor affecting policy implementation. Firm government commitment to achieving a reform programme is an essential aspect of success. Some of the difficulties experienced in introducing health system reform in many CCE countries can be viewed as a function of political will and political stability. Many governments have been short-lived, while rapid changes in administration have led to a succession of different reform proposals being put forward. In several CEE and CIS countries, there has also been a tendency to try to replace the systems established under the former regimes with entirely different approaches, creating the danger of discarding the good with the bad *(474)*.

Lack of political leadership can be a further complication. Some political leaders have only a general idea of their objectives, and may consequently be persuaded to introduce poorly thought-out policies. If there is a political vacuum, a variety of agencies, organizations and groups will seek to push the reform agenda towards changes that are more acceptable to themselves. Multiple approaches to policy formulation and implementation can lead to inaction *(475)*; alternatively, reform may reflect the partisan interests of particular groups of stakeholders such as insurance companies or the medical profession.

It is important to identify a leader who is committed to reform. The Netherlands and Spain both turned to personalities outside the health sector to lead the search for acceptable solutions, in order to generate consensus for change and demonstrate the objective basis for reform. Dekker, an industrialist, in the Netherlands and Abril, a politician, in Spain produced detailed proposals for their respective health systems that attracted widespread attention and provoked debate. The use of outsiders to analyse the health care system may be a good tactic for stimulating discussion, but it can also carry the risk that those with vested interests in maintaining existing arrangements may close ranks against the proposed changes.

STRATEGIC ALLIANCES

Governments depend on a range of actors or stakeholders for policy implementation. This is even more true when they embrace decentralization as a major strategy. If restructuring results in a more passive approach, it will increase the government's dependence on others to put its policies into practice. This is particularly important in the eastern part of the Region, where governments are enacting reforms that reduce their own powers while allowing powerful new stakeholders such as the pharmaceutical and insurance companies to participate.

It may not be entirely clear whether these new actors will facilitate or impede the policy process. A key to successful implementation is maximizing the potential of "policy friends" by establishing alliances of people, organizations and agencies that support the proposed changes, and rendering the influence of "policy foes" less effective through such measures as the flexible interpretation of concessions, inducements and incentives. One approach that has met with some success is to lure two influential groups of stakeholders into confrontation with each other. It could be argued that one contribution to the success of the reforms in New Zealand and the United Kingdom was the creation of a situation in which one set of actors – managers – perceived particular advantages for themselves in terms of self-esteem, enhanced prestige and influence in supporting the changes, to the extent that they chose to discount the concerns of others *(476)*.

PUBLIC SUPPORT

The general population is a particular set of stakeholders that can influence change. Persuading the general citizenry of the need for reform can have an important enabling effect. By contrast, ignoring public views, even when this facilitates change, may slow down or even stall reform in the long term.

This seems especially true when the reforms being implemented lead to a growing conflict between social and market values – one factor in the stop-go reform process in the Netherlands *(466)*. Public views have also tempered the way in which health systems reform has been implemented in the United Kingdom, particularly the shift in policy from covert privatization to one that stressed the importance of a managed market *(70)*. In some countries, the backlash against reform highlights the danger for governments and politicians in taking it for granted that their reform proposals have public support.

One valuable technique is the use of symbolism in presenting reforms. This can be a helpful tool in implementing health systems reform or, at least, in securing support for it. Symbolism may include the use of language that, while appealing to the population, is not precise in its meaning or interpretation. The difficulty with symbolism is that, while people may support the vision, implementing it will depend very much on the power and range of different interests and whether or not they share the objectives. The public must therefore perceive a genuine problem and a need for change, and be offered credible solutions.

The media can often be effective in promoting reforms and in seeking public support. For example, the state's publicity drive was one of the factors that helped transform part of the health sector in north-east Brazil *(477)*. In Mexico, a survey that established considerable public support for health reform was deliberately used to offer the people a voice and make them protagonists for reform *(478)*. In Turkey, officials used the media to promote reform and raise public support, as well as to influence public opinion against the medical profession, who were opposing the changes.

MANAGING THE PROCESS

Managing policy implementation requires a range of skills. One involves assessing the environment or circumstances in which the policy will operate, not only to identify possible obstacles that could impede implementation but also to find factors to facilitate the process. The experiences recounted above illustrate how some governments can understand and influence the environment in favour of reform.

The technical ability to manage implementation involves another set of essential skills. Key elements include setting objectives, allocating responsibility, using mechanisms such as legislation or financial incentives, and pacing the process.

Setting reform objectives

Defining explicit objectives at the outset helps to give a clear sense of direction and facilitates social consensus. In some countries, however, policy-makers have conducted the debate at a symbolic level, keeping the actual goals implicit in order to divert political attention. While this approach may speed the initial process, in the long term it is also likely to generate opposition that may defeat the objectives. Whether or not the objectives are expressed in clear, unambiguous language, or defined in ways open to different interpretations, will partly depend on whether the government has a strong political mandate and is confident that it can carry through reform even in the face of opposition.

Allocating managerial responsibility

European countries differ in the organizational and managerial arrangements introduced to run the reform process. Some countries have had no clear procedures. For example, countries as diverse as Germany, the Russian Federation and the United Kingdom did not establish formal mechanisms, relying instead on a combination of legislation (see below) and professional group support (often secured with specific incentives) to achieve their objectives. Turkey took a different approach, establishing a small unit specifically for implementation. Its mandate was to pursue health reform through technical means, promoting the need for reform (the public relations and marketing aspects), developing consultative procedures, and cultivating alliances with groups favourably disposed to reform. This approach can work well, as long as the body responsible for managing the process retains political support and has access to adequate managerial, financial and legislative tools.

Enabling legislation

Passing appropriate legislation in the early stages of the process can significantly facilitate reform, although having legislation in place does not guarantee automatic implementation, as the experience of many CEE countries aptly demonstrates. The health system reforms in much of northern Europe relied on legislative legitimacy for their implementation. In Germany, for example, the speed with which health system reforms were implemented depended on the nature of the underlying legislation and related regulations. Reforms underpinned by specific regulations were easier to implement, while those that depended on negotiations between different groups were much more difficult to effect.

The usefulness of this tool, however, depends on the characteristics of the health system. Legislation has been less effective in some southern European countries. Also, in some cases overelaborate laws and regulations can slow down and restrict implementation. Croatia is a good example; here, basic, flexible legislation facilitated change. While legislation is important, however, it needs to be supported by other measures if it is to produce the desired outcome.

Financial incentives

Financial incentives have been successful in improving the chances of implementation, both as one-off incentives and for continuing control. One approach involves allocating "seed money" to trigger change or fund pilot innovations. In the United Kingdom, the government made resources available to hasten the introduction of hospital resource management systems (479) and encouraged GPs to become fundholders by offering financial support for computerizing their office management and patient records systems (480).

Pacing reform: "big bang" or incrementalism?

There is considerable debate about the relative merits of a swift and radical reform compared with more incremental approaches. The ability to introduce rapid reforms depends mainly on the configuration of the governance structures and on political will, but is also influenced by contextual circumstances such as the state of the economy or the degree of support from key stakeholders. Rapid reforms with the top-down imposition of a grand plan, as in the Czech Republic, New Zealand and the

United Kingdom, have been effective in bringing about change in a short time. Yet implementing reforms that lack a minimum social consensus may incur both a popular and a professional backlash. Also, when swift and radical change is based on ideology and the impact of the chosen strategies is not carefully considered in advance – a common scenario in current European reforms – it may not be either politically or technically sustainable in the long term.

A more incremental approach, whereby change is tested locally before being extended to the country as a whole, may be more effective *(463)*. This yields more evidence about the effectiveness of different approaches, allowing better decision-making. In the long run, an incremental approach may lead to more socially sustainable policies than the wholesale changes introduced in "big-bang" reforms. Sweden provides an example of the advantages of locally tested reforms, major organizational changes being first introduced by individual county councils. Italy refined the application of a hospital budgeting system based on diagnosis-related groups through several pilot projects prior to full implementation. A local testing approach may be a more effective model for the CEE and CIS countries, which are in the process of restructuring their health care systems but where the political infrastructure is weak *(449)*.

A local testing or incremental approach, however, also has a number of drawbacks. A slow pace of reform allows key groups of stakeholders to organize before change is introduced, and thus to build up resistance. This can be seen in the reform process in the Netherlands, where the slow implementation of the Dekker proposals allowed time for a wave of mergers between health insurance companies and among some larger hospitals, in order to protect their market share if the proposals became policy *(466)*.

Consequently, incremental implementation requires a greater degree of consensus among key health sector actors. An incremental framework is also more likely to succeed if similar reform processes are under way in other social service sectors, generating a critical mass that can make reform visible. While the best approach in each country will ultimately depend on its particular circumstances, there does appear to be a consensus about the advantages of building flexibility into the implementation process. One possible solution may be to combine a "big-bang" approach politically, for the passage of reform legislation, with steady implementation inside health sector institutions. The test of any approach, of course, will be its capacity to achieve systematic and sustainable reform. Here, as elsewhere in health care reform, the challenge is to develop evidence-based policy-making as a counterbalance to political expediency.

Policy-makers should be prepared to modify the strategy when aspects go wrong, as long as such modifications do not affect the consistency of reform. Given the need for flexibility, a well defined role for the health ministry following implementation is essential.

TECHNICAL INFRASTRUCTURE AND CAPACITY

Implementation depends on good information, as well as on relevant technical skills. The countries that have made the most progress with health systems reform are mostly those in northern and western Europe that already had information systems in place to monitor progress, together with the managerial and technical skills required to effect the policies. Countries that lacked one or both of these requirements have typically made little progress. For instance, the Czech Republic, Hungary and Slovenia appear to have been more successful, partly because they built on existing capacity rather than trying to dismantle and rebuild. They chose to involve particular interest groups, such as the medical associations, in building capacity and worked with external agencies to train the cadres who would be given responsibility for implementing reforms. They also worked to build up capacity in auditing and financial management.

In short, if the infrastructure and the technical and managerial capacities necessary for health systems reform are not developed in conjunction with legislation and political frameworks, it is unlikely that implementation can be either successful or sustained.

Strategies for implementation

Implementation should be viewed as integral to the reform process, not simply as an administrative or managerial afterthought *(481)*. The same degree of thought and effort that goes into developing policies should also go into developing an implementation strategy. Reform implementation, however, is neither an exact science nor an automatic process. There is no agreed set of strategies that, if faithfully followed, will ensure success. Furthermore, each country's individual history, economic position and type of government, and/or the relative power of stakeholders, need to be taken into consideration. It is difficult, therefore, if not counterproductive, to argue that certain strategies will succeed in all circumstances. Thus, the approach taken here is to indicate a series of general strategies that have proved effective in particular country situations.

DEVELOPING AN ACTION PLAN

Several countries have prepared a master plan or action plan to oversee implementation, the key areas being: accountability and responsibility; the management structure for implementation; an analysis of resources (financial, human and technical) and sources of funding; and the stages of implementation in terms of when the various steps affecting implementation will begin and how they will proceed.

This approach, derived from rational planning theory, can be useful inasmuch as it provides a clear set of guidelines for overseeing implementation. Nevertheless, policy-makers must be prepared to build flexibility into managing this process – particularly with regard to the pace of reform and the degree of adherence to a previously agreed schedule.

THE ACCORDION METHOD FOR EFFECTING CHANGE

The iterative and multidirectional features of reform implementation are considered in the Accordion Method for effecting change *(482)*. The Accordion Method employs two overarching strategies: consensus building (resistance reduction) and building implementation.

The strategies of consensus building embrace a number of actions, which may include the following.

- To minimize apprehension about cultural or social change, the key actors or stakeholders should be consulted to find out how they think the proposed changes would affect them. Their concerns should be acknowledged, and ways sought to address their anxieties.

- An understanding of the need for and effects of change should be created. This should include an explanation of the purpose of the changes, since the gap between perception and reality can be large and may increase hostility and/or resistance.

- Positive support for change should be generated, making clear to stakeholders the benefits that change will bring to them and to the health system as a whole.

- Political alliances should be built that support change, if possible excluding those stakeholders who are resistant to change. If this is not possible, ways should be found to influence their behaviour, either indirectly through incentives or by rewarding groups that support reform, or directly through payments or other benefits.

- Early in the process, stakeholders should be told the reasons for expected outcomes, and the likely impact of change. A detailed plan of the change process should be drawn up, assigning tasks and responsibilities, indicating resources required, identifying needs for training and related capacity building, and setting out a series of milestones against which to monitor progress.

The parallel strategy of building implementation into the policy process overlaps many of the actions described in consensus building. There are, however, certain measures necessary for rapid implementation.

- Changes should be spread over a reasonable period of time, beginning with the least contentious. As confidence develops, the more controversial elements can be introduced. This approach has been successful in Germany and Hungary.

- The implementation of any policy must be planned in parallel with its development. Implementation can be facilitated if the policy is designed as a series of interrelated projects, each with its own implementation strategy.

- Key actors and stakeholders affected by the policy, whether supportive or not, should be involved in its implementation. One way of building consensus would be by rewarding support. Those who resist change should not be penalized, however, as this could lead to further entrenchment of their position.

- Procedures should be established both for monitoring progress and for evaluating the effects of the changes according to agreed objectives. Stakeholders will expect to see the promised benefits and may withdraw their support if these do not materialize. Early feedback on the changes enables remedial action to be taken as necessary.

The Accordion Method does not come with a guarantee of success. What it does offer is a framework or protocol that may enable governments and others to effect changes to the health care system that will produce tangible benefits for their populations. Thus, two important aspects that should be built into any process are:

- performance monitoring mechanisms, where no formal evaluation of the reforms is planned; and
- clear, open and consistent mechanisms for feedback on planned reforms, in order to help minimize uncertainty.

CHECK-LIST OF ACTIONS

A series of actions that could facilitate implementation is summarized in Table 32 The inherent value of this list is that policy-makers may select those features that enable them to develop policies that are sufficiently robust to survive implementation.

These actions, which embrace both consensus building and implementation tactics, are grouped together under four discrete but related headings:

- *capacity/resources*: the technical, managerial and financial infrastructures necessary for implementation;
- *cultural/social factors* that can inhibit or facilitate the development and implementation of health systems reform;
- *political alliances*: the process of forming relationships that will work towards successful change; and
- *systemic action*: the procedural tasks that will enhance acceptance and implementation of change.

These actions are also classified according to three key capacities for managing reform: looking outwards, looking inwards and looking ahead (Brinkerhoff, D.W., unpublished data, 1995).

Looking outwards is a reminder that policy-makers must look beyond the boundaries of their individual agencies and become aware of who and what may affect what they seek to do. Looking outwards includes recognizing important stakeholders, facilitating participation, building alliances and partnerships, setting clear and feasible objectives, and forging coalitions for change.

Looking inwards refers to those crucial but often overlooked internal structures, systems and procedures. It means developing and/or maintaining the technical support necessary for implementation.

Table 32. Check-list of actions for implementation

Capacity/Resources	Cultural/social factors	Political alliances	Systemic action
Looking outwards			
Provide opportunity for study visits for key stakeholders.	Open up reform debate and policy development process.	Establish stakeholder activity.	Set clear, concise goals.
	Encourage health providers to innovate.	Involve trade unions and related agencies.	Describe expected results.
		Be prepared to compromise.	Identify key stakeholders.
Looking inwards			
Create acceptable finance-generating mechanisms.	Avoid overreliance on market principles.	Restrict lobbying of health providers and suppliers.	Set identifiable, measurable targets.
Set out a clear scope and purpose for tax system.	Establish clear lines of accountability.	Consider ideological and constitutional constraints.	Avoid overcomplex management systems.
Establish fiscal and auditing procedures.			Leave technical matters to managers.
Focus on efficiency and effectiveness of changes.			
Align goals with financial resources.			
Build capacity through training.			
Establish local knowledge base and performance system.			

Looking ahead

Separate reform financing from other activities.

Create mechanisms for resolving conflict.

Prepare for turnover of key actors.

Establish regular feedback on progress.

Pace reform through small, irreversible steps.

Avoid overdependence on key stakeholders.

Map agendas of key stakeholders.

Develop regulations through legislation.

Balance financial and technical goals.

Develop new roles when necessary.

Looking ahead has been described as the capacity to keep an eye on the long term while managing the short term. This means that policy-makers must not lose sight of the long-term goals, and that short-term policy changes must be consistent with these goals.

ANALYSIS FOR CHANGE

The analysis of health care reform has tended to focus on technical features of policy, neglecting contextual factors, the roles of actors and the policy-making process. This might help to explain why some policy changes have not been implemented effectively, and why some expected policy outcomes have not been achieved. Table 33 suggests a number of policy analysis instruments that can support the planning of reform implementation.

Many health care reforms are difficult to execute because policy-makers have not identified the features that facilitate implementation. By undertaking the macro-level analysis of any particular reform, some actions may be taken before implementation is expected. For example, it may be preferable to introduce a marginal change (using existing administrative procedures) that can be put into effect quickly, rather than a more radical change that offers space for resistance because new methods have to be devised for implementing it. On the other hand, as noted above, radical change introduced quickly may be successful.

Similarly, making values explicit helps policy-makers (and researchers) to recognize their own and others' perspectives, and to understand how they may be influencing policy, or conflicting with each other. In general, making values explicit helps in the design of policy but, as discussed above, it may generate resistance in some cases and can be counterproductive.

By undertaking stakeholder analysis, it is possible to map the contours of likely support and opposition, and act to change the map. In political mapping, completing a stakeholder analysis is just one of six steps that need to be taken to influence implementation *(483)*. The first is to assess the objectives of each identified organization, in terms of what the organization will gain from a particular decision and the organizational priority (high, medium or low) for each objective identified. Based on the information collected on organizational structures, the next step is to produce a policy network map that identifies connections and alliances among the organizations involved in the specific health decision.

Having identified and analysed the positions of stakeholders, policy-makers can employ several tactics. They may ignore the stakeholder (taking the risk that implementation may be derailed); they may take the public relations approach (building images, "selling" the need for policy change and wooing opinion leaders); they may use "implicit negotiation" (anticipating objections and designing policies that meet those objections); and finally they may use "explicit negotiation" by working with stakeholders on the policy design *(484)*.

Analysis of financial, technical and managerial resources should be part of planning the execution of any policy. Proponents of reform have to take into account two scenarios of reaction or response to policy change. The first is: when the policy

Table 33. Instruments in policy analysis to support implementation

Area of analysis	Planning action
Analyse the ease of implementing policy change.	Analyse conditions for facilitating change and, where possible, make adjustments (one implementing agency, clear goals, one objective, simple technical features, marginal change, short duration, visible benefits, clear costs).
Make values that underlie policy explicit.	Identify macro- and micro-level values underlying policy decisions. If values conflict with policy, support will have to be mobilized.
Undertake stakeholder analysis.	Review interest groups (and individuals) likely to resist or promote change in policy at national and institutional levels. Plan how to mobilize support by consensus building or by rallying coalitions.
Analyse available financial, technical and managerial resources.	Consider costs and benefits of external funds; assess "rent seeking" behaviour; review salary levels; review incentives to change behaviour; assess need for training, for new information systems or for other resources; assess inducements and sanctions.
Build process of strategic implementation.	Involve planners and managers in analysing how to execute policy; identify networks of supporters for policy change; manage uncertainty; promote public awareness; institute mechanisms for consultation, monitoring and "fine tuning".

is "high politics" and visible, the stakes are critical for government and political élites, and the resources needed to sustain the reform are considerable. Here, skill in political management is essential. The second is when the stakes are lower and, while the resources necessary are also considerable, the brunt is borne at a relatively local level. Here, guaranteeing successful implementation depends on incentives, management skills, training and information *(469)*.

Building a strategic implementation process means involving planners and managers in monitoring and controlling the progress of reform, for example, by establishing milestones or benchmarks against which progress will be measured, by looking at variations from budgets and other resources, and by monitoring results *(484)*. It can also mean identifying and supporting clinical (or other) champions. Lomas *(485)* has shown that, when acknowledged leaders accept innovation, others follow. Indeed, the success of much implementation will depend on identifying strategies that help to change behaviour, having codes of practice that establish expected standards of service provision, or inventing incentives for change. As noted earlier, such public campaigns in Brazil and Mexico have helped explain the reasons for reform and publicized its benefits *(477,478)*.

Planning implementation may also mean managing uncertainty: uncertainties about the working environment, meaning that more information is needed; uncertainties about guiding values, meaning that objectives need to be rethought or clarified; and uncertainties about related decisions, meaning that more coordination is necessary *(486)*.

Policy analysis thus provides a number of different instruments that can be useful at different stages of the policy process: from getting an issue on to the agenda to planning how a particular policy will be implemented. Health care reform is on the policy agenda in most countries. The next stage is ensuring it is implemented according to the original intentions.

8 The Way Forward

Drawing conclusions about current patterns in European health care reform can be a complicated process. In a multifaceted sector such as health and medical services, and in a geographical area as huge as the European Region, each main policy direction often has several counter-trends. Moreover, the reform of health care systems should be understood as only one component of a broader intersectoral strategy to maximize health gain for the entire population. The evidence in this volume indicates that, despite this diversity, a number of general observations about health care reform can validly be made.

Experience to date suggests that health system reform, if it is to be successful, must encompass considerably more than just cost-containment. While financial pressures influence policy-making in all parts of the Region, effective and sustainable reform also requires that health care services constitute a social good, and that specific policy measures can increase health gain and the overall health status of the population. In practice, while cost-containment may be a necessary component of health system reform, it is not sufficient in itself. Indeed, reforms that apply economic theory inappropriately to the production of a complex social good such as health care can generate financially as well as medically and socially counterproductive outcomes.

Pursuing supply-side reforms

This study has drawn on several different conceptual frameworks to analyse health reform strategies in Europe. These include the impact of specific strategies on the equity, efficiency and effectiveness of health systems; a consideration of whether strategies affect the funding, allocation or production aspects of health services; and the degree to which particular strategies concentrate on the patient, the third-party insurer, the third-party purchaser or the service provider. The policy impact of these different levels of analysis can be summarized in a conceptual shorthand that compresses the various categories into two traditional economic parameters: policy interventions instituted on the demand side as against those instituted on the supply side of the health care system.

This conceptual shorthand is contingent upon two theoretical distinctions. The first redefines the term "supply" to capture current practice in European health systems more effectively. In other studies, the application of economic theory to health care has typically assumed a two-part model of a health care system: a production dimension composed of provider institutions, and a finance dimension composed of purchasers of care. The analytical model adopted for this study utilizes a three-part framework: the funding of care (how the money is raised), the production of care (how it is spent) and the allocation mechanism (how the funds are distributed to providers) *(487)*. This three-part model more closely reflects the nature of the reform changes that can be observed in many health systems in the western part of Europe, where the absence of change in health system funding has been combined with substantial change in the allocation mechanisms by which funds are distributed to providers. Moreover, in tax-based health systems, the change in allocation mechanisms has typically been instituted by, and is accountable to, a public authority that also administers the provider institutions. Consequently, for the purposes of this summary, the supply side has been defined as incorporating both the allocation mechanism and the production of services.

The second distinction concerns the difference between two types of demand for health services: aggregate population-based, and individual patient-based. Aggregate population-based demand can be altered by policy decisions that change the total need for curative health services, for example, through health promotion strategies that reduce tobacco and alcohol use and increase physical exercise, or through the wider provision of primary and preventive health care services. While health policy can target either one or both types of demand for health care, many recent health system reforms have focused predominantly on individual patient-based demand.

The WHO study suggests that recent efforts by policy-makers to intervene on this individual patient-based demand side of the health system have not worked well. Measures shifting costs to the patient, such as cost-sharing arrangements or limiting the public package of care, have led to equity problems and provoked popular resistance. Despite these drawbacks, in some of the CEE and most of the CIS countries economic exigencies have required this form of demand-side reform. In many of these countries, however, the collection rate for premium payments has not approached budgeted levels. In western Europe, policy-makers tend not to rely on patient-based demand-side mechanisms or, where they do, they soften their impact to such a degree that the measures have little effect. One example is co-payments, which, to prevent interference with equity, are typically buffered by exemptions for vulnerable groups and/or high users, as well as by income transfer payments to the less well-off. Although priority setting between clinical services continues to be discussed in the western part of Europe, in practice governments have been willing to restrict payments for only a few marginal procedures, such as cosmetic repair of varicose veins and *in vitro* fertilization. Where policy-makers have sought to adopt "basic packages" of care services, governments' unwillingness to restrict access has resulted in 90–95% of all services being labelled "basic".

Similarly, efforts to create stronger incentives for third-party insurers by introducing competition between them may appear attractive in economic theory, but carry substantial negative consequences for the social dimensions of the health system. Where governments have sought to introduce competitive incentives into the funding side of their health systems, concerns about adverse selection ("cream skimming") have compelled them to restrict the entrepreneurial freedom of private insurers. Here, as with other patient-based demand-side measures, if competitive incentives are strong enough to have a financial impact, they tend to be politically unsustainable because they inflict too much damage on important social objectives.

Conversely, efforts to act on the supply side of health systems, on a continuum that moves from resource allocation to the production of health services, have been relatively successful and, for all their complexities, relatively sustainable. In the 1980s, allocation interventions were predominantly regulatory in nature and focused on the macro level, such as in setting expenditure ceilings. In the reforms of the 1990s, the policy tool kit has been expanded to incorporate market-influenced incentive mechanisms as well as standard regulatory measures. Among the "planned market" mechanisms included in this supply-side grouping are contracting and/or commissioning in publicly operated health systems, and performance-related payment systems for professional and institutional providers. Two other areas of recent innovation include giving hospital budgets to PHC providers or boards, and regulatory measures for controlling pharmaceutical expenditures such as reference pricing, positive lists and indicative budgets. Capital planning measures can also be included here, such as efforts to regionalize the delivery of such complex acute procedures as coronary bypass surgery.

Recent reform interventions on the production and provision of services have been quite successful in emphasizing changes at the institutional level, particularly in improving managerial efficiency and in focusing on the quality and effectiveness of medical interventions. The list of interventions at this level is extensive. It comprises a wide variety of outcome-related activities, including: quality assurance initiatives and continuous quality of care development, technology assessment and medical practice guidelines; restructuring hospital configuration and improving institutional governance, for example, by decentralizing operating authority to self-governing hospitals and public firms; and shifting medical interventions into less intensive, more appropriate sectors, for example, by enhancing the role of primary and community care.

Reorienting state regulation

The ability of governments to achieve a sustainable balance between multiple health sector objectives depends on the development of an appropriate mix of supply-side interventions at the micro (institutional) as well as the macro (system) level. As noted above, this mix increasingly includes a carefully constrained role for certain market-oriented incentives as well as traditional regulatory instruments. The effort to decentralize responsibility for publicly owned hospitals to regional and municipal levels of government has been one of the more successful policy initiatives across Europe in the 1990s. In addition, decentralization has increasingly incorporated managerial autonomy for hospitals in the form of self-governing trusts and public firms. Conversely, it has become increasingly apparent that health ministries should not directly manage hospitals themselves, as is still the case in some countries in southern Europe and in the CEE and CIS countries. The role of the state in the health sector is becoming one of strategic planning, monitoring, outcome-oriented regulation and, where appropriate, designing particular subsector markets for service providers. To adapt a metaphor used by public policy analysts (96) the state is learning to do "more steering and less rowing" on the supply side of the health sector. Similarly, on the demand side, the state must continue to take an active role in steering the funding process. If solidarity is to be maintained, there is little room for relaxation of the state's role as regulator and guarantor of universal coverage. Indeed, in the western part of Europe, the long-term success of national policy-makers in capping system-level costs suggests that these countries have adopted many of the necessary policy instruments for controlling the flow of funds into the health care system.

With regard to patients' concerns, the challenge for policy-makers is to channel the desire for patient power in directions that reinforce the mix of regulatory and incentive strategies selected to achieve both solidarity and cost constraint. Experience in several countries suggests that patient choice can contribute to the efficiency and effectiveness of fixed expenditure ceilings and tight provider budgets, as long as choice is *not* linked to a pure fee-for-service payment system. On this issue, policy-makers require mechanisms that constrain patient choice within the broader borders of a supply-side strategy, rather than allowing it to become a fully fledged and disruptive demand-side force. This approach has been employed successfully during the 1990s in several western European health systems, and recent experience suggests that a more disciplined approach to patient choice is equally as essential in the CEE and CIS countries.

STABILIZING THE POLICY PENDULUM

One of the more persistent metaphors for public policy generally is the pendulum. Dissatisfied with an initial position, policy-makers set out to make fundamental changes, i.e. to swing to the opposite point on the pendulum's trajectory. As more is learned about that opposite point, in particular its shortcomings and dilemmas, movement then begins back towards the original position.

In European health system reform in the 1990s, as in other public policy arenas, the challenge for policy-makers lies in overcoming the tendency for policy to swing between the two extremes. The way forward inevitably incorporates elements of both the original position and of radical reform.

Currently, the various countries of the European Region are in different stages of this cycle. Several western European countries are embarking on major experiments. Conversely, in the countries of northern Europe that began their reforms the earliest, there is now a substantial movement back from the most radical position – market-oriented incentives – closer to the original position of publicly planned coordination and cooperation. Similarly, in some CIS countries, there is a tendency to compare the current extremely difficult conditions with the health systems of the Soviet period – which at least functioned – and to hesitate about how to proceed.

In addition to efforts to stabilize the pendulum, effective policy-making should take into consideration the substantial diversity across Europe in such essential policy-related areas as cultural patterns, social values and the socioeconomic level of development. This diversity helps to explain why reform strategies that work in one country cannot be imported into other countries without substantial adaptation. Reflecting the different policy contexts, it is likely that the overall mix of strategies will have to be defined specifically for each country.

At the current stage of health sector development, therefore, it is at best premature to talk about common policy strategies that are appropriate and applicable across the entire European Region, or even in geographical subregions. Recent discussions about so-called "convergence" between the health systems of developed countries appear to have overemphasized specific technical mechanisms (e.g. purchasing and contracting) rather than the purposes to which these instruments are put in different systems. Probing more deeply, political differences in terms of health policy and social differences in terms of cultural values suggest that there is still considerable divergence in health systems in both the western and eastern parts of the Region, as well as between them.

MANAGING CHANGE

The conclusion that policy-makers should draw from this assessment of the policy pendulum, from the difficulties of policy transferral and from the lack of convergence is not that health reform is futile, or that there are no good answers. In fact, as the European experience with health reform has indicated, and as the success of recent supply-side initiatives demonstrates, health reform can succeed as well as fail; it can be moderate as well as radical; it can strengthen PHC and equity as well as harm them, and it can reinforce the moral underpinnings of the welfare state as well as erode them.

The ability to achieve health system objectives rests with the capacity of policy-makers to respond flexibly and creatively to the policy environments they confront. While learning from other countries about reform experiences is an essential element of this process, so is adapting and adjusting reform mechanisms to fit the local situation. While the basic principles of health reform are valid across national borders, their application will depend on individual countries' needs and expectations. As Chapter 7 suggests, the manner in which reform is introduced is nearly as important as which reforms are adopted. The way forward is clearly a complicated one but it is, in fact, forward. A glance back at how health care has changed in the European Region over the last decade confirms how much can be accomplished in the coming years.

References

1. CASSELS, A. *Health sector reform: key issues in less developed countries.* Geneva, World Health Organization, 1995 (document WHO/SHS/NHP/95.4).
2. *The reform of health care systems: a review of seventeen OECD countries.* Paris, Organisation for Economic Co-operation and Development, 1994 (Health Policy Studies, No. 5).
3. BERMAN, P. Health sector reform: making health development sustainable. *Health policy*, **32**: 3–13 (1995).
4. MAXWELL, R.J. *Health and wealth: an international study of health spending.* Cambridge, MA, Lexington Books, 1981.
5. PAUL, S. *Capacity building for health sector reform.* Geneva, World Health Organization, 1995 (document WHO/SHS/NHD/95.8).
6. SALTMAN, R.B. & VON OTTER, C. *Planned markets and public competition. Strategic reform in northern European health systems.* Buckingham, Open University Press, 1992.
7. SALTMAN, R.B. The context for health reform in the United Kingdom, Sweden, Germany, and the United States. *Health policy* (in press).
8. BENSON, J.K. The interorganizational network as a political economy. *Administrative science quarterly*, **20**: 229–249 (1975).
9. HABERMAS, J. *Théorie de l'agir communicationnel.* Paris, Fayard, 1987.
10. SEN, A. *Inequality reexamined.* Cambridge, MA, Harvard University Press, 1992.
11. CLARK, D.G. Autonomy, personal empowerment and quality of life in long-term care. *Journal of applied gerontology*, **7**(3): 279–297 (1988).
12. CANGUILHEM. *Le normal et le pathologique.* Paris, Presses Universitaires de France, 1966.
13. GUATTARI, F. Pour une refondation des pratiques sociales. *Le monde diplomatique*, (463): 26 (1992).
14. EVANS, R.G. & STODDART, G.L. Producing health, consuming health care. *In:* Evans, R.G. et al., ed. *Why are some people healthy and others not?* Berlin, de Gruyter, 1994.
15. FISCHER, F. *Technocracy and the politics of expertise.* Newbury Park, Sage, 1990.
16. SALTMAN, R.B. Emerging trends in the Swedish health system. *International journal of health services*, **21**(4): 615–623 (1991).
17. BOURDIEU, P. *Raisons pratiques.* Paris, Editions de Minuit, 1994.
18. CONTANDRIOPOULOS, A.P. Réformer le système de santé: une utopie pour sortir d'un status quo impossible. *Ruptures*, **1**(1): 8–26 (1994).
19. ROBINSON, R. & LE GRAND, J. Contracting and the purchaser–provider split. *In:* Saltman, R.B. & von Otter, C., ed. *Implementing planned markets in health care.* Buckingham, Open University Press, 1995.
20. *EBRD transition report.* London, European Bank for Reconstruction and Development, 1996.

21. WELLINGS, K. Assessing AIDS/HIV prevention. What do we know in Europe. General population. *Sozial- und Präventivmedizin*, **39**(Suppl.): 14–46 (1994).

22. MURRAY, C.J.L. Quantifying the burden of disease: the technical basis for disability-adjusted life years. *Bulletin of the World Health Organization*, **72**(3): 429–445 (1994).

23. BARNUM, H. Evaluating healthy days of life gained from health projects. *Social science and medicine*, **24**: 833–841 (1987).

24. MURRAY, J.L. & BOBADILLA, J.L. Epidemiological transitions in the formerly socialist economies: divergent patterns of mortality by cause of death. *In:* Bobadilla, J.L. & Costello, C., ed. *Mortality profiles and adult health interventions in the Newly Independent States.* Washington, DC, National Academy of Sciences, 1996.

25. BOWLING, A. *Measuring health: a review of quality of life measuring scales.* Buckingham, Open University Press, 1991.

26. GUDEX, C. *QALYs and their use by the health service.* York, Centre for Health Economics, 1988 (Discussion Paper No. 20).

27. MURRAY, C. & LOPEZ, A. *Global comparative assessments in the health sector. Disease burden, expenditures and intervention packages.* Geneva, World Health Organization, 1994.

28. WORLD BANK. *World development report 1993. Investing in health.* New York, Oxford University Press, 1993.

29. GUNNING-SCHEPERS, L.J. ET AL. Population interventions reassessed. *Lancet*, **1**: 479–481 (1989).

30. CHENET, L. ET AL. Changing life expectancy in central Europe: is there a single reason. *Journal of public health medicine*, **18**(3): 329–336 (1996).

31. CHENET, L. ET AL. Changing life expectancy in the 1980s: why was Denmark different? *Journal of epidemiology and community health*, **50**(4): 404–407 (1996).

32. BOBAK, M. & MARMOT, M. East–west mortality divide and its potential explanations: proposed research agenda. *British medical journal*, **312**: 421–425 (1996).

33. EURONUT-SENECA. Nutrition and the elderly in Europe. *European journal of clinical nutrition*, **45**(Suppl.): 326–345 (1991).

34. EVANS, R.G. ET AL., ED. *Why are some people healthy and others not?* Berlin, de Gruyter, 1994.

35. SMITH, D.G. ET AL. The magnitude and causes of socio-economic differentials in mortality: further evidence from the Whitehall Study. *Journal of epidemiology and community health*, **44**: 265–270 (1990).

36. WILKINSON, R.G. Income distribution and life expectancy. *British medical journal*, **304**: 165–168 (1992).

37. KAPLAN, G.A. ET AL. Inequality in income and mortality in the United States. Analysis of mortality and potential pathways. *British medical journal*, **312**: 999–1003 (1996).

38. BEN-SHLOMO, Y. ET AL. Does the variation in the socioeconomic characteristics of an area affect mortality? *British medical journal*, **312**: 1013–1014 (1996).

39. HAJDU, P. ET AL. Changes in premature mortality differentials by marital status in Hungary and in England and Wales. *European journal of public health*, **5**: 259–264 (1995).

40. BOSMA, J.H.A. *A cross-cultural comparison of the role of some psychosocial factors in the etiology of coronary artery disease. Follow-up to the Kaunas–Rotterdam intervention study (KRIS)*. Maastricht, Maastricht University Press, 1994.

41. *HIV/AIDS surveillance in Europe*. Saint-Maurice, European Centre for the Epidemiological Monitoring of AIDS, 1996.

42. LALONDE, M. *A new perspective on the health of Canadians: a working document*. Ottawa, Information Canada, 1974.

43. KARLEN, A. *Plague's progress: a social history of man and disease*. London, Victor Gollancz, 1995.

44. *World population prospects 1950–2025*. New York, United Nations, 1992.

45. INDREDAVIK, B. ET AL. Benefit of a stroke unit: a randomized controlled trial. *Stroke*, **22**: 1026–1031 (1991).

46. DE LORGERIL, M. ET AL. Mediterranean alpha-linoleic acid-rich diet in secondary prevention of coronary heart disease. *Lancet*, **343**: 1454–1459 (1994).

47. AUSTOKER, J. Diet and cancer. *British medical journal*, **308**: 1610–1614 (1994).

48. *OECD health data 96*. Paris, Organisation for Economic Co-operation and Development, 1996.

49. *OECD health data 95*. Paris, Organisation for Economic Co-operation and Development, 1995.

50. ABEL-SMITH, B. Who is the odd man out? *Health and society*, **63**(1): 1–17 (1985).

51. ABEL-SMITH, B. *Cost containment and new priorities in health care: a study of the European Community*. Aldershot, Avebury Ashgate, 1992.

52. *Trends in health status, services, and finance – the transition in central and eastern Europe*. Washington, DC, World Bank, 1996 (Technical Paper, No. 341).

53. UNITED NATIONS DEVELOPMENT PROGRAMME. *Human development report 1996*. Oxford, Oxford University Press, 1996.

54. SMEE, C. Self-governing trusts and GP fundholders. The British experience. *In:* Saltman, R. & von Otter, C., ed. *Implementing planned markets in health care*. Buckingham, Open University Press, 1995, pp. 177–208.

55. WHITEHEAD, M. Is it fair? Evaluating the equity implications of the NHS reforms. *In:* Robinson, R. & Le Grand, J., ed. *Evaluating the NHS reforms*. London, King's Fund Institute, 1994, pp. 208–242.

56. DIDERICHSEN, F. Market reforms in health care and sustainability of the welfare state: lessons from Sweden. *Health policy*, **32**: 141–153 (1995).

57. DAHLGREN, G. *Framtidens sjukvårdsmarknader* [Future health care markets]. Stockholm, Natur och Kultur, 1994.

58. DUNNING, A. *Choices in health care: a report by the government committee on choices in health care. Executive summary*. Rijswijk, Ministry of Welfare, Health and Culture, 1992.

59. WENNBERG, J.E. Dealing with medical practice variations: a proposal for action. *Health affairs*, **3**(2): 6–31 (1984).

60. SALTMAN, R. & VON OTTER, C., ED. *Implementing planned markets in health care.* Buckingham, Open University Press, 1995.

61. SALTMAN, R.B. Patient choice and patient empowerment in northern European health systems: a conceptual framework. *International journal of health services*, **24**(2): 201–229 (1994).

62. ENTHOVEN, A. *Reflections on the management of the NHS.* London, Nuffield Provincial Hospitals Trust, 1985.

63. SALTMAN, R.B. & VON OTTER, C. Revitalizing public health care systems. A proposal for public competition in Sweden. *Health policy*, **7**: 21–40 (1987).

64. LE GRAND, J. & BARTLETT, W. *Quasi-markets and social policy.* London, Macmillan, 1993.

65. YOUNG, D.W. & SALTMAN, R.B. *The hospital power equilibrium – physician behaviour and cost control.* Baltimore, MD, Johns Hopkins University Press, 1985.

66. MCLACHLAN, G. & MAYNARD, A. *The public/private mix for health.* London, Nuffield Provincial Hospitals Trust, 1982.

67. DE ROO, A.A. Contracting and solidarity: Market-oriented changes in Dutch health insurance schemes. *In:* Saltman, R.B. & von Otter, C., ed. *Implementing planned markets in health care.* Buckingham, Open University Press, 1995, pp. 45–64.

68. HUNTER, D.J. & GUENTERT, B. The financing of health care. *In:* Harrington, P. & Ritsatakis, A., ed. *European Health Policy Conference: Opportunities for the Future, Copenhagen, 5–9 December 1994. Vol. IV. Health care reforms for health gain.* Copenhagen, WHO Regional Office for Europe, 1995 (document EUR/ICP/HFAP 9401/CN01 (IV)), pp. 15–27.

69. HAM, C. *Management and competition in the new NHS.* Oxford, Radcliffe Medical Press, 1994.

70. HAM, C. & BROMMELS, M. Health care reform in the Netherlands, Sweden, and the United Kingdom. *Health affairs*, **13**(5): 105–19 (1994).

71. *Renewing the NHS.* London, Parliamentary Labour Party, 1995.

72. VON OTTER, C. Applying market theory to health care. *In:* Hunter, D., ed. *Paradoxes of competition in health care.* Leeds, University of Leeds, 1991.

73. JOST, T.S. ET AL. The British health care reforms, the American health care revolution, and purchaser/provider contracts. *Journal of health politics, policy and law*, **20**(4): 885–908 (1995).

74. KETTL, D.F. *Sharing power: public governance and private markets.* Washington, DC, Brookings Institution, 1993.

75. RONDINELLI, D. Government decentralisation in comparative theory and practice in developing countries. *International review of administrative sciences*, **47**: 133–145 (1981).

76. SALTMAN, R.B. & AKANOV, A. *Decentralization: the case of Kazakhstan.* Geneva, World Health Organization, 1996 (document).

77. CHEEMA, G. & RONDINELLI, D. *Decentralisation and development.* Newbury Park, Sage, 1983.

78. RONDINELLI, D. ET AL. *Decentralisation in developing countries.* Washington, DC, World Bank, 1983 (Staff Working Paper No. 581).

79. COLLINS, C.D. & GREEN, A.T. Decentralisation and primary health care: some negative implications in developing countries. *International journal of health services*, **24**(3): 459–475 (1994).

80. BORGENHAMMER, E. *At vårda liv: organisation, etik, kvalitet* [Looking after life: organization, ethics, quality]. Stockholm, SNS Förlag, 1993.

81. REGAN, D.E. & STEWART, J. An essay in the government of health: the case for local authority control. *Social policy and administration*, **16**: 19–43 (1982).

82. GOLINOWSKA, S. & TYMOWSKA, K. Poland. *In:* Johnson, N. *Private markets in health and welfare.* Oxford, Berg, 1995.

83. ANELL, A. Implementing planned markets in health care: the case of Sweden. *In:* Saltman, R.B. & von Otter, C., ed. *Implementing planned markets in health care.* Buckingham, Open University Press, 1995, pp. 209–226.

84. FREIRE, J.M. Health care reforms in Spain. *In:* Artundo, C. et al., ed. *Health care reforms in Europe.* Madrid, Ministry of Health and Consumer Affairs, 1993.

85. HUNTER, D. ET AL. Optimal balance of centralized and decentralized management responsibilities. *In:* Saltman, R.B. et al., ed. *Critical challenges for European health policy.* Buckingham, Open University Press (in press).

86. MARTIKAINEN, A. & UUSIKYLÄ, P. *Restructuring health policies – the Finnish case.* Helsinki, University of Helsinki, 1996.

87. OROSZ, E. *Decentralization and health care system change in Hungary.* Budapest, Eötvös Loránd University, 1995.

88. HUNTER, D.J. The case for closer cooperation between local authorities and the NHS. *British medical journal*, **310**: 1587–1589 (1995).

89. BARR, N. *The economics of the welfare state.* London, Weidenfeld and Nicolson, 1987.

90. MUSGROVE, P. *Public and private roles in health.* Washington, DC, World Bank, 1996.

91. RUBÁŠ, L. *Health care transformation in the Czech Republic: analysis of the present situation and objectives for the future.* Prague, Committee for Social Policy and Health, Parliament of the Czech Republic, 1994.

92. CHINITZ, D. Israel's health policy breakthrough: the politics of reform and the reform of politics. *Journal of health politics, policy and law*, **20**(4): 909–932 (1995).

93. LIGHT, D.W. The radical experiment: transforming Britain's national health system to interlocking markets. *Journal of public health policy*, **13**(2): 146–155 (1992).

94. ÖRN, P. Socialstyrelsens utredning om Medanalys: flera hundra förfalskade provsvar lämnade laboratorieföretaget [The assessment of MEDANALYS by the Ministry of Social Affairs: several hundred falsified sample results left the laboratory]. *Läkartidningen*, **93**(7): 532 (1996).

95. WHITE, J. *Competing solutions.* Washington, DC, Brookings Institution, 1995.
96. OSBORNE, D. & GAEBLER, T. *Reinventing government.* Reading, MA, Addison Wesley, 1993.
97. ORESKOVIC, S. The miracle of centralisation. *Eurohealth*, **1**(1): 25–26 (1995).
98. TCHERNJAVSKII, V.E. & KOMAROV, Y. *Decentralization and changes in the functioning of health care system in the Russian Federation.* Moscow, MedSocEcon-Inform, 1996.
99. MILLS, A. Decentralisation and accountability in the health sector from an international perspective: what are the choices? *Public administration and development*, **47**: 281–292 (1994).
100. STEWART, J. *Accountability to the public.* London, European Policy Forum, 1992.
101. NHS EXECUTIVE. *Local freedoms, national responsibilities.* Leeds, NHS Executive, 1994.
102. CARLSEN, F. Hospital financing in Norway. *Health policy*, **28**(2): 79–88 (1994).
103. ARNSTEIN, S.R. A ladder of citizen participation. *American Institute of Planners journal*, **35**(4): 216–224 (1966).
104. McKEE, M. ET AL. Leap of faith over the data tap. *Lancet*, **345**(8963): 1449–1450 (1995).
105. *Local voices: views of local people in purchasing for health.* London, NHS Executive, 1992.
106. FLUSS, S.J. *Patients' rights, informed consent, access and equality.* Sweden, Nerenias and Santeris Publishers, 1994.
107. MARTENSTEIN, L.F. The codification in the Netherlands of the principal rights of patients: a critical review. *European journal of health law*, **2**: 33–44 (1995).
108. DEPARTMENT OF HEALTH. *Being heard: the report of a review committee on NHS complaints procedures.* London, H.M. Stationery Office, 1994.
109. DEPARTMENT OF HEALTH. *Acting on complaints.* London, H.M. Stationery Office, 1995.
110. DEPARTMENT OF HEALTH. *Consumers and research in the NHS: an R and D contribution to consumer involvement in the NHS.* Leeds, NHS Executive, 1995.
111. GROENEWEGEN, P.P. ET AL. *Remunerating general practitioners in western Europe.* Aldershot, Avebury Ashgate, 1991.
112. STÆHR JOHANSEN, A. Primary care in Denmark. *In:* Alban, A. & Christiansen, T., ed. *The nordic lights: new initiatives in health care systems.* Odense, Odense University Press, 1995, pp. 81–105.
113. JONSSON, E. *Konkurrens inom sjukvården. Vad säger forskningen om effekterna?* [Competition within health care. What does research say about the effects?]. Stockholm, SPRI, 1993.
114. VAN DE VEN, W.P.M.M. ET AL. Risk-adjusted capitation: recent experiences in the Netherlands. *Health affairs*, **13**(5): 120–136 (1994).
115. BRUSTER, S. ET AL. Survey of hospital patients. *British medical journal*, **309**: 1542–1546 (1994).
116. BOSANQUET, N. Improving health. *In:* Jowell, R. et al., ed. *British social attitudes: the 11th report.* Aldershot, Dartmouth, 1994.

117. CARTWRIGHT, A. & WINDSOR, J. *Outpatients and their doctors.* London, H.M. Stationery Office, 1992.

118. COULTER, A. General practice fundholding. *European journal of public health*, **5**(4): 233–239 (1995).

119. *Fundholding: the main report.* London, Audit Commission, 1996.

120. MAHON, A. ET AL. Choice of hospital for elective surgery referral: GPs' and patients' views. *In:* Robinson, R. & LeGrand, J., ed. *Evaluating the NHS reforms.* London, King's Fund Institute, 1994, pp. 108–129.

121. LEAVY, R. ET AL. Consumerism and general practice. *British medical journal*, **298**: 737–739 (1989).

122. JONES, D. ET AL. Monitoring changes in health services for older people. *In:* Robinson, R. & Le Grand, J., ed. *Evaluating the NHS reforms.* London, King's Fund Institute, 1994.

123. CALNAN, M. ET AL. *Going private: why people pay for their care.* Buckingham, Open University Press, 1993.

124. FLYNN, R. Managed markets: consumers and producers in the national health service. *In:* Burrows, R. & Marsch, A., ed. *Consumption and class, divisions and change.* Basingstoke, Macmillan, 1992.

125. SYKES, W. ET AL. *Listening to local voices: a guide to research methods.* Leeds, Nuffield Institute for Health Services Studies, 1992.

126. WINKLER, F. Consumerism in health care: beyond the supermarket model. *Policy and politics*, **15**(1): 1–8 (1987).

127. BOWLING, A. *What people say about prioritising health services.* London, King's Fund Institute, 1993.

128. HEGINBOTHAM, C. Rationing. *British medical journal*, **304**(6825): 496–499 (1992).

129. *Perspectives on health promotion.* Ottawa, Canadian Public Health Association, 1995.

130. DEKKER, E. Health care reforms and public health. *European journal of public health*, **4**(2): 281–286 (1994).

131. *Health promotion and health care system reforms: a consensus statement. First meeting of the European Committee for Health Promotion Development, Dublin.* Copenhagen, WHO Regional Office for Europe, 1995 (document EUR/ICP/HEP/011).

132. LEVIN, L.S. & ZIGLIO, E. Health promotion as an investment strategy: considerations on theory and practice. *Health promotion international*, **11**: 33–40 (1996).

133. WHITE, M. ET AL. Hungary: a new public health. *Lancet*, **341**: 43–44 (1993).

134. *Expert Committee on Public Health Administration. First report.* Geneva, World Health Organization, 1952 (WHO Technical Report Series, No. 55).

135. WINSLOW, C.E.A. *Evolution and significance of the modern public health campaign.* New York, Arno, 1923.

136. AMERICAN INSTITUTE OF MEDICINE. *The future of public health.* Washington, DC, National Academy Press, 1988.

137. ACHESON, E.D. *Public health in England. Report of the committee of enquiry into the future development of the public health function.* London, H.M. Stationery Office, 1988.

138. FRENK, J. The new public health. *In: The crisis of public health: reflections for the debate.* Washington, Pan American Health Organization, 1992, pp. 68–85.

139. KUNST, A.E. & MACKENBACH, J.P. *Measuring socioeconomic inequalities in health.* Copenhagen, WHO Regional Office for Europe, 1995 (document EUR/ICP/RPD 416).

140. DUBOS, R. *Mirage of health.* New York, Harper Colophan, 1979.

141. DEPARTMENT OF HEALTH AND SOCIAL SECURITY. *Inequalities in health: report of a research working group (The Black Report).* London, H.M. Stationery Office, 1980.

142. *Targets for health for all.* Copenhagen, WHO Regional Office for Europe, 1985 (European Health for All Series, No. 1).

143. Ottawa Charter for Health Promotion. *Health promotion,* **1**(4): iii–v (1986).

144. TSOUROS, A.D. The WHO Healthy Cities Project: state of the art and future plans. *Health promotion international,* **10**(2): 133–141 (1995).

145. PUSKA, P. ET AL. *Community control of cardiovascular diseases: the North Karelia project.* Copenhagen, WHO Regional Office for Europe, 1981.

146. SECRETARY OF STATE FOR HEALTH. *The health of the nation.* London, H.M. Stationery Office, 1992.

147. ROBINSON, M. ET AL. *Health of the nation: every government department's business.* London, RSM Press, 1996.

148. MCCARTHY, M. & REES, S. *Health systems and public health medicine in the European Community.* London, Royal College of Physicians, 1992.

149. DESENCLOS, J.-C. ET AL. Variations in national infectious disease surveillance in Europe. *Lancet,* **341**: 1003–1006 (1993).

150. DIXON, R.E. Costs of nosocomial infections and benefits of infection control programs. *In:* Wenzel, R.P., ed. *Prevention and control of nosocomial infections.* Baltimore, Williams & Williams, 1987, pp. 19–25.

151. ROBERTS, J.A. & SOCKETT, P.N. The socio-economic impact of human *Salmonella enteriditis* infection. *International journal of food microbiology,* **21**: 117–129 (1994).

152. O'BRIEN, J.M. ET AL. Tempting fate: control of communicable disease in England. *British medical journal,* **306**: 1461–1464 (1993).

153. HEINZ-TROSSEN, A. *Zur Reglementierung der Prostiten – insbesondere zur Arbeit der Gesundheitsämter der Bundesrepublik Deutschland West.* Bonn, Öffentliches Gesundheitswesen, 1991.

154. ROSEWITZ, B. & WEBBER, D. *Reformversuche und Reformblokaden im deutschen Gesundheitswesen.* Frankfurt-am-Main, Campus-Verlag, 1990.

155. JESSE, M. & MARSHALL, T. *Health care systems in transition: Estonia.* Copenhagen, WHO Regional Office for Europe, 1996 (document).

156. VAN DE VEN, W.P.M.M. ET AL. Forming and reforming the market for third-party purchasing of health care. *Social science & medicine,* **39**(10): 1405–1412 (1994).

157. ROSE, G. Sick individuals and sick populations. *International journal of epidemiology*, **14**: 32–38 (1985).

158. BACH, S. Managing a pluralist health system: the case of health care reform in France. *International journal of health services*, **24**(4): 593–606 (1994).

159. GRAF VON DER SCHULENBURG, J.-M. Forming and reforming the market for third-party purchasing of health care: a German perspective. *Social science & medicine*, **39**(10): 1473–1481 (1994).

160. NONNEMAN, W. & VAN DOORSLAER, E. The role of the sickness funds in the Belgian health care market. *Social science & medicine*, **39**(10): 1483–1495 (1994).

161. MCKEE, M. ET AL. Health sector reform in the Czech Republic, Hungary and Romania. *Croatian medical journal*, **35**: 238–244 (1994).

162. STEENSBERG, J. Post-Soviet public health administration in Estonia. *World health forum*, **15**: 335–338 (1994).

163. BELLER, M. Epidemiology and public health in the Yogodnoye district. *Alaska medicine*, **34**: 21–27 (1992).

164. BOJAN, F. ET AL. Status and priorities of public health in Hungary. *Zeitschrift für Gesundheitswissenschaften*, **1**(Suppl.): 48–55 (1994).

165. SHAPIRO, S. ET AL. Ten-to-fourteen-year effect of screening on breast cancer mortality. *Journal of the National Cancer Institute*, **69**: 349–355 (1982).

166. TABAR, L. ET AL. Reduction in mortality from breast cancer after mass screening with mammography. *Lancet*, **1**: 829–832 (1985).

167. MCKEE, M. ET AL. Preventing sudden infant deaths – the slow diffusion of an idea. *Health policy* (in press).

168. MCKEE, M. ET AL. Public health medicine training in the European Community: is there scope for harmonization? *European journal of public health*, **2**: 45–53 (1992).

169. APPLEBY, J. *Financing health care in the 1990s*. Buckingham, Open University Press, 1992.

170. ABEL-SMITH, B. ET AL. *Choices in health policy: an agenda for the European Union*. Luxembourg and Aldershot, Office for Official Publications of the European Communities and Dartmouth Publishing Company, 1995.

171. ABEL-SMITH, B. & MOSSIALOS, E. Cost containment and health care reform: a study of the European Union. *Health policy*, **28**(2): 89–132 (1994).

172. RUBIN, R.J. & MENDELSON, D.N. *A framework for cost-sharing policy analysis*. Basle, Pharmaceutical Partners for Better Health Care, 1995.

173. FELDMAN, R. & DOWD, B. What does the demand curve for medical care measure? *Journal of health economics*, **12**(2): 193–200 (1993).

174. PREKER, A.S. & FEACHEM, R.G.A. *Searching for the silver bullet: market mechanisms and the health sector in central and eastern Europe*. Washington, DC, World Bank, 1995.

175. AKIN, J. ET AL. *Financing health services in developing countries: an agenda for reform. A World Bank policy study*. Washington, DC, World Bank, 1987.

176. JIMENEZ, E. *Pricing policy in the social sectors: cost recovery for education and health in developing countries*. Baltimore, MD, Johns Hopkins University Press, 1987.

177. MOONEY, G. & RYAN, M. Agency in health care: getting beyond first principles. *Journal of health economics*, **12**(2): 125–135 (1993).
178. LABELLE, R. ET AL. A re-examination of the meaning and importance of supplier-induced demand. *Journal of health economics*, **13**(3): 347–368 (1994).
179. PAULY, M.V. Editorial. A re-examination of the meaning and importance of supplier-induced demand. *Journal of health economics*, **13**(3): 369–372 (1994).
180. FUCHS, V.R. Physician-induced demand: a parable. *Journal of health economics*, **5**(4): 367 (1986).
181. MOONEY, G. *Key issues in health economics.* Hemel Hempstead, Harvester Wheatsheaf, 1994.
182. EVANS, R.G. *Strained mercy: the economics of Canadian health care.* Toronto, Butterworths, 1984.
183. RICE, T. Demand curves, economists, and desert islands: a response to Feldman and Dowd. *Journal of health economics*, **12**(2): 201–204 (1993).
184. McCLELLAN, M. The uncertain demand for medical care: a comment on Emmett Keeler. *Journal of health economics*, **14**(2): 239–242 (1995).
185. EVANS, R.G. ET AL. *User fees for health care: why a bad idea keeps coming back.* Toronto, Canadian Institute for Advanced Research Program in Population Health, 1993.
186. FAHS, M.C. Physician response to the United Mine Workers' cost-sharing program: the other side of the coin. *Health services research*, **27**(1): 25–45 (1992).
187. STODDART, G.L. ET AL. *Why not user charges? The real issues.* Ontario, The Ontario Premier's Council on Health, Well-being and Social Justice, 1993.
188. *The reform of health care: a comparative analysis of seven OECD countries.* Paris, Organisation for Economic Co-operation and Development, 1992 (Health Policy Studies, No. 2).
189. RODWIN, V.G. & SANDIER, S. Health care under French national health insurance. *Health affairs*, **12**(3): 111–131 (1993).
190. *German health reforms: changes result in lower health costs in 1993.* Washington, DC, United States General Accounting Office, 1994 (Report GAO/HEHS-95-27).
191. NOLAN, B. Economic incentives, health status and health services utilisation. *Journal of health economics*, **12**(2): 151–169 (1993).
192. JÖNSSON, B. & GERDTHAM, U.G. Cost sharing for pharmaceuticals: the Swedish reimbursement system. *In*: Mattison, N., ed. *Sharing the costs of health: a multicountry perspective.* Basle, Pharmaceutical Partners for Better Health Care, 1995.
193. BALABANOVA, D. Health care reforms in Bulgaria: current problems and options for development. *Eurohealth*, **1**(2): 25–28 (1995).
194. PREKER, A.S. & HERBERT, W.B. Healing the wounds. *In:* Paine, L., ed. *New world health.* London, Sterling Publications, 1995, pp. 15–18.
195. VON BREDOW, L. The reform of health care in the Czech Republic. *Eurohealth*, **1**(2): 22–25 (1995).

196. KINCSES, G. *The role of co-payment. The possibilities and barriers of adaptation in central–eastern Europe.* Budapest, National Information Center for Health Care, 1995.

197. ABEL-SMITH, B. & FALKINGHAM, J. *Financing health services in Kyrgyzstan: the extent of private payments.* London, London School of Economics, 1995.

198. RASELL, M.E. Cost sharing in health insurance – a reexamination. *New England journal of medicine*, **332**(17): 1164–1168 (1995).

199. NEWHOUSE, J.P. A design for a health insurance experiment. *Inquiry*, **11**(1): 5–27 (1974).

200. MANNING, W.G. ET AL. Health insurance and the demand for medical care: evidence from a randomized experiment. *American economic review*, **77**(3): 251–277 (1987).

201. VAN DOORSLAER, E. & WAGSTAFF, A. Equity in the finance of health care: methods and findings. *In*: van Doorslaer, E. & Wagstaff, A. *Equity in the finance and delivery of health care: an international perspective.* Oxford, Oxford University Press, 1993.

202. KLEIN, R. On the Oregon trail: rationing health care. *British medical journal*, **302**: 1–2 (1991).

203. HUNTER, D. *Rationing dilemmas in health care.* Birmingham, National Association of Health Authorities and Trusts, 1993.

204. DANIELS, N. *Just health care.* Cambridge, Cambridge University Press, 1985.

205. CHURCHILL, L.R. *Rationing health care in America.* South Bend, IN, University of Notre Dame Press, 1987.

206. HARRIS, J. QALYfying the value of life. *Journal of medical ethics*, **13**: 117–123 (1987).

207. KLEIN, R. Dimensions of rationing: who should do what? *British medical journal*, **307**(6899): 309–311 (1993).

208. HEGINBOTHAM, C. & HAM, C. *Purchasing dilemmas.* London, King's Fund Institute, 1992.

209. MAYNARD, A. Developing the health care market. *Economic journal*, **101**: 177–186 (1991).

210. HEGINBOTHAM, C. Health care priority setting: a survey of doctors, managers and the general public. *In*: Smith, R., ed. *Rationing in action.* London, BMJ Publishing Group, 1993.

211. SWEDISH PARLIAMENTARY PRIORITIES COMMISSION. *Priorities in health care.* Stockholm, Ministry of Health and Social Affairs, 1995.

212. HAM, C.J. ET AL. *Priority setting for health gain.* London, Department of Health, 1993.

213. BARKER, J. *Local NHS health care purchasing and prioritising from the perspective of Bromley residents – a qualitative study.* Bromley, Bromley Health Authority, 1995.

214. BOWIE, C. ET AL. Consulting the public about health service priorities. *British medical journal*, **311**: 1155–1158 (1995).

215. KLEIN, R. & REDMAYNE, S. *Patterns of priorities.* Birmingham, National Association of Health Authorities and Trusts, 1992.

216. HOUSE OF COMMONS HEALTH COMMITTEE. *Priority setting in the NHS: purchasing.* London, H.M. Stationery Office, 1995 (Report HC 134–1).
217. APPLEBY, J. ET AL. *Acting on the evidence.* Birmingham, National Association of Health Authorities and Trusts, 1995.
218. COCHRANE LIBRARY, OXFORD. *Cochrane Collaboration.* London, BMJ Publishing Group, 1996 (database).
219. DEPARTMENT OF HEALTH. *Government response to the first report for the health committee session 1994–95.* London, H.M. Stationery Office, 1995.
220. BRINDLE, D. Fresh limits on NHS feared. *The guardian,* 30 August 1995, p. 1.
221. KLEIN, D.H. Who should live and who should die? *Inquiry,* **31**(3): 239–240 (1994).
222. KITZHABER, J.A. Prioritising health services in an era of limits: the Oregon experience. *British medical journal,* **307**: 373–377 (1993).
223. *Prioritization of health services.* Portland, Oregon Health Services Commission, 1991.
224. NATIONAL ADVISORY COMMITTEE ON CARE. *Third report: core services of 1995/ 96.* Wellington, Health and Disability Support Services, 1994.
225. CUMMING, J. Core services and priority setting: the New Zealand experience. *Health policy,* **29**: 41–60 (1994).
226. HAM, C.J. Health care rationing. *British medical journal,* **310**: 1483–1484 (1995).
227. BODENHEIMER, T. & GRUMBACH, K. Financing universal health insurance: taxes, premiums, and the lessons of social insurance. *Journal of health politics, policy and law,* **17**(3): 438–462 (1992).
228. GLASER, W.A. *Health insurance in practice.* San Francisco, Jossey-Bass, 1991.
229. ROEMER, M.I. *National health systems of the world.* Oxford, Oxford University Press, 1991.
230. ELLENCWEIG, A.Y. & CHINITZ, D.P. Israel's health system reform. *European journal of public health,* **3**(1): 85–91 (1993).
231. BECKMAN, M. & ZARKOVIC, G. Transition to health insurance in former socialist countries. *In: The process and management of change – transition to a health insurance system in the countries of central and eastern Europe. Proceedings of the second meeting of the Working Party on Health Care Reforms in Europe, Essen, Germany, 19–21 October 1993.* Copenhagen, WHO Regional Office for Europe, 1995 (document EUR/ICP/PHC 216(C)).
232. STRUK, P. & MARSHALL, T. *Health care systems in transition: Czech Republic.* Copenhagen, WHO Regional Office for Europe, 1996 (document).
233. MASSARO, T.A. ET AL. Health system reform in the Czech Republic. Policy lessons from the initial experience of the general health insurance company. *Journal of the American Medical Association,* **271**(23): 1870–1874 (1994).
234. SKACKOVÁ, D. & MARSHALL, T. *Health care systems in transition: Slovakia.* Copenhagen, WHO Regional Office for Europe, 1996 (document).
235. TOMES, I. Albania – social insurance in Albania: a system in transition. *International social security review,* **47**(1): 73–79 (1994).
236. *The process of restructuring Hungarian health care – 1990–94.* Budapest, Ministry of Welfare, 1994.

237. TCHERNJAVSKII, V.E. & MARSHALL, T. *Health care systems in transition: Russian Federation.* Copenhagen, WHO Regional Office for Europe, 1994 (document).

238. TRAGAKES, E. Health care reforms in the CCEE/NIS: issues of spending, health insurance and efficiency. *In:* Harrington, P. & Ritsatakis, A., ed. *European Health Policy Conference: Opportunities for the Future, Copenhagen, 5–9 December 1994. Vol. V. Health challenges in central and eastern Europe and the newly independent states.* Copenhagen, WHO Regional Office for Europe, 1995 (document EUR/ICP/HFAP 94 01/CN01 (V)), pp. 55–74.

239. ENSOR, T. Health system reform in former socialist countries of Europe. *International journal of health planning and management*, **8**: 169–187 (1993).

240. CHINITZ, D. ET AL. Balancing competition and solidarity in health financing. *In:* Saltman, R.B. et al., ed. *Critical challenges for European health policy.* Buckingham, Open University Press (in press).

241. CURTIS, S. ET AL. Health care reforms in Russia: the example of St Petersburg. *Social science & medicine*, **40**(6): 755–765 (1995).

242. PREKER, A.S. ET AL. *Health status, health services and health expenditure: trends during the transition in CEE.* Washington, DC, World Bank, 1995.

243. VULIC, S. & MARSHALL, T. *Health care systems in transition: Croatia.* Copenhagen, WHO Regional Office for Europe, 1997 (document).

244. VIENONEN, M., ED. The Fifth Meeting of the Expert Network on Health and Health Care Financing Strategies, Ljubljana, Slovenia, 14–16 November 1995. *Antidotum*, Suppl. No. 1, 1996.

245. HARCUS, I. *European health care insurance – growing opportunities in the private sector.* London, Financial Times Business Information, 1994 (Financial Times Management Report).

246. FELDBAUM, E.G. & HUGHESMAN, M. *Healthcare systems: cost containment versus quality.* London, Financial Times Business Information, 1993 (Financial Times Management Report No. 147).

247. MARGA, I. & MARSHALL, T. *Health care systems in transition: Latvia.* Copenhagen, WHO Regional Office for Europe, 1996 (document).

248. ASHFORD, D.E. *The emergence of the welfare state.* New York, Oxford University Press, 1986.

249. ESPING-ANDERSEN, G. *The three worlds of welfare capitalism.* Princeton, NJ, Princeton University Press, 1990.

250. CULYER, A.J. Health, health expenditures, and equity. *In:* van Doorslaer, E. et al., ed. *Equity in the finance and delivery of health care. An international perspective.* Oxford, Oxford University Press, 1993, pp. 299–319.

251. PAULY, M.V. Overinsurance and public provision of insurance: the role of moral hazard and adverse selection. *Quarterly journal of economics*, **88**: 44–62 (1974).

252. ROTHSCHILD, M. & STIGLITZ, J. Equilibrium in competitive insurance markets: an essay on the economics of imperfect information. *Quarterly journal of economics*, **90**: 629–649 (1976).

253. WAGSTAFF, A. ET AL. Equity in the finance of health care: some international comparisons. *Journal of health economics*, **11**(4): 361–387 (1992).

254. FRIEDMAN, M. & FRIEDMAN, R. *Free to choose.* New York, Free Press, 1981.

255. BERG, A. ET AL. *Public perception of the health system following implementation of the National Health Insurance Law: selected preliminary findings from a survey of the general population (an executive summary of a research report).* Jerusalem, Brookdale Institute, 1996.

256. WASEM, J. Der kassenartenübergreifende Risikostrukturausgleich – Chancen für eine neue Wettbewerbsordnung in der GKV. *Sozialer Fortschritt*, **42**: 31–39 (1993).

257. SCHNEIDER, M. Health care cost containment in the Federal Republic of Germany. *Health care financing review*, **12**(3): 87–101 (1991).

258. DE SWAAN, A. *De mens is de mens een zorg* [People are a concern to people]. Amsterdam, Muelenhoff, 1989.

259. HARRISON, A. *From hierarchy to contract.* Newbury, Policy Journals, 1993.

260. KONGSTVEDT, P.R. *The managed health care handbook.* Gaithersburg, MD, Aspen, 1993.

261. *Changing health care in the Netherlands.* The Hague, Ministry of Welfare, Health and Cultural Affairs, 1988.

262. SHEIMAN, I. Forming the system of health insurance in the Russian Federation. *Social science & medicine*, **10**: 1425–32 (1994).

263. HAM, C. Contestability: a middle path for health care. *British medical journal*, **312**: 70–71 (1996).

264. GLASER, W. *Paying the doctor.* San Francisco, Jossey-Bass, 1970.

265. CONTANDRIOPOULOS, A.P. ET AL. Systèmes de soins et modalités de rémunération. *Sociologie du travail*, **1**(90): 95–115 (1990).

266. POUVOURVILLE, G. Le paiement de l'acte médical: une comparaison avec la France, les Etats-Unis et le Québec. *Journal d'économie médicale*, **5**(1): 5–20 (1987).

267. HICKSON, G.B. ET AL. Physician reimbursement by salary or fee-for-service: effect on physician practice behaviour in a randomized prospective study. *Pediatrics*, **80**(3): 344–350 (1987).

268. VAYDA, E. A comparison of surgical rates in Canada and in England and Wales. *New England journal of medicine*, **289**: 1224–1229 (1973).

269. VAYDA, E. ET AL. A decade of surgery in Canada, England and Wales, and the United States. *Archive of surgery*, **117**: 846–853 (1982).

270. RICE, T. The impact of changing Medicare reimbursement rates on physician-induced demand. *Medical care*, **21**: 803–815 (1983).

271. RICE, T. Physician initiated demand for medical care: new evidence from the Medicare program. *Advances in health economics and health services research*, **5**: 129–160 (1984).

272. LABELLE, R. ET AL. *Financial incentives and medical practice: evidence from Ontario on the effect of changes in physician fees on medical care utilization.* Ontario, Centre for Health Economics and Policy Analysis, 1990.

273. ROCHAIX, L. *Adjustment mechanisms in physicians' services markets.* Thesis, Department of Economics, University of York, 1991.

274. ROCHAIX, L. Financial incentives for physicians: the Quebec experience. *Health economics*, **2**: 163–176 (1993).

275. KEELER, E.B. & BRODIE, M. Economic incentives in the choice between vaginal delivery and Caesarean section. *Milbank quarterly*, **71**(3): 365–404 (1993).

276. DONALDSON, C. & GERARD, K. Paying general practitioners: shedding light on the review of health services. *Journal of the Royal College of General Practitioners*, **39**(320): 114–117 (1989).

277. LUFT, H.S. How do health maintenance organizations achieve their savings? *New England journal of medicine*, **298**: 1336–1343 (1978).

278. GREENFIELD, S. ET AL. Variations in resource utilization among medical specialties and systems of care: results from the Medical Outcomes Study. *Journal of the American Medical Association*, **267**: 1624–1630 (1992).

279. STEARNS, S. ET AL. Physician responses to fee-for-service and capitation payment. *Inquiry*, **29**: 416–425 (1992).

280. ELLIS, R.P. & McGUIRE, T.G. Optimal payment systems for health services. *Journal of health economics*, **9**: 375–396 (1990).

281. DELNOIJ, D.M.J. *Physician payment systems and cost control.* Utrecht, NIVEL, 1994.

282. ROCHAIX, L. *The French health care system at the crossroads. Proceedings of the Second European Conference in Health Economics.* Paris, CREDES-CES, 1992.

283. HUGHES, D. & YULE, B. The effect of per-item fees on the behaviour of primary health care. *Journal of health economics*, **11**(4): 413–438 (1992).

284. ROBINSON, J.C. Payment mechanisms, nonprice incentives, and organisational innovation in health care. *Inquiry*, **30**(3): 328–333 (1993).

285. HILLMAN, A.L. ET AL. How do financial incentives affect physicians' clinical decisions and the financial performance of health maintenance organizations? *New England journal of medicine*, **321**: 86–92 (1989).

286. HEMENWAY, D. ET AL. Physicians' responses to financial incentives. Evidence from a for-profit ambulatory care center. *New England journal of medicine*, **322**(15): 1059–1063 (1990).

287. STODDART, G.L. Reflections on incentives and health system reform. *In:* Lopez-Casasnovas, G., ed. *Incentives in health systems*, Berlin, Springer-Verlag, 1991, pp. 75–95.

288. PETERSEN, L.K. *Hospital financing in Denmark.* Paris, Organisation for Economic Co-operation and Development, 1995.

289. *Strategy for health.* Warsaw, Ministry of Health and Social Welfare, 1994.

290. SOURTY-LE GUELLEC, M.-J. Hospital financing in France. *In*: Wiley, M.M., ed. *Hospital financing in seven countries.* Washington, DC, Government Printing Office, 1995.

291. LEIDL, R. Hospital financing in Germany. *In*: Wiley, M.M., ed. *Hospital financing in seven countries.* Washington, DC, Government Printing Office, 1995.

292. WILEY, M.M. Budgeting for acute hospital services in Ireland: the case-mix adjustment. *Journal of the Irish Colleges of Physicians and Surgeons*, **24**: 283–290 (1995).

293. MAPELLI, V. *Hospital financing in Italy.* Paris, Organisation for Economic Co-operation and Development, 1995.

294. SOLSTAD, K. & NYLAND, K. *Financing acute hospitals in Norway.* Paris, Organisation for Economic Co-operation and Development, 1995.

295. PFEIFFER, K.P. The model of a new hospital financing system in Austria – its possible effects on hospitals. *In:* Schwartz, F.W. et al., ed. *Fixing health budgets: experience from Europe and North America.* London, Wiley and Sons, 1996.

296. JAMSEN, R. & KLEMOLA, K. *Financing acute hospitals in Finland.* Paris, Organisation for Economic Co-operation and Development, 1995.

297. BARTLETT, W. & LE GRAND, J. The performance of trusts. *In:* Robinson, R. & Le Grand, J., ed. *Evaluating the NHS reforms.* London, King's Fund Institute, 1994, pp. 54–73.

298. WILEY, M.M. *Hospital financing and payment systems: a review of selected OECD countries.* Paris, Organisation for Economic Co-operation and Development, 1995.

299. MOSSIALOS, E. & ABEL-SMITH, B. Pharmaceuticals. *In:* Baldwin, R., ed. *Regulation in question: the growing agenda.* London, London School of Economics, 1995.

300. AARON, H. Economic aspects of the role of the government in the health care. *In:* van der Gaag, J. & Perlman, M., ed. *Health, economics and health economics.* Amsterdam, North-Holland, 1981.

301. ARROW, K. Uncertainty and the welfare economics of medical care. *American economic review,* **53**(6): 941–73 (1963).

302. CULLIS, J. & WEST, P. *The economics of health: an introduction.* New York, New York University Press, 1979.

303. ABEL-SMITH, B. *Value for money in health services: a comparative study.* London, Heinemann, 1976.

304. TEELING-SMITH, G. *Medicines for the year 2000.* London, Office of Health Economics, 1979.

305. WELLS, N. *Pharmaceuticals among the sunrise industries.* London, Croom Helm, 1986.

306. BARRIE, G.J. *Patents and pharmaceuticals.* New York, New York University Press, 1977.

307. COOPER, M.C. *Prices and profits in the pharmaceutical industry.* Oxford, Pergamon Press, 1966.

308. INTERMINISTERIAL PRICES COMMITTEE. *Activity report.* Rome, Ministry of Health, 1995.

309. VARTHOLOMEOS, J. & TINIOS, P. The structure and reform of social security and the demand for pharmaceuticals in Greece. *In:* Mossialos, E. et al., ed. *Cost containment, pricing and financing of pharmaceuticals in the European Community: the policy-makers' view.* Athens, LSE Health and Pharmetrica S.A., 1994.

310. *Facts 1994: medicine and dental care.* Copenhagen, MEFA, 1994.

311. MOSSIALOS, E. & ABEL-SMITH, B. *Cost containment in the pharmaceutical sector in the EU Member States.* London, London School of Economics, 1996.

312. *Beoordeling ABDA-Prijsvergelijking Geneesmiddelen* [Evaluation of the ABDA drug prices evaluation study]. The Hague, Government Research Institute (IOO), 1995.

313. *Vergleich europäischer Arzneimittelpreise* [Comparison of European pharmaceutical prices]. Eschborn, Bundesvereinigung Deutscher Apothekerverbände, 1993.

314. BURSTALL, M. Cost and utilization of pharmaceuticals in the United Kingdom. *Health policy* (in press).

315. BALL, B. The current market for generics in Europe. *In: Proceedings of a Meeting on Recent Changes Affecting the Development and Marketing of Generic Medicines, London, 27–28 September, 1994.* Basle, International Pharmaceutical Congress, 1995, pp. 60–83.

316. DUKES, M.N. Change and growth in generic markets in developed and developing countries. Proceedings of the Conference "Medicines and the new economic environment", Madrid, 29–31 March 1995. *Pharmacoeconomics* (in press).

317. *Good pharmacy practice (GPP) in community and hospital pharmacy settings.* Geneva, World Health Organization, 1996 (document WHO/PHARM/DAP/96.1).

318. WALT, G. Implementing health care reforms: a framework for discussion. *In:* Saltman, R.B. et al., ed. *Critical challenges for European health policy.* Buckingham, Open University Press, 1995.

319. THOMAS, L. *The lives of a cell.* New York, Bantam Books, 1975.

320. WEISBROD, B.A. The health care quadrilemma. An essay on technological change, insurance, quality of care, and cost containment. *Journal of economic perspectives*, **29**: 523–552 (1991).

321. *Working for patients.* London, H.M. Stationery Office, 1989.

322. McPHERSON, K. ET AL. Small area variations in the use of common surgical procedures: an international comparison of New England, England, and Norway. *New England journal of medicine*, **307**: 1310–1314 (1982).

323. WENNBERG, J.E. Population illness rates do not explain population hospitalisation rates: a comment on Mark Blumberg's thesis that morbidity adjusters are needed to interpret small area variations. *Medical care*, **25**: 354–359 (1987).

324. McPHERSON, K. Why do variations occur? *In*: Mooney, G. & Andersen, T.F., ed. *The challenges of medical practice variations.* London, Macmillan, 1990.

325. CHALMERS, I. & ALTMAN, D., ED. *Systematic reviews.* London, BMJ Publishing Group, 1995.

326. BLACK, N.A. ET AL. A randomised controlled trial of surgery for glue ear. *British medical journal*, **300**: 1551–1556 (1990).

327. HUNTER, D.J.W. ET AL. Health care sought and received by men with urinary symptoms and their views on prostatectomy. *British journal of general practice*, **45**: 27–30 (1995).

328. MULROW, C.D. Rationale for systematic reviews. *In:* Chalmers, I. & Altman, D.G., ed. *Systematic reviews.* London, BMJ Publishing Group, 1995, pp. 1–8.

329. ENKIN, M. ET AL. *Guide to effective care in pregnancy and childbirth.* Oxford, Oxford University Press, 1995.

330. BERGREM, H. ET AL. *Five years with the St Vincent Declaration: report based on 1994 questionnaires completed by the St Vincent Declaration liaison persons of WHO/EURO Member States.* Copenhagen, WHO Regional Office for Europe, 1995 (document ICP/NCD 602).

331. PETERSEN, P.E. Effectiveness of oral health care – some Danish experiences. *Proceedings of the Finnish Dental Society*, **88**: 1–2 (1992).

332. STÆHR JOHANSEN, K. The OBSQID project: obstetrical quality development through integrated use of telematics. *Technology and informatics*, **14**: 59–62 (1994).

333. BANTA, H.D. & LUCE, B. *Health care technology and its assessment, an international perspective.* Oxford, Oxford University Press, 1993.

334. Editorial. "Miraculous" developments from health services research. *British medical journal*, **312**(7024): 131 (1996).

335. GILLIS, C.R. & HOLLIS, D.J. Survival outcome of care by specialist surgeons in breast cancer: a study of 3786 patients in the west of Scotland. *British medical journal*, **312**(7024): 145–148 (1996).

336. *Health for all targets: the health policy for Europe.* Copenhagen, WHO Regional Office for Europe, 1991 (European Health for All Series, No. 4).

337. HAVELIN, L.I. ET AL. The effect of cement types on early revision of Charnley total hip prostheses. *Journal of bone and joint surgery*, **77-A**: 1543–1550 (1995).

338. ANDREASEN, A.H. ET AL. Improvement in outcome of breast cancer in Denmark. *In:* Roger France, F.H. et al., ed. *Case-based telematic systems.* Amsterdam, IOS Press, 1994.

339. FREEMANTLE, N. & MAYNARD, A. Something rotten in the state of clinical and economic evaluations? *Health economics*, **3**: 63–67 (1994).

340. STOCKING, B. *Expensive health technology: regulatory and administrative mechanisms in Europe.* Oxford, Oxford University Press, 1988.

341. BATTISTA, R.N. ET AL. Lessons from the eight countries. *Health policy*, **30**(1): 397–421 (1994).

342. PECKHAM, M. Research and development for the national health service. *Lancet*, **338**: 367–371 (1991).

343. MAXWELL, R. Quality assessment in health. *British medical journal*, **288**: 1470–1471 (1984).

344. BLOMHØJ, G. ET AL. *Continuous quality development: a proposed national policy.* Copenhagen, WHO Regional Office for Europe, 1993 (document EUR/ICP/CLR 059).

345. BLACK, N. Research, audit and education. *British medical journal*, **304**: 698–700 (1992).

346. BLACK, N. Quality assurance of medical care. *Journal of public health medicine*, **12**: 87–104 (1990).

347. DONABEDIAN, A. *A guide to medical care administration.* Washington, DC, American Public Health Association, 1969.

348. MCKEE, M. & HUNTER, D. Mortality league tables: do they inform or mislead? *Quality health care*, **4**: 5–12 (1994).

349. MANT, J. & HICKS, N. Detecting differences in quality of care. The sensitivity of measures of process and outcome in treating myocardial infarction. *British medical journal*, **311**: 793–796 (1995).

350. BERGREM, H. ET AL. Diabetes care in Europe. The St Vincent Declaration coming of age? *Diabetes, nutrition and metabolism*, **9**: 330–336 (1996).

351. *Medical audit, a first report: what, why and how?* London, Royal College of Physicians, 1989.

352. ANKONÉ, A. & SPREEUWENBERG, C. Artsen werken samen van Ierland tot Kyrgyzstan [Doctors collaborate from Ireland to Kyrgyzstan]. *Medisch Contact*, **48**(6): 165–167 (1993).

353. SCRIVENS, E. ET AL. Accreditation: what can we learn from the Anglophone model? *Health policy*, **34**: 153–226 (1995).

354. ZAVARTNIK, J.J. Strategies for reaching poor blacks and Hispanics in Dade County, Florida. *Cancer*, **72**(3): 1088–1092 (1993).

355. BLACK, N. & JOHNSTON, A. Volume and outcome in hospital care: evidence, explanations and implications. *Health services management research*, **3**(2): 108–114 (1990).

356. SOWDEN, A.J. ET AL. Volume and outcome in coronary artery bypass graft surgery: true association or artefact? *British medical journal*, **311**: 151–155 (1995).

357. HALEY, L.R.W. *Managing hospital infection control for cost-effectiveness: a strategy for reducing infectious complications.* Chicago, American Hospital Publishing Inc., 1986.

358. STÆHR JOHANSEN, K. WHOCARE: hospital infection surveillance and feedback programme. *Healthcare computing*, **859**: 366 (1992).

359. EDDY, D. Practice policies, what are they? *Journal of the American Medical Association*, **263**: 877–880 (1990).

360. GRIMSHAW, J.M. & RUSSELL, I.T. Achieving health gain through clinical guidelines: II – ensuring that guidelines change medical practice. *Quality in health care*, **3**: 45–52 (1994).

361. LOMAS, J. ET AL. Do practice guidelines change practice? The effect of a consensus statement on the practice of physicians. *New England journal of medicine*, **321**: 1306–1131 (1989).

362. KOSECOFF, J. ET AL. Effects of the National Institutes of Health Consensus Development Program on physician practice. *Journal of the American Medical Association*, **258**: 2708–2713 (1987).

363. MCKEE, M. & CLARKE, A. Guidelines, enthusiasms, uncertainty, and the limits to purchasing. *British medical journal*, **310**(6972): 101–104 (1995).

364. OXMAN, A. ET AL. No magic bullets: a systematic review of 102 trials of interventions to improve professional practice. *Canadian Medical Association journal*, **153**(10): 1423–1431 (1995).

365. JENSEN, L.P. & SCHROEDER, T.V. How can vascular registers help us to improve risk benefit relations in vascular surgery. The Danish experience. *In:* Swedenborg, J. & Blohmé, L., ed. *Risk benefit aspects of vascular surgery.* Stockholm, Karolinska Institute, 1994.

366. European Forum of Medical Associations and WHO. *Policy of medical associations regarding quality of care development. Workshop on the project to develop policies and mechanisms for national medical associations regarding quality of care development, Utrecht, 28–29 January 1993.* Copenhagen, WHO Regional Office for Europe, 1993 (document EUR/ICP/HSC 021(C)BD/01/A)

367. McCarthy, G.J. Involving physicians in TOM. To gain physician support for quality management, hospital administrators must treat physicians as customers. *Health progress,* **74**(10): 33–35 (1993).

368. Krueger, N.E. & Mazuzan, J.E., Jr. A collaborative approach to standards, practices. Setting the stage for continuous quality improvement. *AORN journal,* **57**(2): 467, 470–475, 478–480 (1993).

369. Borgions, J. et al. *Développement continu de la qualité des soins: proposition de politique nationale.* Brussels, Ministère de la santé publique et de l'environnement; Copenhagen, WHO Regional Office for Europe, 1995 (document).

370. Sorli, J. et al. *Quality in health care: a proposed national policy.* Ljubljana, Ministry of Health, 1996.

371. *The obstetrical quality development through integrated use of telematics project: European consensus conference on quality assurance indicators for perinatal care.* Copenhagen, WHO Regional Office for Europe, 1993 (document EUR/ICP/CLR 066).

372. Piwernetz, K. et al. DiabCare quality network in Europe. *St Vincent Declaration newsletter,* **7**: 15–16 (1995).

373. Møller, I. et al. *Manual on quality assurance indicators in oral health care. The ORATEL Project: telematic system for quality assurance in oral health care, CEC Project A2029.* Copenhagen, WHO Regional Office for Europe, 1992 (document EUR/ICP/ORH 120).

374. Stæhr Johansen, K. Continous surveillance of surgical wound infections. *In: Hospital management international 1989.* London, International Hospital Federation, 1989, pp. 365–367.

375. *Quality assurance indicators in mental health care. Report on a WHO consensus meeting.* Copenhagen, WHO Regional Office for Europe, 1994 (document EUR/ICP/CLR 062).

376. Warner, M. *Implementing health care reforms through substitution.* Cardiff, Welsh Institute for Health and Social Care, 1996.

377. Expert Advisory Group on Cancers. *A policy framework for commissioning cancer services. A report by the Expert Advisory Group on Cancers to the Chief Medical Officers of England and Wales.* London, Department of Health, 1995.

378. van Beekum, D. & Haerkens, E. Moving technology from the hospital to the home: a systematic approach. *In:* Costin, D. & Warner, M.M., ed. *From hospital to home care: the potential for acute service provision.* London, King's Fund Institute, 1992.

379. Lee, S. *Hospital care in Europe: the challenge of a changing role.* London, Financial Times Business Information, 1995 (Financial Times Management Report).

380. GASPOZ, J.M. ET AL. Cost–effectiveness of a new short-stay unit to "rule out" acute myocardial infarction in low risk patients. *Journal of the American College of Cardiology*, **24**: 1249–1259 (1994).

381. BRILLMAN, J.C. & TANDBERG, D. Observation unit impact on emergency department admission for asthma. *American journal of emergency medicine*, **12**: 11–14 (1994).

382. CONNETT, G.J. ET AL. Audit strategies to reduce hospital admissions for acute asthma. *Archives of diseases in childhood*, **69**: 202–205 (1993).

383. ROSSI, P. ET AL. Improving quality in emergency services to reduce hospital admission. *Quality assurance in health care*, **5**: 127–129 (1993).

384. SWIFT, P.G. ET AL. A decade of diabetes: keeping children out of hospital. *British medical journal*, **307**: 96–98 (1993).

385. KORNOWSKI, R. ET AL. Intensive home-care surveillance prevents hospitalization and improves morbidity rates among elderly patients with severe congestive heart failure. *American heart journal*, **129**: 762–766 (1995).

386. ELLENCWEIG, A.Y. ET AL. The effect of admission to long-term care program on utilization of health services by the elderly in British Columbia. *European journal of epidemiology*, **6**(2): 175–183 (1990).

387. CHANG, J.I. ET AL. Patient outcomes in hospital-based respite: a study of potential risks and benefits. *Journal of the American Board of Family Practitioners*, **5**: 475–481 (1992).

388. STUCK, A.E. ET AL. A trial of annual in-home comprehensive geriatric assessments for elderly people living in the community. *New England journal of medicine*, **333**: 1184–1189 (1995).

389. PATHY, M.S.J. ET AL. Randomised trial of case finding and surveillance of elderly people at home. *Lancet*, **34**: 890–893 (1992).

390. PAYNE, S.M.C. Identifying and managing inappropriate hospitalisation. *Health services research*, **22**: 709–769 (1987).

391. WESTPHAL, M. ET AL. Changes in the average length of stay and average charges generated following institution of PSRO. *Health services research*, **14**: 253–265 (1979).

392. WICKIZER, T.M. ET AL. Does utilisation review reduce unnecessary hospital care and contain cost? *Medical care*, **27**: 632–647 (1989).

393. WERNEKE, U. & MACFAUL, R. A criticism of the paediatric appropriateness evaluation protocol. *Archives of disease in childhood* (in press).

394. INGLIS, A.L. ET AL. Appropriateness of hospital utilization. *Medical care*, **33**: 952–957 (1995).

395. BARÉ, M.L. ET AL. Appropriateness of admissions and hospitalisation days in an acute-care teaching hospital. *Revue d'épidémiologie et de santé publique*, **43**: 328–336 (1995).

396. VICTOR, C.R. & KHAKOO, A.A. Is hospital the right place? A survey of inappropriate admissions to an inner London NHS trust. *Journal of public health medicine*, **16**: 286–290 (1994).

397. VICTOR, C. ET AL. The inappropriate use of acute hospital beds in an inner London District Health Authority. *Health trends*, **25**: 94–97 (1993).

398. NAMDARAN, F. ET AL. Bed blocking in Edinburgh hospitals. *Health bulletin*, **50**(3): 223–227 (1992).

399. MCCLARAN, J. ET AL. Chronic status patients in a university hospital: bed-day utilization and length of stay. *Canadian Medical Association journal*, **145**: 1259–1265 (1991).

400. APOLONE, G. ET AL. A survey of the necessity of the hospitalisation day in an Italian teaching hospital. *Quality assurance in health care*, **3**: 1–9 (1991).

401. HYNES, M. ET AL. Patients 21 days or more in an acute hospital bed: appropriateness of care. *Irish journal of medical sciences*, **160**: 389–392 (1991).

402. ANDERSON, P. ET AL. Use of hospital beds: a cohort study of admission to a provincial hospital. *British medical journal*, **297**: 910–912 (1988).

403. COID, J. & CROME, P. Bed-blocking in Bromley. *British medical journal*, **292**: 1253–1256 (1986).

404. POPPLEWELL, P.Y. ET AL. Peer review of utilisation of medical beds at Flinders Medical Centre. *Australia and New Zealand journal of medicine*, **14**: 226–230 (1984).

405. SEYMOUR, D.G. & PRINGLE, R. Elderly patients in a general surgical unit: do they block beds? *British medical journal*, **284**: 1921–1923 (1982).

406. MURPHY, F.W. Blocked beds. *British medical journal*, **1**: 1395–1396 (1977).

407. RUBIN, S.G. & DAVIES, G.H. Bed blocking by elderly patients in general hospital wards. *Age and ageing*, **4**: 142–147 (1975).

408. DEPARTMENT OF HEALTH. *Economies of scope and scale in health services: summary of evidence.* Leeds, NHS Executive, 1995.

409. *Report of an independent review of specialist services in London. Cardiac services. Renal Services. Neurosciences.* London, H.M. Stationery Office, 1993.

410. OFFICE OF TECHNOLOGY ASSESSMENT. *The quality of medical care: information for consumers.* Washington, DC, Government Printing Office, 1988.

411. LUFT, H.S. ET AL. *Hospital volume, physician volume and patient outcomes: assessing the evidence.* Ann Arbour, MI, Health Administration Press Perspectives, 1990.

412. HARDING, M. ET AL. Management of a malignant teratoma: does referral to a specialist unit matter? *Lancet*, **341**: 999–1002 (1993).

413. MCARDLE, C. & HOLE, D. Impact of variability amongst surgeons on postoperative morbidity and mortality and ultimate survival. *British medical journal*, **302**: 1901–1905 (1991).

414. CROMWELL, J. ET AL. Learning by doing in CABG surgery. *Medical care*, **28**(1): 6–18 (1990).

415. KELLY, J.V. & HELLINGER, F.J. Heart disease and hospital deaths: an empirical study. *Health services research*, **22**(3): 369–395 (1987).

416. *Report of the national confidential enquiry in perioperative deaths.* London, Royal College of Surgeons, 1992.

417. HANNAN, E.L. ET AL. Improving the outcomes of CABG surgery in New York State. *Journal of the American Medical Association*, **271**: 10 (1994).

418. FRAM, A. ET AL. Is there a rationale for regionalizing organ transplantation services? *Journal of health politics, policy & law,* **14**: 1 (1989).

419. LAWTON, R. ET AL. The effects of patient, hospital and physician characteristics on length of stay and mortality. *Medical care,* **29**(3): 251–253 (1991).

420. GARNICK, D.W. ET AL. Surgeon volume vs hospital volume: which matters more? *Journal of the American Medical Association,* **262**: 4 (1989).

421. KELLY, J.V. & HELLINGER, F.J. Physician and hospital factors associated with mortality of surgical patients. *Medical care,* **24**: 9 (1986).

422. BANTA, H.D. Future health care technology and the hospital. *Health policy,* **14**(1): 61–73 (1990).

423. *Alma-Ata 1978: primary health care.* Geneva, World Health Organization, 1978 (Health for All Series, No. 1).

424. WHITE, K.L. *Healing the schism: epidemiology, medicine and the public's health.* New York, Springer-Verlag, 1991.

425. McKEOWN, T. *The role of medicine: dream, mirage or nemesis.* Oxford, Basil Blackwell, 1979.

426. TARIMO, E. & WEBSTER, E.G. *Primary health care: concepts and challenges in a changing world. Alma-Ata revisited.* Geneva, World Health Organization, 1994 (document WHO/SHS/CC/94.2).

427. MULLAN, F. Community-oriented primary health care: an agenda for the 80's. *New England journal of medicine,* **307**: 1076–1078 (1982).

428. WRIGHT, R.A. Community-oriented primary care. The cornerstone of health care reform. *Journal of the American Medical Association,* **269**(19): 2544–2547 (1993).

429. GODINHO, J. ET AL. Tipping the balance towards primary health care: a research project of the Commision of the European Communities. *European journal of public health,* **2**(3–4): 129–219 (1992).

430. MARINKER, M. *The end of general practice. The 1994 Bayliss Lecture.* London, Private Patient Plan Ltd., 1994.

431. STARFIELD, B. ET AL. The influence of patient–practitioner agreement on the outcome of care. *American journal of public health,* **71**: 117–123 (1981).

432. *The challenge for nursing and midwifery in the 21st century – the Heathrow debate.* London, Department of Health, 1994.

433. SALISBURY, C.J. & TETTERSELL, M.J. Comparison of the work of a nurse practitioner with that of a general practitioner. *Journal of the Royal College of General Practitioners,* **38**: 314–316 (1988).

434. SPITZER, W.O. ET AL. The Burlington randomized trial of the nurse practitioner. *New England journal of medicine,* **290**(5): 251–256 (1974).

435. FELDMAN, M.J. ET AL. Studies of nurse practitioner effectiveness. *Nursing research,* **36**(5): 303–308 (1987).

436. AUDIT COMMISSION. *The virtue of patients: making best use of ward nursing resources.* London, H.M. Stationery Office, 1991.

437. CARR-HILL, R. ET AL. *Skill mix and the effectiveness of nursing care.* York, Centre for Health Economics, University of York, 1992.

438. NATIONAL HEALTH SERVICE. *Evaluation of nurse practitioner pilot projects.* London, Touche Ross & Co., 1994.

439. SHI, L. ET AL. A rural-urban comparative study of nonphysician providers in community and migrant health centers. *Public health reports,* **109**(6): 809–815 (1994).

440. OFFICE OF TECHNOLOGY ASSESSMENT. *Nurse practitioners, physician assistants and certified nurse-midwives: a policy analysis, health technology case study.* Washington, DC, Government Printing Office, 1986.

441. COOPER, M.H. Jumping on the spot – health reform New Zealand style. *Health economics,* **3**: 69–72 (1994).

442. CHERNICHOVSKY, D. & CHINITZ, D. The political economy of health system reform in Israel. *Health economics,* **4**: 127–141 (1995).

443. DE LEEUW, E. & POLMAN, L. Health policy making: the Dutch experience. *Social science & medicine,* **40**(3): 331–338 (1995).

444. JOHNSON, N., ED. *Private markets in health and welfare.* Oxford, Berg, 1995.

445. JAMES, J.H. Reforming the British National Health Service: implementation problems in London. *Journal of health politics, policy and law,* **20**(1): 191–210 (1995).

446. WALT, G. & GILSON, L. Reforming the health sector in developing countries: the central role of policy analysis. *Health policy,* **9**(4): 353–370 (1994).

447. CUMPER, G.E. Should we plan for contradiction in health services? The Jamaican experience. *Journal of health policy,* **8**(2): 113–121 (1993).

448. IMMERGUT, E. *Health politics: interests and institutions in Western Europe.* Cambridge, Cambridge University Press, 1992.

449. WLODARCZYK, C. Expert network on health and health care financing strategies in countries of central and eastern Europe, or on the advantages of neighbourly cooperation in health care reforms. *Antidotum,* **1**(Suppl.): 8–21 (1993).

450. HEGINBOTHAM, C. & MAXWELL, R. Managing the transitions: a Western European view of health care development in Eastern Europe. *European journal of public health,* **1**(1): 36–44 (1991).

451. PIERSON, P. *Dismantling the welfare state?* Cambridge, Cambridge University Press, 1994.

452. MOHAN, J. *A national health service?* New York, St Martin's Press, 1995.

453. PEABODY, J.W. ET AL. Health system reform in the Republic of China. Formulating policy in a market-based health system. *Journal of the American Medical Association,* **273**(10): 777–781 (1995).

454. FIGUERAS, J. ET AL. Health care systems in Southern Europe: is there a Mediterranean paradigm? *International journal of health sciences,* **5**(4): 135–146 (1994).

455. MARTINEZ, J. & SANDIFORD, P. *Health sector reforms in central America.* Liverpool, Liverpool School of Tropical Medicine, 1995.

456. MILLS, A. ET AL., ED. *Health system decentralization; concepts, issues and country experience.* Geneva, World Health Organization, 1990.

457. MARMOR, T. & HAMBURGER, T. The missing alternative: how Washington élites pushed single-payer reform plans off the agenda. *In:* Marmor, T., ed. *Understanding health care reform.* New Haven, Yale University Press, 1994.

458. Borissov, V. & Rathwell, T. Health care reforms in Bulgaria: an initial apprais-al. *Social science & medicine*, **42**(11): 1501–1510 (1995).

459. Cleaves, P. Implementation amidst scarcity and apathy: political power and policy design. *In:* Grindle, M., ed. *Politics and policy implementation in the Third World*. Princeton, NJ, Princeton University Press, 1980.

460. Klein, R. Big bang health care reform – does it work? The case of Britain's 1991 National Health Service reforms. *Milbank quarterly*, **73**(3): 299–337 (1995).

461. Gladstone, D. & Goldsmith, M. Health care reform in the UK: working for patients? *In:* Seedhouse, D., ed. *Reforming health care: the philosophy and practice of international health reform*. Chichester, John Wiley, 1995, pp. 71–84.

462. Ashton, T. From evolution to revolution: restructuring the New Zealand health system. *In:* Seedhouse, D., ed. *Reforming health care: the philosophy and prac-tice of international health reform*. Chichester, John Wiley, 1995, pp. 85–93.

463. Borren, P. & Maynard, A. The market reform of the New Zealand health care system: searching for the Holy Grail in the Antipodes. *Health policy*, **27**(3): 233–52 (1994).

464. Robinson, R. & Le Grand, J., ed. *Evaluating the NHS reforms*. London, King's Fund Institute, 1994.

465. Johansson, L. Decentralization from acute to home care settings in Sweden. *Health policy* (in press).

466. Groenewegen, P.P. The shadow of the future: institutional change in health care. *Health affairs*, **13**(5): 137–148 (1994).

467. Harrison, S. & Pollitt, C. *Controlling health professionals. The future of work and organization in the National Health Service*. London, Open University Press, 1994 (State of Health Series).

468. Wilding, P. *Professional power and social welfare*. Henley-on-Thames, Routledge and Kegan Paul, 1984.

469. Grindle, M. & Thomas, J. *Public choices and policy change*. Baltimore, MD, Johns Hopkins University Press, 1991.

470. Brommels, M. Contracting and political boards in planned markets. *In:* Salt-man, R.B. & von Otter, C., ed. *Implementing planned markets in health care*. Buckingham, Open University Press, 1995, pp. p. 86–109.

471. Richardson, J. *Policy styles in Western Europe*. London, George Allen and Unwin, 1982.

472. Steinmo, S. & Watts, J. It's the institutions, stupid! Why comprehensive na-tional health insurance always fails in America. *Journal of health politics, poli-cy and law*, **20**(2): 329–372 (1995).

473. Zarkovic, G. et al. *Reform of the health care systems in former socialist coun-tries: problems, options, scenarios*. Neuherberg, Institut für Medizinische In-formatik und Systemforschung (Medis), 1994.

474. Mierzewski, P. Reform experiences. Facing the challenges. *Antidotum*, **1**(Suppl.): 68–70 (1993).

475. JONCZYK, J. The Polish dilemma and proposals for change. *Antidotum*, **1**(Suppl.): 81–84 (1993).

476. PECK, E. Power in the National Health Service: a case study of a unit considering NHS trust status. *Health services management research*, **4**(2): 120–130 (1991).

477. TENDLER, J. & FREEDHEIM, S. Trust in a rent-seeking world: health and government transformed in Northeast Brazil. *World development*, **22**: 1771–1791 (1994).

478. *Health and the economy – overview.* Mexico City, Fundación Mexicana para la Salud, 1995.

479. KEEN, J. ET AL. Doctors and resource management: incentives and goodwill. *Health policy*, **24**(1): 71–82 (1993).

480. GLENNERSTER, H. ET AL. *Implementing GP fundholding.* Buckingham, Open University Press, 1995.

481. BARRETT, S. & HILL, M. Policy, bargaining and structure in implementation theory: towards an integrated perspective. *Policy and politics*, **12**(3): 219–240 (1984).

482. ANSOFF, I. & McDONNELL, C. *Implementing strategic management.* Hemel Hempstead, Prentice Hall, 1990.

483. REICH, M.R. *Political mapping of health policy.* Boston, Harvard University, 1993.

484. FREEMAN, R.E. *Strategic management.* London, Pitman, 1990.

485. LOMAS, J. Retailing research: increasing the role of evidence in clinical services for childbirth. *Milbank quarterly*, **71**(3): 439–475 (1993).

486. FRIEND, J. & HICKLING, A. *Planning under pressure.* Oxford, Pergamon Press, 1993.

487. SALTMAN, R.B. A conceptual overview of recent health care reforms. *European journal of public health*, **4**(2): 287–293 (1994).

Annex – Authors, paper titles and contributions

ANELL, ANDERS; BARNUM, HOWARD
The allocation of capital and health sector reform.

BANTA, DAVID; GULÁSCI, LÁSZLÓ
Outcomes of health care in Europe.

BOBADILLA, JOSÉ LUIS
Setting health priorities in the newly independent states.

BURY, JACQUES
Contribution from training and research in public health.

CALNAN, MICHAEL; HALIK, JANOZ; SABBAT, JOLANTA
Citizen participation and patient choice in reformed health systems.

CAMPBELL, SALLY
The role of nursing in primary health care.

CHINITZ, DAVID; PREKER, ALEXANDER; WASEM, JÜRGEN
Balancing competition and solidarity in health financing.

CONTANDRIOPOULOS, ANDRÉ-PIERRE; LAURISTAN, MARJU; LEIBOVICH, ELLEN
Values, norms and the reform of health care systems.

DOYLE, NICK; LETHBRIDGE, JANE
Public health, health promotion and intersectoral action.

EDWARDS, NIGEL; HENSHER, MARTIN; WERNEKE, URSULA
Changing hospitals in Europe.

FAWCETT-HENESY, AINNA
Changing the boundaries of care: substitution of health services across the acute primary care interface.
Primary health care nursing in Europe: facing the changes.

FUENZALIDA-PUELMA, HERNÁN
Regulation of health insurance.

GARCÍA-BARBERO, MILAGROS
An education and training strategy for HFA.

GERVAS, JUAN
Cross-national analysis of "WHO country profiles" on general practice in Europe.

GUDEX, CLAIRE; SØRENSEN, JAN
Evaluating the impact of health care reforms on health and clinical outcome.

GÜNTERT, BERNHARD
Strengthening decentralised provider management.

HAM, CHRIS; HONIGSBAUM, FRANK
Priority setting and rationing health services.

HUNTER, DAVID; VIENONEN, MIKKO; WLODARCZYK, CEZARY
Optimal balance of centralized and decentralized management responsibilities.

JOLLY, DOMINIQUE
Evolution of hospitals in Europe: past, present and future.

KANAVOS, PANOS
Health expenditures in CEE: friend or foe?

KOKKO, SIMO; HÁVA, PETR; ORTÚN, VICENTE; LEPPO, KIMMO
The role of the state and health care reforms.

KUTZIN, JOSEPH; KINCSES, GYULA
What is the appropriate role for patient cost sharing in European health care systems?

LOVELACE, CHRISTOPHER; SEDGWICK, JOAN
Policy strategies and reform trends in Canada and New Zealand.

MCKEE, MARTIN
Health challenges and their implications for health services.
Improving quality of care.

MCKEE, MARTIN; BOJAN, FERENC
Reforming public health services.

MOSSIALOS, ELIAS
The usual suspect and the failure of cost containment: a study of regulating expenditure on medicines in selected European countries.

PHILALITHIS, ANASTAS
   Primary health care: policy and development.

PREKER, ALEXANDER; GOLDSTEIN, ELLEN; CHELLARAJ, GNANARAJ;
   ADEYI, OLUSOJI
   Central and eastern Europe: trends in health status, health services and health finance during the transition.

RATHWELL, THOMAS
   Review of implementation of health care reforms in the European Region.

RATHWELL, THOMAS; WALT, GILL
   An action plan for implementing health system reform.

ROCHAIX, LISE; MAREK, MICHAEL
   Performance-tied payment systems for physicians: evidence from selected countries.

SAVAS, SERDAR; SHEIMAN, IGOR; MAARSE, HANS; TRAGAKES, ELLIE
   Contracting models and provider competition in Europe.

STÆHR JOHANSEN, KIRSTEN; ANDERSEN, JØRGEN STEEN;
   ROGER FRANCE, FRANCIS; BABIC, DRAZEN
   Fostering quality of care development.

STOBBELAAR, FRANS
   Ensuring value for money from pharmaceuticals in CEE and NIS countries.

TRAGAKES, ELLIE
   Comparative review of health care financing systems in the European Region.

TRAGAKES, ELLIE; VIENONEN, MIKKO
   Health care reforms in the European scene.

TSOUROS, AGIS; LIPP, ALISTAIR
   "Leadership for health": reforming public health services.

VAN DER VELDEN, KOOS
   The contribution of general practice to health: can GPs move from primary care to primary health care.

WALT, GILL
   Implementing health care reforms: a framework for discussion.

WARNER, MORTON
Implementing health care reforms through substitution. Implications for the primary health care sector.

WILEY, MIRIAM
Financing operating costs for acute hospital inpatient services in selected countries in the European Region.